Small Animal
DENTISTRY

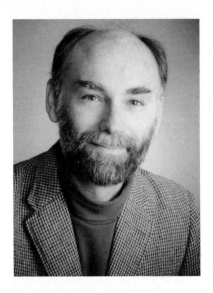

COLIN E. HARVEY

A graduate of the School of Veterinary Science at the University of Bristol, England, in 1966, Dr. Harvey completed internship and residency training in small animal surgery at the University of Pennsylvania, receiving the Diploma of the American College of Veterinary Surgeons in 1972. Progressively narrowing his area of specialization to the head and neck, (for the last several years, limited to oral, dental, and nasal diseases), he worked with dentists and physicians at the University of Pennsylvania and Hahneman University. Currently, Dr. Harvey is professor of surgery and dentistry at the University of Pennsylvania School of Veterinary Medicine. Since 1983 he has had a secondary appointment in the department of periodontics at the School of Dental Medicine, University of Pennsylvania.

Dr. Harvey is a Fellow of the Royal College of Veterinary Surgeons (UK), Fellow of the College of Physicians (Philadelphia), Charter Fellow of the Academy of Veterinary Dentistry, and Charter Diplomate and past President of the American Veterinary Dental College.

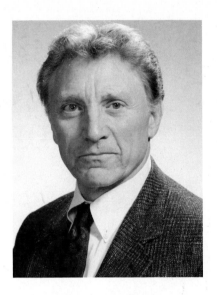

PETER P. EMILY

A graduate of the Creighton University School of Dentistry in 1959, Dr. Emily received postgraduate training in oral pathology, periodontics, and endodontics at the Denver General Hospital and University of Pennsylvania. His active interest in veterinary dentistry started in 1962, and he continues to be a consultant to veterinarians in many parts of the United States and several foreign countries. Dr. Emily has been a judge at dog shows for many years and is a consultant in dentistry to the American Kennel Club and Senior Dog Judges Association. He conducts intramural and continuing education courses at Colorado State University and the University of Missouri and in many parts of the world.

Dr. Emily is an Honorary Member of the Academy of Veterinary Dentistry and of the American Veterinary Dental College. An annual award presented by the American Veterinary Dental College is named in his honor. Dr. Emily was the recipient of the American Animal Hospital Association 1992 Award of Merit for outstanding contributions to veterinary medicine.

Small Animal
DENTISTRY

COLIN E. HARVEY
BVSc, FRCVS, DipACVS, DipAVDC

Professor of Surgery and Dentistry
University of Pennsylvania
Schools of Veterinary Medicine and Dental Medicine
Philadelphia, Pennsylvania

PETER P. EMILY
DDS, Cert Perio, Hon Mem AVDC

Dental and Veterinary Dental Practitioner
Director of Animal Dentistry
Colorado State University and University of Missouri;
Veterinary Dental Consultant
Denver Zoological Gardens;
Private Practice
Lakewood, Colorado

With 783 illustrations and 125 in full color

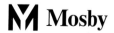

St. Louis Baltimore Boston Chicago London Philadelphia Sydney Toronto

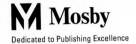

Mosby
Dedicated to Publishing Excellence

Publisher: George Stamathis
Editor-in-Chief: Don Ladig
Executive Editor: Linda L. Duncan
Developmental Editor: Melba Steube
Project Manager: Patricia Tannian
Production Editor: John Casey
Designer: Julie Taugner
Manufacturing Supervisor: Betty Richmond

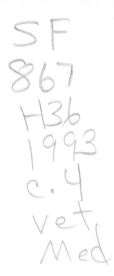
Printed in the United States of America

Mosby–Year Book, Inc.
11830 Westline Industrial Drive
St. Louis, Missouri 63146

Library of Congress Cataloging in Publication Data

Harvey, Colin E.
    Small animal dentistry / Colin E. Harvey, Peter P. Emily.
        p.   cm.
    Includes bibliographical references and index.
    ISBN 0-8016-6076-9
    1. Veterinary dentistry.   2. Dogs—Diseases.   3. Cats—Diseases.
I. Emily, Peter.   II. Title.
SF867.H36   1993
636.7′08976—dc20   93-16959
                                                         CIP

93 94 95 96 97 GW/UN/MY 9 8 7 6 5 4 3 2

*Dedicated to continued rapid improvement
in a field too long neglected.*

*May the patients who contributed
to the early steep slope part of the learning curve
not have suffered in vain.*

Foreword

Veterinary dentistry has gained rapid acceptance today and is now respected as a scientific discipline around the world. This important medical field was undeservedly neglected for many decades until recently. Students now rightly demand instruction and practical training in this field. Practicing veterinarians in every part of the world attend lectures and refresher courses, demonstrating the importance of veterinary dentistry for them.

No longer is treatment of a single tooth sufficient reason to publish a lavishly illustrated paper. Now, books, journals, and videotapes offer the student and practitioner plenty of information on well-accepted techniques that can be profitably made use of in everyday practice.

This book ranks high among many similar publications of veterinary dentistry. Its authors have included their great experience of many decades as veterinary dentists in this comprehensive and well-illustrated reference book. Outstanding perspective of the subject is achieved because one of the authors is a (human) dentist, the other a veterinary dentist. Both authors strongly recommend refraining from employing methods as they are used in human dentistry without careful consideration. In spite of numerous similarities, differences between human and animal teeth are significant, and understanding the differences is essential to selecting the correct technique for treating animals.

May this book meet with the success it deserves. Its authors, as well as myself, have devoted their lives to improving the practice of veterinary dentistry.

Professor Karl Zetner
University of Vienna, Austria

Preface

Welcome to the rapidly expanding world of veterinary dentistry. Until the last 100 years, veterinary dental knowledge consisted largely of detailed descriptions of the dental changes that could be used to age animals, initially in the horse (e.g., Girard in 1828 and Simonds in 1854). The first text devoted to veterinary dentistry was published in 1889 (Hinebauch), and a second one was published in 1905 (Merillat). Both books concentrated largely on the horse and contained little information on small animal dentistry. The horse remained the major focus of veterinary dentistry for most of the first half of the twentieth century. Becker's book, published in 1938, added innovative techniques and considerable detail in equine dentistry. The major work in comparative dental pathology in the first half of this century was the monumental contribution of Colyer *Variations and Diseases of the Teeth of Animals,* published in 1936 (a revised edition by Miles and Grigson was published in 1990). One notable contribution to the canine literature at this time was Mellanby's detailed series of papers in 1929 on the effect of dietary changes on developing dentition and dental diseases.

Progress in small animal dentistry became more rapid as a result of the pioneering work of Joseph Bodingbauer in Vienna, starting in the 1930s. The Veterinarmedizinischen Universitat in Vienna has continued as a major force in veterinary dentistry, with the passing of the mantle from Bodingbauer to Erich Eisenmenger, and since the 1970s, to Karl Zetner. Karl is acknowledged worldwide as a leader in this field in both education and research. Many of the techniques discussed in this book are beautifully illustrated in a series of videotapes produced by Karl Zetner.

Other European centers of research in small animal dentistry in the latter half of the twentieth century include the Universities of Zurich and Hannover, as well as a dedicated and growing core of specialized practitioners, such as Peter Fahrenkrug.

The advancement of small animal dentistry in the United States from the early 1970s onwards was catalyzed by the pioneering work of Donald Ross and formation of the American Veterinary Dental Society (AVDS) in 1976. The AVDS, organized by Benjamin H. Colmery, fostered a group of inspired practitioners who collaborated in publication of a Dentistry issue of the Veterinary Clinics—Small Animal Practice in 1986 (edited by Pat Frost) and created the Academy of Veterinary Dentistry (1987) and the American Veterinary Dental College (1988). The group included Gary Beard, Peter Emily, Tom Mulligan, and Chuck Williams, who, as lectures of continuing education seminars and with the support of Henry Schein, Inc., have done so much to popularize ongoing instruction and practice in small animal dentistry in the last 5 years.

A critical review of the literature in comparative periodontal disease was published by Page and Schroeder in 1982 and is an excellent introduction to the literature published in human dental journals. A new series of veterinary dental texts appeared in the 1980s, concentrating on small animal dentistry: Zetner's *Tierarztliche Zahnheilkunde* (1982), Tholen's *Concepts in Veterinary Dentistry* (1983), *Fahrenkrug's Handbuch der Zahnbehandlung in der Kleintierpraxis* (1984), Harvey's *Veterinary Dentistry* (1985), d'Authevile and Barrairon's *Odontostomatologie Veterinarie* (1985), and Klinge's *Hund-tandvard* (1987). Some of these books were written by or with contributions and assistance from human dentists. Human dental and oral surgical techniques were described for use in animals, and huge leaps were made in understanding what we could do and how to do it.

Until recently the use of techniques developed for use on human teeth and mouths was accepted with little question in small animal dentistry. Probably the most important recent change is the questioning of this overall acceptance of use of human dental techniques. Much practical and research-generated information on this topic is now available and is incorporated into this book to put the techniques borrowed from human dentistry into context. Thus we can truly start to think of the content of this book as "small animal dentistry."

Important differences between human and carnivore dentistry include anatomy (dental arch and root apex), function (jaw occlusal pressure and direction of available jaw movement), physiology (salivary and oral pH), practicality of oral home care, and microbiology (significant similarities and differences, including importance of viruses in feline oral disease).

This book can include only the information available to the authors at the time of writing. In some areas the state-of-the-art information has not changed greatly in the last 5 years. In others, change is occurring rapidly, and areas of current frustration, such as gingivitis-stomatitis and dental resorptive lesions in cats, may be less problematic in the near future.

Although it is often difficult to obtain detailed follow-up of veterinary dental procedures because of the need for anesthesia to obtain correctly positioned radiographs, we have tried to illustrate long-term results when practical—everything looks good at the end of the procedure (in most cases, anyway!), but the veterinary dental literature is short on follow-up results. We have also chosen to include some examples of when things do not go right—not all of them are from the "Elsewhere Veterinary Hospital"! Comments and suggestions for improvement of this book are welcomed by the authors.

Colin E. Harvey
VHUP 3113
3850 Spruce Street
Philadelphia, PA 19104

Peter P. Emily
1051 Independence Street
Lakewood, CO 80215

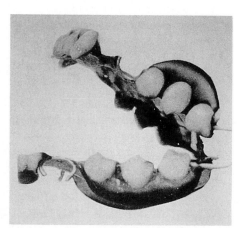

False teeth made for a dog—a case report from the 1897 *J Comp Ther.*

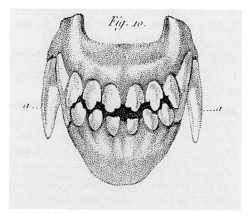

Rostral dentition of the dog from a plate illustrating aging changes. From Girard NF, Girard J: *Traite de l'age du cheval, augmentee de l'age du boeuf, du mouton, du chien et du cochon,* ed 3, Paris, 1834, Bechet Jeune.

► HISTORICAL REFERENCES

Becker E: *Neuzeitliche Untersuchung und Behandlung der Zahn-krankheiten beim Pferd*, Hannover, 1938, M&H Schaper.

Colyer F: *Variations and diseases of the teeth of animals*, London, 1936, John Bale, Sons and Danielsson.

d'Authevile P, Barrairon E: *Odontostomatologie veterinaire*, Paris, 1985, Maloine SA.

Eisenmenger E, Zetner K: *Tierarztliche Zahnheilkunde*, Berlin, 1982, Paul Parey.

Fahrenkrug P: *Handbuch der Zahnbehandlung in der Kleintier-praxis*, Hasloh, 1984, published by the author.

Frost P, editor: Dentistry. *Vet Clin North Am, Sm Anim Pract* 16:785, 1986.

Girard J, Girard NF: *Traite de l'age du cheval, augmentee de l'age du boeuf, du mouton, du chien et du cochon*, ed 3, Paris, 1834, Bechet Jeune.

Harvey CE, editor: *Veterinary dentistry*, Philadelphia, 1985, WB Saunders.

Hinebauch TD: *Veterinary dental surgery*. Lafayette, Ind, 1889, published by the author.

Klinge B: *Hund-tandvard*, Malmo, 1987, Invest-Odont.

Mellanby M: Diet and the teeth: an experimental study. Part A. Dental structure in dogs (pp. 1-308); Part B. Diet and dental disease in dogs (pp. 1-69). Diet and dental structure in mammals other than the dog (pp. 70-94). London, 1929-1930, Medical Research Council, Her Majesty's Stationery Office.

Merillat LA: *Animal dentistry and diseases of the mouth*. Chicago, 1905, Alexander Eger.

Miles AEW, Grigson C: *Colyer's variations and diseases of the teeth of animals*, Cambridge, 1990, Cambridge University Press.

Page RC, Schroeder HE: *Periodontitis in man and other animals: a comparative review*, Basel, 1982, Karger.

Simonds JB: *The age of the ox, sheep, and pig*, London, 1854, WS Orr & Co.

Tholen MA: *Concepts in veterinary dentistry*, Edwardsville, Kan, 1983, Veterinary Medicine Publishing Practice Co.

Acknowledgments

This is a cross-cultural book. Each of us brings an in-depth background from one culture and has learned much from practitioners and researchers in other cultures.

Colin Harvey wishes to acknowledge the members of the dental and dental hygienist professions who have contributed to his dental education, in particular: Laura Braswell, Peter Emily, Peter Fahrenkrug, Bonnie Flax, David Garber, Amy Golden, Keith Grove, Ben Hammond, Louis Rossman, Deborah Sams, Allan Shaw, Roberta Thorne, Carl Tinkelman, Marsha Venner, and Sam Yankell. Veterinarians and other scientists who have helped to move his informal dental education along include: Thomas Eriksen, Philippe Hennet, Larry Laster, Ayako Okuda, Fran Shofer, Frank Verstraete, and the many veterinarians in dental practice who have been willing to accept challenges, have observed the results, and have shared their experiences.

Peter Emily wishes to acknowledge the contributions of his colleagues in the CE Seminars Veterinary Dental Programs (Gary Beard, Tom Mulligan, Chuck Williams) and the support he has received from Colorado State University and Dr. Eric Pope at the University of Missouri.

Both authors have benefited greatly from the opportunity to work with and spend endless hours of convivial discussion of veterinary dentistry with Karl Zetner. Both authors also wish to acknowledge the pivotal importance of Gerry Selin in the recent explosive development of veterinary dentistry—a hands-on discipline requires hands-on training if it is to produce competent practitioners—and at a global level, Gerry Selin saw the need and made it happen.

Parts of the text were read and suggestions for improvement offered by Drs. Sydney Evans, Michael Goldschmidt, Philippe Hennet, Gail Smith, and Ms. Bonnie Flax, RDH; their help is appreciated and any remaining errors or omissions are the responsibility of the authors.

Acknowledgments in books such as this often include a statement that preparing it was a pleasure. In fact, it is hard work, but the work was made much less onerous with the willing and very capable assistance of William Alston, Doug Thayer, Joseph Magrane, and the artistic skills of Dennis Giddings. Sandy Reinhardt and the staff at Mosby were very helpful.

Some figures included in this book first appeared in *Veterinary Dentistry,* edited by C.E. Harvey and published by W.B. Saunders in 1985. These include figures provided by C.F. Burrows, A.S. Dorn, D. Garber, W. Miller, L. Rossman, and J.P. Weigel. Other figures from previously published material are included, with permission of the copyright owners cited in the legend.

Contents

1

Function, Formation, and Anatomy of Oral Structures in Carnivores

► FUNCTION

Functions of the oral structures include the introduction of food and fluids into the alimentary canal, protection against external forces such as predators or societal rivals, protection against microbial organisms and other potentially injurious ingested material, grooming, evaporative heat loss (particularly in dogs), sexual enhancement by licking and taste stimulation, and communication (for example, lip raising or teeth baring).

Food first must be identified, usually by olfactory or visual stimulation. Carnivorous species frequently must subdue their food source, usually with their canine teeth. To so do, they must be able to open the mouth wide enough for the upper and lower teeth to encompass the prey. A wide opening also is necessary to permit the sectorial (carnassial) teeth to engage part of the prey so that it can be cut into pieces small enough to swallow. Some carnivores, such as cats, are primarily predators. Others, such as dogs, are primarily carrion eaters and may be omnivorous. These differences are reflected in the presence or absence of crushing (molar) teeth.

Carnivores have limited ability to move the jaws other than in an open-close plane (that is, the temporomandibular joint is a hinge joint that is not capable of much lateral excursion or protrusive or retrusive movements). This allows the temporomandibular joint to be surrounded by strong ligaments that prevent disruption of the joint when extreme occlusive forces are applied during struggling by prey or for cracking of bones and tearing of flesh.

Once a piece of food material small enough to swallow is separated from the carcass, the food goes directly to the pharynx. The placement of the food bolus in the mouth (prehension) and the process of drinking (lapping) are accomplished by actions of the tongue, an organ that can stretch, shorten, tip up, or curl down at will.

A bolus that is ready for passage to the pharynx and beyond is pushed caudally by the tongue. This initiates deglutition (swallowing), a complex reflex action that prevents inundation of the airway. The bolus must pass through the airway, between the nasopharynx and larynx. The process starts by action of the muscles attached to the bones that form the hyoid arch, causing the larynx to be pulled rostrally. By a simple hinge mechanism, this action causes the epiglottis to cover the laryngeal opening (glottis). The tongue moves caudally, forming the bolus and pumping it caudally. As the bolus reaches the pharynx, the muscles in the soft palate and nasopharyngeal wall

1

contract to form a sphincteric ring, closing off the nasopharynx. The bolus cannot escape into the larynx, nasopharynx, or oral cavity (which is closed off by the contracted tongue making contact with the roof of the mouth). The cranial esophageal sphincter (cricopharyngeal muscle) relaxes, and the pharyngeal muscles contract from rostral to caudal, pushing the bolus into the esophagus. Once the bolus has crossed the pharynx, the cricopharyngeal muscle contracts, preventing regurgitation of material into the pharynx. The nasopharyngeal sphincter muscles and hyoid muscles then relax; this restores the airway lumen by opening the nasopharynx and causes the epiglottis to lift from the glottis.

The passage of food material is assisted by the secretions of the salivary glands, which lubricate the food. Salivary secretion is coordinated with prehension and deglutition, although a basal secretion flow continuously moistens the oropharyngeal mucosa. Parasympathetic fibers in the trigeminal and facial (chorda tympani) nerves cause secretion in response to olfactory, visual, and gustatory stimulation.

Grooming is accomplished by the tongue and the incisor teeth. Heat loss in dogs, which have few sweat glands in their skin, is achieved principally by evaporation of nasal and salivary secretions during panting. The lateral nasal gland, which secretes a serous fluid at a rate that is proportional to ambient temperature, is the major source of fluid for evaporative loss, although the salivary and scattered mucosal glands in the oral cavity also contribute. Panting is an efficient one-way system (in through the nose, out through the mouth) effected by contraction of the hyoepiglottic muscle, which causes the epiglottis and soft palate to separate during expiration.

Protection against microbial invasion is provided at three levels. The primary layer is the film of oral fluid created by salivary secretions, which bathes the oral mucosal surfaces with a fluid rich in antibacterial barriers. These biochemical antibacterial substances include mucin, lactoferrin, lysozyme, and lactoperoxidase. Saliva also contains immunoglobulins, predominantly IgA synthesized by plasma cells associated with the salivary glands. The "minor" glands are more involved than the "major" glands (mandibular, parotid, sublingual, and zygomatic), perhaps because

the shorter ducts result in greater antigenic stimulation. The second layer provides mechanical protection by the tough oral epithelium. The third layer consists of the rich vascular supply and aggregation of immunoreactive cells in the supporting connective tissues. The immunologic function of the lymphatic tissue ring in the oropharynx and nasopharynx is particularly important as a source of antigenic stimulation for circulating antibody production.

Taste is of unknown clinical importance in veterinary species; the macrosmatic (highly developed sense of smell) carnivorous species probably depend as much or more on olfaction (sense of smell) than on gustation (sense of taste) as an appetite stimulant. Because food is provided for companion animals by their owners, the effects of loss of olfaction or gustation are rarely evident clinically.

▶ FORMATION

The gastrointestinal tract consists of a blind-ended tube formed by entodermal proliferation very early in embryonic development. Two depressions form over the cranial and caudal extensions of the primitive gut. The cranial depression, the stomodeum, sinks in until only a thin layer of tissue, the oral plate, separates the primitive gut lumen from the external environment. The oral plate then ruptures to establish continuity; it is located at the level of what will be the oropharynx in the adult. Thus the oral cavity and most of the oropharynx and related structures are formed from stomodeal ectoderm and supporting mesenchymal connective tissue.

At the time that the oral plate ruptures, the stomodeum is still very shallow compared with the complex oral cavity present at birth. Structures that will form the jaws and face subsequently grow forward. The mandible and maxilla start as paired processes. The mandibular processes grow together and join to form the mandibular arch, although in the dog and the cat, the symphysis remains fibrous throughout life. Development of the upper jaw is more complicated. The maxillary processes grow together, but they do not join. They fuse with the premaxilla that forms from paired nasomedial processes. Disruption of development of any of the multiple sites of origin of the upper jaw can result in complex congenital anomalies. The area formed by the midnasal process (the premaxilla, which is the site of origin of the upper incisor teeth) is called the *primary palate*. The palate may fail to fuse—either in the midline or on one or both sides—with the structures formed from the maxillary processes (the maxilla and all the upper teeth other than the incisors), which is called the *secondary palate*. The palate itself is formed in three parts. One part is a triangular rostral contribution from the conjoined midnasal processes forming the premaxilla, which becomes the area rostral to and including the incisive papilla. The larger portion of the palate is formed by two shelflike projections that grow medially from the maxillary processes and join to separate the nasal cavity from the oral cavity.

The tongue arises from a midline prominence and two lateral swellings that form most of its substance. The origins of the muscles of the tongue are occipital somite myotomes that migrate forward, carrying with them the hypoglossal nerve, which thus takes a long loop across the lateral tissues of the pharynx. The sensory supply of the tongue is derived from the trigeminal, facial, glossopharyngeal and vagus nerves, which are the nerves associated with the first through fourth branchial arches that form the epithelial surface of the tongue.

Teeth arise from thickenings on the jaws called *dental ledges* (Fig. 1-1). Ectodermal epithelial cells push into the underlying mesenchymal tissues to form a labiogingival lamina, which forms the lips, and a dental lamina. The long dental lamina then splits to form separate buds, the enamel organs. These differentiate into cup-shaped structures with an inner ameloblast layer surrounding a papilla of mesenchymal cells that proliferate to form the dentin and pulp of the tooth. Nerves and vessels proliferate, sending branches into each papilla, and mandibular or premaxillary/maxillary bone proliferates so that the calcified structures of the jaws are in place. Both deciduous and permanent teeth buds form within a short time of each other in utero. The buds that will form the permanent teeth start as small buds from the deciduous tooth bud and remain dormant for some time, until jaw length has provided space for them to develop. Thus, for permanent teeth that have a deciduous

counterpart, absence of the deciduous tooth bud means absence of the permanent tooth also.

Dentin is formed by odontoblasts, the outermost layer of the mesenchymal dental papilla. Dentin matrix is secreted and later strengthened by deposition of calcium salts. Cytoplasmic strands of the odontoblast cells remain embedded in the dentin. The tissues remaining in the pulp are blood vessels, nerves, and supporting connective tissue. The tissues that form the pulp canal and roots of the teeth are described in more detail in Chapter 6. The dental pulp tissues remain active during life, initially causing lengthening of the root, followed by development ("closure" or "apexification") of the apex (tip) of the root and, later, progressive narrowing of the pulp chamber and root canal. Apical closure usually is evident by about 18 months in dogs and cats, with subsequent root canal narrowing occurring most rapidly up to about 3 years of age.

Teeth erupt because of progressive growth of roots. Lengthening of the root after eruption results from activity of cells in Hertwig's root sheath, a ring of tissue at the apex of the root in young teeth. This tissue lies to the outside of the root dentin and thus may survive pulpal necrosis (see Chapter 6).

Enamel is formed by ameloblasts in the inner lining of the ectodermally generated enamel organ; a prism of calcified organic matrix forms perpendicular to each ameloblast, providing the strong rigid smooth surface of the tooth. Crown formation is completed entirely within the bone of the jaws, well before root lengthening commences.

Cementum formation does not occur until the tooth is almost full grown and is in position. Before eruption the tooth is surrounded by a specialized layer of mesenchymal tissue, the dental sac. Part of this is lost during eruption, but the deeper part forms cementum on the dentin surface of the root, much as periosteum forms bone. Between the periosteum of the surrounding bone and the cementoblasts of the dental sac remnant—and embedded in the organic matrix of the two structures—are the periodontal fibers formed from connective tissue within this narrow space. These tissues are described in greater detail in Chapter 4.

Permanent teeth erupt at specific times for particular teeth in each species. This varies somewhat, par-

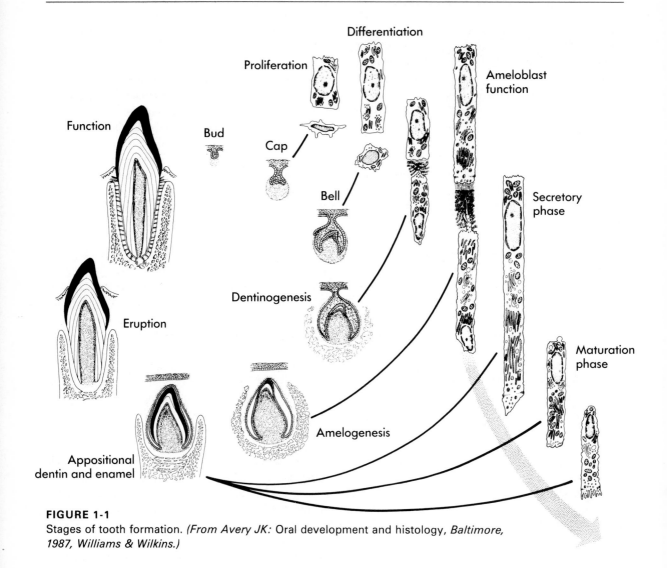

FIGURE 1-1
Stages of tooth formation. *(From Avery JK:* Oral development and histology, *Baltimore, 1987, Williams & Wilkins.)*

ticularly for a species such as the dog where there is a very wide range in body size among breeds. Even without a permanent tooth erupting beneath it, the deciduous tooth normally is shed on schedule as a result of internal resorption. During eruption the root of the developing permanent tooth lengthens and pushes against the deciduous tooth, disrupting its blood supply. The root of the deciduous tooth is resorbed, and the tooth becomes so weakly held in position that occlusal pressure dislodges it from the mouth. The gingival tissue is cut or torn by the de-

veloping crown during eruption. Between the time of initial penetration by the crown tip and eruption to full-crown height, the gingival tissues are unable to heal to the enamel. The result may be bleeding, sometimes accompanied by inflammation (pericoronitis), although this is rarely of clinical importance in dogs and cats. Growth of the root of the permanent tooth continues until the crown is in fully erupted position, at which time the gingival epithelium and connective tissue heal to form the normal gingival attachment at the cementoenamel junction.

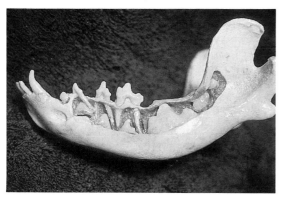

FIGURE 1-2
Dissected mandible of a 2- to 3-month-old dog
showing the developing permanent teeth embedded
in the jaws.

Growth of the upper and lower jaws is relatively independent each of the other. This can cause occlusion abnormalities of the teeth if opposing quadrants occlude in abnormal relationship and cause dental interlock (see Chapter 8). The succession of deciduous by permanent teeth provides functional dentition of a size suitable for the jaw at the time of eruption, as well as replacement at a later time by a larger set of teeth appropriate for the larger jaws of the mature animal (Fig. 1-2). Abnormal dental interlock can occur with deciduous or permanent teeth. Growth of the mandible can continue in giant-breed dogs well beyond the time of skeletal maturity of limb bones.

The salivary glands and ducts develop from invaginations of oral epithelium. Myoepithelial cells, autonomic nerves, and vessels develop to form the functional unit. Salivary secretion is abundant in carnivores: the mandibular, sublingual, and parotid glands can be resected or ligated bilaterally with no discernible clinical abnormality.

▶ ANATOMY

Lips

The opening of the lips is wide in carnivores, extending to the level of the first molar teeth so that the mouth can be opened adequately to accommodate large sections of food material that will be separated into swallowable chunks. The lips themselves are soft and fleshy; they are covered by normal hairy skin on the external surface and by nonkeratinized squamous epithelium on the inner surface. Between the epithelial surfaces lie the facial muscles, connective tissue and vessels, and the large trigeminal nerve branches serving the vibrissae. As with all oral cavity surfaces, the mucosal surfaces of the lips normally are moistened continuously by salivary gland secretions. The upper lip overhangs the junction of the lower lip and oral tissues, so that the oral epithelium is not normally visible except during eating and drinking or, in dogs, during panting.

In the dog the lower lip is rather loosely attached to the mandible and, in giant-breed dogs, may form a furrow that allows salivary secretions to leak from the mouth. There is a short, firmer attachment (frenulum) of the lower lip to the mandible at about the level of the first premolar tooth that causes an indentation of the skin; it is this area that forms a valley of skin that becomes diseased in lip-fold dermatitis in spaniels and sometimes in other breeds. This frenulum also may be of clinical significance in periodontal disease (see Chapter 4). There is a less obvious frenulum on the upper lip opposite the second or third upper premolar close to where the infraorbital nerve and vessels emerge from the infraorbital foramen. The lips, and less frequently the tongue, often are partially pigmented, except in chows and related breeds in which the entire oral epithelial surface is pigmented.

If the upper lip is lifted and curled out, the openings of two salivary ducts can be seen: (1) the parotid papilla as a single papilla on the mucosa that lies opposite the upper carnassial tooth and (2) the zygomatic duct openings as a line of several papillae on a ridge of mucosa caudal and medial to the parotid papilla and opposite the last molar tooth.

Teeth

When the lips are raised or the mouth is open, the teeth are the most obvious structures visible because of the contrasting color of enamel against the other oral structures. The surface of normal teeth of dogs is dense white and smooth; the teeth of cats often are slightly yellow compared with those of the dog.

The following dental formula applies to the dog:

$$\text{Deciduous} - 2\ (I\frac{3}{3},\ C\frac{1}{1},\ P\frac{2}{2},\ M\frac{1}{1}) = 28$$

$$\text{Permanent} - 2\ (I\frac{3}{3},\ C\frac{1}{1},\ P\frac{4}{4},\ M\frac{2}{3}) = 42$$

The following dental formula applies to the cat:

$$\text{Deciduous} - 2\ (I\frac{3}{3},\ C\frac{1}{1},\ P\frac{3}{2}) = 26$$

$$\text{Permanent} - 2\ (I\frac{3}{3},\ C\frac{1}{1},\ P\frac{3}{2},\ M\frac{1}{1}) = 28$$

Eruption times vary within a narrow range in normal dogs; congenital anomalies and systemic disease can cause eruption to be outside the normal range; eruption schedules for each tooth are shown in Table 1-1. Factors that affect the time of eruption include general health and nutritional state, sex, body size, and season of birth. Teeth of female dogs erupt earlier than those of males, teeth of larger breed dogs erupt earlier, and teeth of dogs born in the summer erupt earlier. Once the teeth are fully erupted, tooth development continues until the root has attained full length and apical closure (see preceding discussion of Hertwig's root sheath activity) and then ceases except for laying down of additional dentin by odontoblast activity on the inner dentinal surface.

TABLE 1-1	Teeth eruption schedules for the dog and cat*			
	Deciduous teeth (weeks)		Permanent teeth (months)	
	Dog	Cat	Dog	Cat
Incisors	3-4	2-3	3-5	3-4
Canines	3	3-4	4-6	4-5
Premolars	4-12	3-6	4-6	4-6
Molars	—	—	5-7	4-5

*Variations occur with breed and size of animal; gingival eruption is followed by extrusion to full crown height over a period of several weeks.

All teeth are similar structurally (Fig. 1-3), although they differ significantly in size, shape, and function. A mature tooth has a crown and one or more roots. The crown is covered with enamel, a very dense, smooth tissue with very little organic content. The root is covered with a thin layer of cementum, a calcified structure into which the periodontal fibers penetrate to hold the tooth in position. The enamel (crown) and cementum (root) meet at the cemento-enamel junction (CEJ). In an extracted tooth, this line is clear because of the color change and roughness of the cementum compared with the enamel. In many teeth there is a bulge of enamel just coronal to the CEJ, which permits the attachment of gingiva in a protected concavity—the "neck" of the tooth. The apex of the root of a mature tooth contains several small foramina ("apical delta") for passage of blood vessels and nerves into the pulp cavity. The pulp cavity is much larger and the dentin is thinner in growing animals. The dentin continues to thicken throughout life.

The surfaces of teeth are identified by specific names. These anatomic terms for the surfaces of teeth are based on the position of that structure in an animal with normal occlusion (Fig. 1-4). Even when the teeth occupy an abnormal position in the mouth, their shape rarely changes except as a result of abnormal wear or trauma:

Coronal—in the direction of the tip of the crown
Apical—in the direction of the tip (apex) of the root
Mesial—facing toward the rostral end of the arch or toward the midline (for incisor teeth)
Distal—facing in the caudal direction of the arch (or laterally for incisor teeth)
Buccal (facial)—facing toward the cheek or lip
Lingual (lower teeth) or palatal (upper teeth)—facing toward the tongue or palate

The four canine teeth, situated at the rostral corners of the jaws, are the largest teeth. The single, slightly curved crown tapers smoothly to a rounded tip in the dog and is more pointed in the cat. The canine teeth crowns often have linear grooves in their surface, particularly in cats. In dogs the canine teeth are oval in cross section, with a distinct ridge on the mesio-lingual and distolingual surfaces so that these ridges form the frame of facets on the lingual-palatal surface

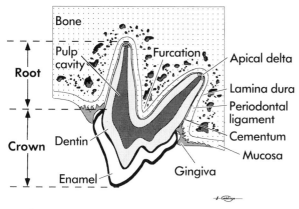

FIGURE 1-3
Anatomic features of a double-rooted tooth.

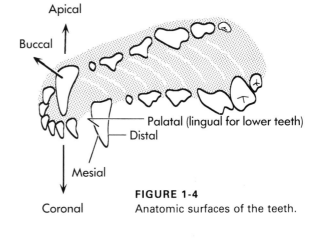

FIGURE 1-4
Anatomic surfaces of the teeth.

of the teeth. With the mouth closed in normal occlusion ("scissors bite"), the lower canine tooth is located between the upper canine tooth and the upper third incisor tooth. The roots of the canine teeth are single but very large and long, often up to twice as long as the crown and wider than the crown in the midsection; they curve caudally so the apex lies deep to the first—and sometimes to the second—premolar teeth. The upper canine tooth root is indicated by a palpable smooth protuberance (jugae) on the surface of the maxilla. There usually is a space (diastema) between the upper canine teeth and the incisor and first premolar teeth.

The six upper and lower incisor teeth sit in curved lines between the canine teeth; the corner incisor is the largest and the central incisor the smallest. At least early in life, they have three cusps at the tip of the crown. The middle cusp is much larger and higher than the two lateral cusps (Fig. 1-5). Attempts to estimate a dog's age by the wear on the cusps of the incisor teeth rarely are successful because of variable wear caused by dietary differences and other chewing behaviors. The incisors of cats have a large central cusp and two lateral protuberances that often are too small to see distinctly. The roots of the incisor teeth are single and narrower, but longer, than the crowns. The lateral cusps of the crowns of the incisor teeth usually contact those of adjacent incisor teeth, although in large, wide-faced dogs there may be an obvious interdental space. The crown tips of the upper

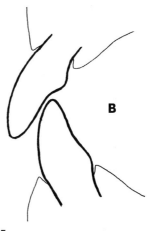

A

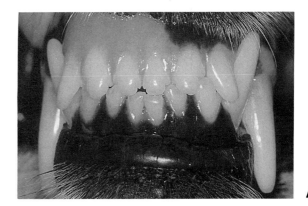

B

FIGURE 1-5
A, Rostral view of the incisor teeth of a dog. **B**, Sagittal section of incisor teeth in occlusion.

incisor teeth lie just rostral to and slightly overlap the tips of the lower incisor teeth when the jaws are closed in a dog with normal occlusion. The tips of the lower incisor teeth occlude against the shelf of enamel on the palatal surface of the upper incisor teeth known as the *cingulum* (Fig. 1-5, *B*). Widespread variation in incisor occlusion occurs among dogs; lower incisor placement well rostral to the upper incisors is considered normal in brachycephalic breeds. These and other patterns are described in Chapter 8. In cats the incisors often are in "level bite;" that is, the incisal edges occlude upon each other.

The numbering of premolar and molar teeth can be confusing. The primitive carnivore has four premolar and three molar permanent teeth in each quadrant. When less than a complete set is present, it is presumed that premolar teeth are absent starting from the rostral end of the jaw and molar teeth from the caudal end. Thus in the dog, with four upper and lower premolar (PM) teeth, two upper molar (M) teeth, and three lower molar teeth, the numbering is simple (see also Fig. 1-6):

Upper— PM1 PM2 PM3 PM4 M1 M2
Lower—PM1 PM2 PM3 PM4 M1 M2 M3

In the cat the numbering seems to make less sense, even though it is anatomically and developmentally correct. The cat has three upper premolars and one molar tooth, and two lower premolars and one molar tooth (see also Fig. 1-7):

Upper—(PM1) PM2 PM3 PM4 M1
Lower—(PM1) (PM2) PM3 PM4 M1

PM4 and M1 are the large carnassial teeth. On the basis of the aforementioned numbering system, the upper carnassial tooth is always PM4 and the lower carnassial tooth is always M1. In this text, for the cat the aforementioned nomenclature will be used. In many instances in other sources, a simpler but anatomically incorrect nomenclature is used for cats: PM1, PM2, PM3, M1 (upper) and PM1, PM2, and M1 (lower).

The largest and most obvious of the cheek (premolar and molar) teeth are the carnassial teeth, which provide a shearing or scissors action for reducing large sections of food to a size suitable for swallowing. These teeth are the upper fourth premolar and lower first molar teeth in both dogs and cats. The crown of the upper carnassial tooth occludes against the crown of the lower carnassial tooth, which normally lies lingual to the upper crown in resting occlusion. The crowns are large and multicusped. The other premolar teeth have a central large cusp and one (mesial) and one or two (distal) smaller cusps. In the dog the upper first molar tooth has three cusps of almost equal size, forming an occlusal surface for crushing/grinding; although caries formation is rare in dogs, the shape of the crown of this tooth makes it most likely to be affected. Other grinding teeth with occlusal tables are the upper second molar, the distal half of the lower first molar, and the second and third molar teeth in dogs. There are no grinding teeth in cats (the very small upper molar tooth has only a small central conical crown and thus could be considered as a grinding tooth, but there is no occluding tooth in the lower jaw to grind against). The crown of the lower molar tooth in cats has a distinctly different shape from any other tooth—approximately equal mesial and distal cusps that are sharply pointed, with a deep cleft between them.

The larger cheek teeth are multirooted, the upper fourth premolar and first and second molars in dogs and the upper fourth premolar in cats having three roots. Generally the roots of multirooted teeth are approximately equal in size and diverge slightly from each other; exceptions are the upper fourth premolar (carnassial) tooth—in which the palatal root is smaller than the mesial and distal roots in both dogs and cats—and the lower molar tooth in cats, in which the mesial root is two or three times as wide as the distal root and the distal root often is directed at a distinct angle caudally.

Deciduous teeth are smaller and slimmer than permanent teeth (see Fig. 8-14). Occlusal contact of deciduous teeth is minimal in dogs and cats, although the deciduous upper first molar tooth in the dog has a trituberculate grinding surface similar to the permanent first upper molar; in the dog this is the only deciduous tooth with three roots. The roots of deciduous teeth are long and slender, although some root resorption often has taken place by the time that it is necessary to examine or extract these teeth clinically.

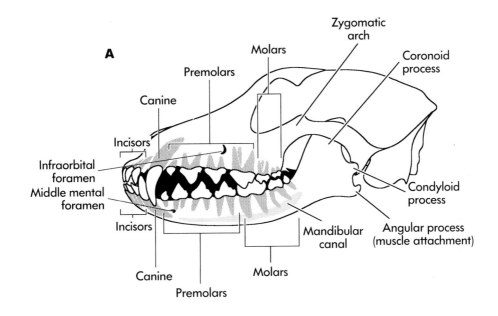

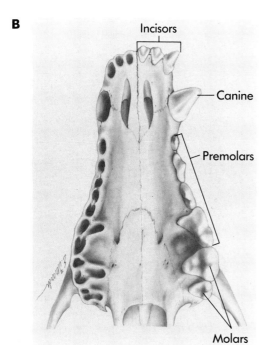

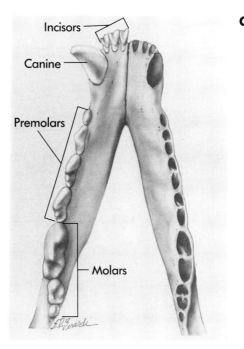

FIGURE 1-6
Lateral and ventrodorsal views of the skull and teeth of a dog showing normal occlusion and roots. **A,** Lateral view of the upper and lower jaws. **B,** Upper jaw with teeth in place on right side and root alveoli on left. **C,** Lower jaw with teeth in place on left side and root alveoli on right.

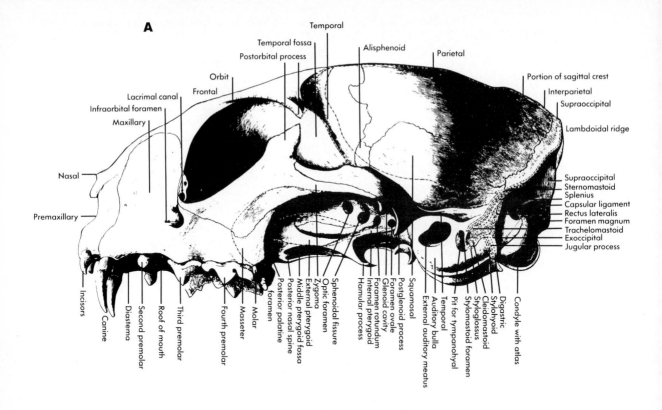

A

Temporal

Temporal fossa

Postorbital process

Alisphenoid

Parietal

Orbit

Portion of sagittal crest

Frontal

Interparietal

Lacrimal canal

Supraoccipital

Infraorbital foramen

Maxillary

Lambdoidal ridge

Nasal

Supraoccipital
Sternomastoid
Splenius
Capsular ligament
Rectus lateralis
Foramen magnum
Trachelomastoid
Exoccipital
Jugular process

Premaxillary

Incisors

Canine

Diastema

Second premolar

Roof of mouth

Third premolar

Fourth premolar

Masseter

Molar

Posterior palatine foramen

Posterior nasal spine

Middle pterygoid

External pterygoid

Zygoma

Optic foramen

Sphenoidal fissure

Hamular process

Internal pterygoid

Foramen rotundum

Foramen ovale

Glenoid cavity

Postglenoid process

Squamosal

Temporal

Auditory bulla

External auditory meatus

Pit for tympanohyal

Stylomastoid foramen

Styloglossus

Cleidomastoid

Stylohyoid

Digastric

Condyle with atlas

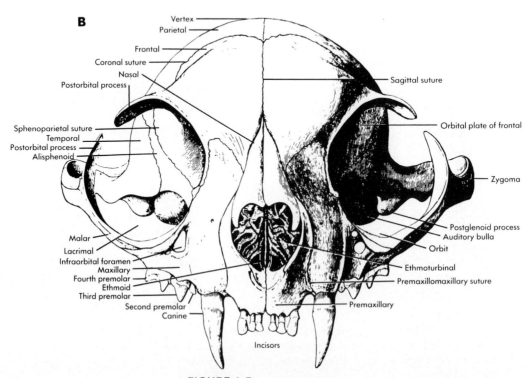

B

Vertex

Parietal

Frontal

Coronal suture

Nasal

Sagittal suture

Postorbital process

Orbital plate of frontal

Sphenoparietal suture

Temporal

Postorbital process

Alisphenoid

Zygoma

Postglenoid process
Auditory bulla
Orbit

Malar

Lacrimal

Infraorbital foramen

Maxillary

Fourth premolar

Ethmoid

Third premolar

Second premolar

Canine

Ethmoturbinal

Premaxillomaxillary suture

Premaxillary

Incisors

FIGURE 1-7
For legend see opposite page.

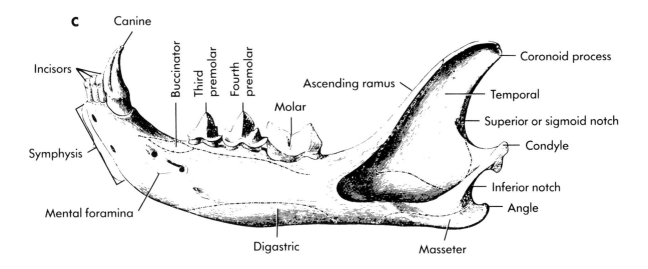

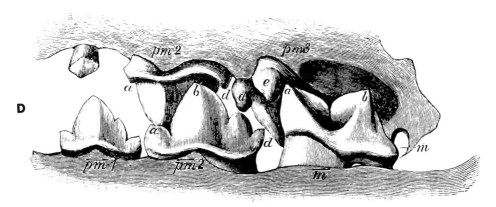

FIGURE 1-7
Lateral (**A** and **C**), frontal (**B**), and medial (**D**) views of the skull and teeth of a cat. *(From Jayne H: The skeleton of the cat, Philadelphia, 1898, JB Lippincott.)*

Jaws

The roots of the teeth, which sit in alveoli or sockets within the mandible, maxilla, or incisive bones, are held in place by the periodontal fibers that penetrate both tooth and bone (see Chapter 4).

The mandible consists of two bones joined rostrally at the symphysis by a fibrous joint. The symphysis extends from the rostral tip of the mandible to the level of the first premolar tooth in the dog, or midway between the canine and third premolar teeth in cats. The teeth are contained in the body of the mandible,

a slightly curved bone with an obvious medullary cavity, with two or three mental foramina piercing the lateral cortex (Figs. 1-6 and 1-7). The largest mental foramen is located ventral to the first premolar tooth in dogs, and the canine-premolar diastema in cats. Another foramen is between the first (central) and second (middle) incisor teeth, and often one more caudal to the large mental foramen. The medullary cavity carries the sensory mental nerves and vessels that supply the teeth and skin of the rostral lip. The (vertical) ramus, which joins the body of the mandible at

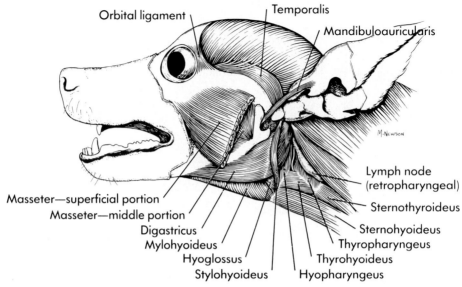

Orbital ligament   Temporalis   Mandibuloauricularis

Masseter—superficial portion
Masseter—middle portion
Digastricus
Mylohyoideus
Hyoglossus
Stylohyoideus

Lymph node (retropharyngeal)
Sternothyroideus
Sternohyoideus
Thyropharyngeus
Thyrohyoideus
Hyopharyngeus

FIGURE 1-8
Lateral view of the muscles of mastication of a dog. *(From Evans HE:* Miller's anatomy of the dog, *ed 3, Philadelphia, 1993, WB Saunders.)*

its caudal end, has three projections (Figs. 1-6 and 1-7). The most dorsal is the coronoid process, a broad but thin, flat area of bone for attachment of the temporal muscle at its dorsal tip and rostral edge (coronoid crest) and the masseter muscle lateroventrally. Projecting caudally is the articular process; the transversely oriented condyle at its caudal end articulates with the temporal bone to form the temporomandibular joint (TMJ). The angular process (muscular process) extends caudoventrally, forming the site of insertion of the pterygoid muscle and additional fibers of the masseter muscle. The muscles of mastication (temporal, medial and lateral pterygoid, and masseter) close the jaws, and when desired by carnivores, with great force (Fig. 1-8). The digastric muscle, a smaller muscle originating on the jugular process of the skull and inserting on the ventral surface of the mandible, opens the jaws. The muscles of mastication, along with the rostral part of the digastric muscle, are supplied by the mandibular branch of the trigeminal nerve. The caudal part of the digastric muscle is supplied by the facial nerve.

The TMJ is formed between the articular process of the mandible and the mandibular fossa of the temporal bone (Figs. 1-6 and 1-7). The joint surface is separated into a dorsal (temporal) and a ventral (mandibular) compartment by an articular disk, a flat fibrocartilaginous plate. The shapes of the mandibular process and the temporal facet do not match exactly, allowing some sliding as well as hinge movements, although sliding movement is less available than for noncarnivorous species. The joint capsule is surrounded by fibrous tissue, formed into a strong ligament laterally.

The incisive, maxillary, and palatine bones form the roof of the mouth and support the upper teeth. Incisor teeth are rooted in the incisive bone; primary palate abnormalities, which consist of hare lip and asymmetric rostral cleft palate, are restricted to the structures supported by this bone (see Chapter 10). Two large openings in the incisive bones—the palatine fissures—often can be palpated as soft areas at the rostral end of the palate; they contain the nasopalatine ducts.

The maxilla carries the canine, premolar, and molar teeth. There is a slight alveolar process (dental ridge); however, the CEJ of the teeth generally is level with the surface of the mucoperiosteum of the palate. The roots of the teeth thus extend into the maxilla proper, rather than being confined to a dental ledge as in species such as humans. Bony prominences (jugae) can be seen or felt on the external surface of the maxilla, or they extend into the nasal spaces. The infraorbital canal, carrying the infraorbital nerves and vessels, is present just dorsal to or between the roots of the upper molar and fourth premolar teeth on the lateral aspect of the maxilla. It opens at the infraorbital foramen at the level of and just dorsal to the distal root of the third premolar tooth (Figs. 1-6 and 1-7).

The palatine bones do not contain teeth. The palatine shelves of the maxillary bone and the palatine bones separate the oral and nasal cavities. Secondary palate abnormalities affect this area as a result of failure to fuse in the midline (see Chapter 10). The soft palate continues caudally from the caudal end of the palatine bones, consisting of nasal epithelium (dorsally) and oral epithelium (ventrally) separated by muscles and loose connective tissue.

Oral Soft Tissues

The gingival tissues and peridontal ligament are described in detail in Chapter 4.

The gingival height differs significantly from tooth to tooth. It is widest over the canine teeth (up to 15 mm in a large dog) and narrowest over the upper second, third, and fourth premolar teeth (in the dog) or upper second and third premolar teeth (in the cat, in which it may measure only 1 to 2 mm) (see Fig. A-1, *B*, p. 49).

Laterally (buccally) the gingiva meets the mucosa of the lips at the mucogingival junction (MGJ). Medially (palatally, lingually, on the upper jaw) the gingiva is continuous without obvious demarcation of the mucoperiosteum of the palate; these tissues are similar histologically. The palatal mucosa is thrown into obvious folds that lie perpendicular to the long axis of the palate (Fig. 1-9, *A*); in the cat these folds often have a line of small caudally facing projections (Fig. 1-9, *B*). At the rostral end of the palate lies an obvious

midline protuberance, the incisive papilla. The nasopalatine ducts open just lateral to this papilla.

On the lower jaw the sublingual mucosa attaches to the gingiva at the MGJ and forms a trough between the mandible and the tongue. The mandibular and sublingual salivary gland ducts run submucosally in this tissue before opening onto the lateral surface of the lingual caruncle lateral to and at the base of the frenulum of the tongue. Large sublingual veins often are visible through the mucosa in this area.

The tongue, although particularly long in dogs, usually is retained in the mouth except when the animal is panting; the tongue may extend out of the mouth in brachycephalic dogs at other times. The dorsal surface of the tongue is covered by a thick mucosa that is formed into papillae (Fig. 1-10). Specialized areas of mucosa form the taste buds, although taste sensation (gustation) is of little clinical significance in companion animals. In the dog the surface of the tongue is soft compared with the rather stiff, rough surface of the tongue of the cat, which has firm papillae that point caudally (Fig. 1-10, *B*). A dorsal midline groove extends along the rostral surface of the tongue. Hairs arranged in a midline row or in two symmetric rows parallel to the midline are seen in an occasional dog (see Fig. A-2, p. 50). In newborn animals the lateral surfaces of the tongue are fimbriated. The rostral end of the tongue is free, and the lingual frenulum ventrally is loose, allowing the tongue to extend a considerable distance. The free rostral end contains a ventral stiffening rod, the lyssa, formed of fat and muscle in a fibrous sheath. The major function of the tongue is to form food boluses and to lap fluids. Its muscular structure is complex. The motor nerve supply is the hypoglossal nerve (XII); the sensory supply is a combination of trigeminal (V), facial (VII), glossopharyngeal (IX), and vagus (X) nerves, combining special sensory responses from the taste buds with normal sensory function.

The salivary glands are separated into *major* and *minor* glands. The major glands are those that can be identified surgically as distinct areas of tissue in specific locations. The major glands are the parotid (serous secretions only), mandibular (seromucous), sublingual (seromucous), and zygomatic (seromucous)

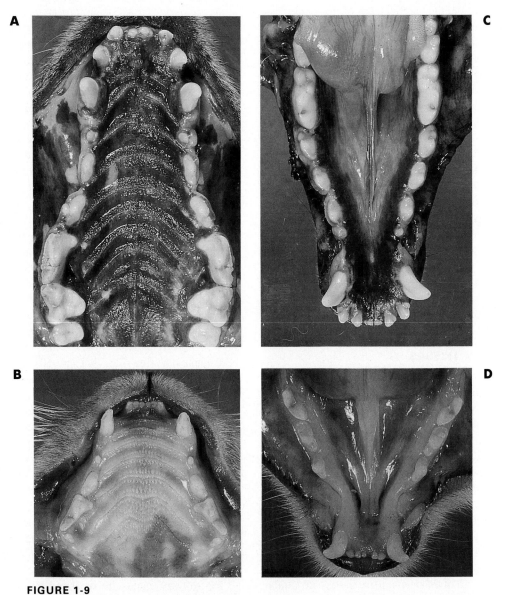

FIGURE 1-9
A, Palate and upper jaw of a dog. **B,** Palate and upper jaw of a cat. **C,** Sublingual area and mandibles of a dog. The tongue is deflected dorsally. **D,** Sublingual area and mandibles of a cat. The tongue is deflected dorsally.

A

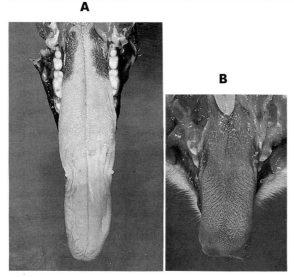

B

FIGURE 1-10
Dorsal view of the tongue of a dog (**A**) and a cat (**B**).

(Fig. 1-11). The minor glands are scattered areas of salivary tissue. The ducts of dorsal and ventral buccal glands may be visible clinically as a series of small red spots in the upper and lower fornices of the lips, extending over the glossopalatine folds. There is an abundance of saliva in normal carnivores; the parotid, mandibular, and sublingual glands can be resected or ligated bilaterally with no untoward clinical effect.

Principal blood supply to the oral region is the external carotid artery via its branches—the maxillary, facial, palatal, and lingual arteries (Fig. 1-12). Awareness of the location of these arteries is essential during major oral surgery. The maxillary artery, which supplies the palate, the mandible, and associated muscles, gives off the infraorbital artery supplying the maxilla. After exiting from the infraorbital foramen, the infraorbital artery runs between the maxilla and skin in an exposed position. The palatine branch of

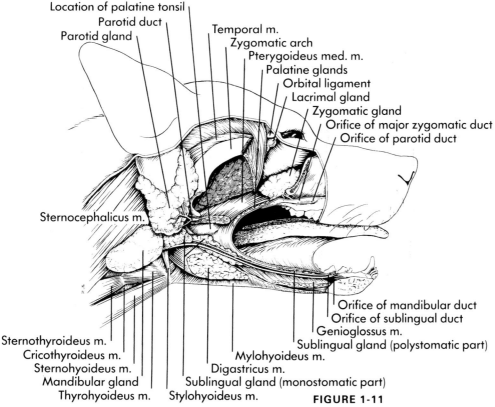

Location of palatine tonsil
Parotid duct
Parotid gland
Temporal m.
Zygomatic arch
Pterygoideus med. m.
Palatine glands
Orbital ligament
Lacrimal gland
Zygomatic gland
Orifice of major zygomatic duct
Orifice of parotid duct
Sternocephalicus m.
Orifice of mandibular duct
Orifice of sublingual duct
Genioglossus m.
Sublingual gland (polystomatic part)
Sternothyroideus m.
Cricothyroideus m.
Sternohyoideus m.
Mandibular gland
Thyrohyoideus m.
Mylohyoideus m.
Digastricus m.
Sublingual gland (monostomatic part)
Stylohyoideus m.

FIGURE 1-11
Lateral view of the salivary glands of a dog. *(From Evans HE: Miller's anatomy of the dog, ed 3, Philadelphia, 1993, WB Saunders.)*

A

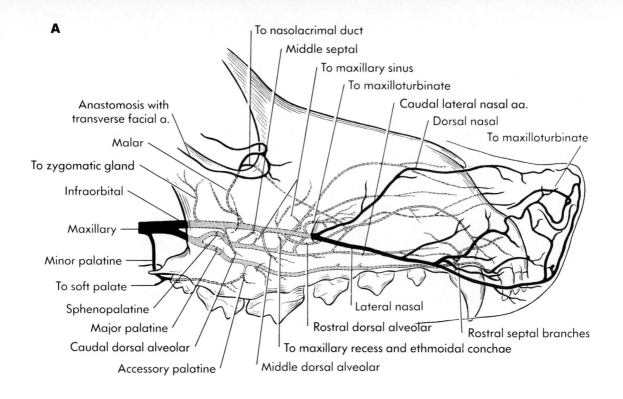

To nasolacrimal duct
Middle septal
To maxillary sinus
To maxilloturbinate
Caudal lateral nasal aa.
Dorsal nasal
To maxilloturbinate

Anastomosis with transverse facial a.
Malar
To zygomatic gland
Infraorbital
Maxillary
Minor palatine
To soft palate
Sphenopalatine
Major palatine
Caudal dorsal alveolar
Accessory palatine

Middle dorsal alveolar
To maxillary recess and ethmoidal conchae
Rostral dorsal alveolar
Lateral nasal
Rostral septal branches

B

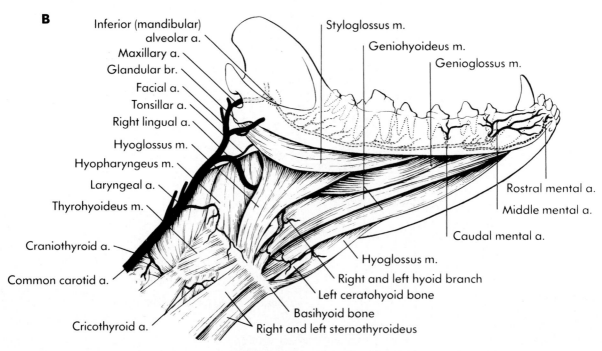

Inferior (mandibular) alveolar a.
Maxillary a.
Glandular br.
Facial a.
Tonsillar a.
Right lingual a.
Hyoglossus m.
Hyopharyngeus m.
Laryngeal a.
Thyrohyoideus m.
Craniothyroid a.
Common carotid a.
Cricothyroid a.

Styloglossus m.
Geniohyoideus m.
Genioglossus m.

Rostral mental a.
Middle mental a.
Caudal mental a.
Hyoglossus m.
Right and left hyoid branch
Left ceratohyoid bone
Basihyoid bone
Right and left sternothyroideus

FIGURE 1-12
For legend see opposite page.

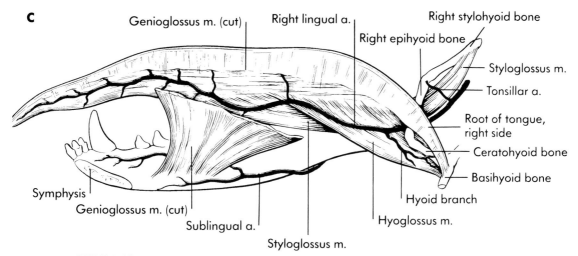

FIGURE 1-12
Lateral views of the arteries of the upper jaw and face (**A**), lower jaw (**B**), and tongue (**C**). *(From Evans HE:* Miller's anatomy of the dog, *ed 3, Philadelphia, 1993, WB Saunders.)*

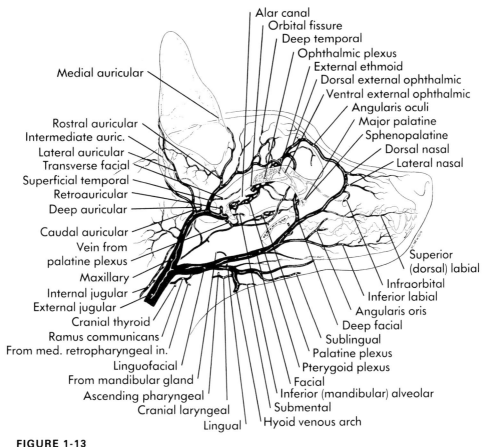

FIGURE 1-13
Veins of the oral and adjacent tissues in the dog. *(From Evans HE:* Miller's anatomy of the dog, *ed 3, Philadelphia, 1993, WB Saunders.)*

the maxillary artery emerges onto the ventral surface of the palatine bone through a foramen that lies midway between the dental arcade and the midline, level with the palatal root of the upper carnassial tooth. The facial artery, together with branches from the infraorbital artery, supplies the lips and superficial facial muscles. The lingual artery supplies the tongue; it runs with the hypoglossal nerve. The collateral circulation system in the dog and cat is very well organized; both common carotid arteries can be ligated in dogs without clinically obvious effects. Venous drainage is via the lingual-facial vein and branches of the maxillary veins; these two systems join to form the external jugular vein (Fig. 1-13). Lymphatic channels are plentiful in the head and neck. The major lymph nodes that drain oral and pharyngeal structures are the facial, parotid, and—of major clinical importance as sites of metastatic disease—the mandibular and retropharyngeal nodes. The facial node, which lies on the maxilla at the level of the upper carnassial tooth, sometimes can be palpated in a dog. The parotid nodes usually are hidden in adjacent soft tissues. The mandibular nodes can be palpated as small paired structures lying lateroventral to the mandibular salivary glands. Lymphatic drainage caudally is via the cervical lymph nodes and tracheal trunks, which terminate either in the thoracic duct or directly into a venous structure at the thoracic inlet.

▶ SUGGESTED READINGS

Arnall L: Some aspects of dental development in the dog: calcification of crown and root of the deciduous dentitions, *J Small Anim Pract* 1:169, 1961.

Arnall L: Some aspects of dental development in the dog: eruption and extrusion, *J Small Anim Pract* 1:259, 1961.

Berman E: The time and pattern of eruption of the permanent teeth of the cat, *Lab Anim Sci* 24:929, 1974.

Evans HE, Christensen GC: *Miller's anatomy of the dog,* ed 2, Philadelphia, 1979, WB Saunders Co.

Hennet P: Apical anatomy of the teeth of dogs, *J Endodontol,* 1991 (in press).

Hennet P, Harvey CE: Apical anatomy of the teeth of cats, *Proc Vet Dent Forum* 5:145, 1991.

Hooft J, Mattheeuws D, Van Bree P: Radiology of deciduous teeth resorption and definitive teeth eruption in the dog, *J Small Anim Pract* 20:175, 1979.

Kremenak CR: Dental eruption chronology in dogs: deciduous teeth gingival emergence, *J Dent Res* 48:1177, 1969.

Lawson DD, Nixon GS, Noble HW, Weipers WL: Dental anatomy and histology of the dog, *Res Vet Sci* 1:201, 1960.

Masson E, Hennet P, Calas P: Apical root canal anatomy in the dog, *Endod Dent Traumatol* 8:109, 1992.

McKeown M: The deciduous dentition of the dog—its form and function, *Irish Vet J* 25:169, 1971.

Morgan JP, Miyabayashi T: Dental radiology: aging changes in permanent teeth of beagle dogs, *J Small Anim Pract* 32:11, 1991.

Newman PM: Canine teeth, *JAVMA* 174:1075, 1979 (letter).

Orsini P, Hennet P: Anatomy of the mouth and teeth of the cat, *Vet Clin North Am, Small Anim Pract* 22:1265, 1992.

Ross DMJ, Neuhaus RG, de Neuhaus IP, Pagliari de Ross MC, Marx G: Chronologie der Zahnentwicklung des Hundes, *Tierarztl Umschau* 34:418, 1979.

Roush JK et al: Normal blood supply to the canine mandible and mandibular teeth, *Am J Vet Res* 50(6):9, 1989.

Smith MM et al: Furcation anatomy of the fourth maxillary premolar in dogs, *Vet Surg* 19:75, 1990.

Stockard CR: The genetic and endocrinic basis for differences in form and behavior, *Am Anat Memoir* 19, Philadelphia, 1941, Wistar Institute.

Wissdorf VH: Beitrag zur Zahnentwicklung und deren Storungen beim Hund, *Effem-Forschung Kleintiernahrung* 18:1, 1984.

2

Oral Examination and Diagnostic Techniques

Oropharyngeal diseases are common in dogs and cats, although signs often are not apparent to the owner until the disease is well advanced. Sometimes the lesion and the diagnosis are obvious (for example, a short, jagged canine tooth with a pink spot in a dog with a history of recent trauma is unlikely to be anything except a fractured tooth). However, signs often are not specific for a particular disease and may result from primary oral disease or from oral effects of systemic or skin disease.

▶ HISTORY

Age, breed, and sequence of development of oral signs often are useful indicators. Information regarding litter mates is also of value for some conditions.

Current History

Even when oral lesions are the primary or only reason for bringing in the animal for examination, a full current history is essential. General health (vomiting, diarrhea, weight loss; coughing, sneezing; polydypsia, polyuria; scratching, rubbing, or chewing the skin or mucocutaneous junction areas) should be questioned. The animal's current environment (inside/outside, allowed to run free), eating and drinking patterns, access to chewing materials, and behavioral idiosyncracies (rock or wood chewing) must be known. Questions must be asked. When eating, has the type of food that the animal is willing or able to eat changed? Is there hesitation during prehension or swallowing, or does food drop out of the mouth? Does the animal move to the food, start to prehend, and then back off? Is there head shaking or bobbing? Clinical signs that may be specific for oral diseases are described next.

▶ SIGNS OF OROPHARYNGEAL DISEASE

In some instances, clinical signs reported by the owner strongly indicate a specific condition. Generally, however, clinical signs indicate only the need for a more thorough examination.

Halitosis

The single most common sign of oral diseases is mouth odor. Halitosis is more readily recognized in dogs because of the close interaction between many owners and their pets. Because cats often are more independent, the owner initially may observe other signs. An unpleasant odor may be caused by local disease, most commonly by periodontal disease (as a result of bacterial activity that releases sulfur compounds), by nonoral diseases such as uremia, respiratory, or gastrointestinal disease, or by diet. When there is acute necrosis in oral tissues, such as with some severe acute inflammatory diseases (ulcerative stomatitis, acute necrotizing ulcerative gingivitis), or rapidly growing tumors (malignant melanoma), the smell may be almost overpowering. A uremic dog with periodontal disease emits a distinctive odor (a combination of ammonia from breakdown of urea in saliva combined with the bacterial activity of periodontal disease).

A smell emanating from the general area of the mouth may not be oral in origin. Lip-fold dermatitis, seen most often in spaniels, is a chronic moist dermatitis or pyoderma that produces a rank smell from the lower lip. It is due to seborrhea and secondary infection exacerbated by the moist environment created by the lip conformation.

Inappetence

Inappetence results from fever and depression or other effects associated with many systemic and oral diseases, as well as from pain associated with inflammation and ulceration in the oral cavity. This may progress to unwillingness or inability to drink, causing dehydration.

Pawing

Pawing at the mouth and rubbing the mouth on furnishings are indications of oral pain or inflammation or inflammation of the mucocutaneous junction or skin of the lips.

Drooling of Saliva

Drooling usually results from reluctance or inability to swallow rather than from increased salivary production. Saliva may be blood stained if ulceration is present in the mouth. It also may be caused by reluctance to close the mouth because of pain from an endodontic abscess or other dental disease or from inability to close the mouth (discussed later).

Dysphagia

Difficulty in or pain on swallowing may result from inflamed, ulcerated, or traumatized tissues that cause local pain or from obstruction to the mechanics of swallowing by a mass lesion, neurologic disease, or cleft palate.

Rapid Jaw and Tongue Movements

Teeth or jaw chattering indicates oral pain (for example, external odontoclastic resorption lesions in cats) or neurologic abnormality (for example, distemper infection). Another cause is a linear foreign body caught around the tongue that the animal is attempting to dislodge. In dogs the tongue often moves rapidly in time with respiratory movements during panting.

Inability or Unwillingness to Open the Mouth

This may result from oral pain that causes guarding or from abscessed tissue in the sublingual or orbital areas. Other causes are mechanical obstruction such as proliferative bone resulting from chronic middle ear disease or zygomatic or coronoid process masses resulting in reduced range of temporomandibular joint motion (for example, callous formation after fracture, especially in a young dog, or multilobular osteomafibroma of the canine skull). In addition, craniomandibular osteopathy can occur in West Highland white dogs, or trismus can result from tetanus or masticatory muscle myositis (eosinophilic or atrophic myositis). An observant owner may note that the dog is unwilling or unable to eat or chew on one side of the mouth. The owner also may notice that a previously compliant dog or cat is unable or unwilling to allow the owner to open its mouth, for example, for toothbrushing.

Inability to Close the Mouth

The mouth may hang open as a result of mandibular trauma, mandibular neuropraxia, temporomandibular joint (TMJ) luxation or dysplasia, or myofacialis in young dogs.

▶ PHYSICAL EXAMINATION

The mouth can be considered a window into the body. The lining of the cheek is a thin semitransparent membrane that permits the observer to view function and changes in the vessels and connective tissue beneath the buccal mucosa. Because it is the largest and most accessible membraneous area, physical examination, whether for an oral problem or not, always should include a close look at the mucosa of the mouth. The skin and nonoral mucocutaneous junction areas also should be examined carefully.

Gentleness and patience are necessary to permit systematic examination. Sedation may be required in a particularly fractious animal or when the oral lesions are painful.

The buccal mucosa of the cheek is examined by lifting the animal's lips before attempting to open the mouth inasmuch as this will reveal any buccal ulcers that would be painful if squeezed against the maxilla (Fig. 2-1). Even in an uncooperative dog that is wearing a muzzle, part of the lining of the cheek pouch is visible, including the lateral gingiva that covers the canine teeth and some adjacent buccal mucosa.

The mucous membranes, which should glisten from coverage by a layer of saliva, may be pigmented. The mucosal surface should be intact and nonpainful to touch. The buccal mucosa and the attached gingiva—the two are separated by an obvious furrow, the mucogingival junction (MGJ)—are compared. The gingival height (from MGJ to the free edge of the gingiva [free gingival margin] where it joins the crown of the tooth) varies from tooth to tooth, being widest over the canine teeth and least obvious at the caudal edge of the last molar tooth (see Fig. A-1, A, p. 49). The gingiva cannot be moved like the buccal mucosa and normally feels very dense (like the rubber in a pencil eraser). There are relatively few sensory nerve endings in the gingiva; thus even in a skittish dog, this is a safe area to depress for observing vascularity and capillary refill time.

Although helpful information can be obtained without opening the animal's mouth, additional knowledge can be gained by further inspection. The mouth will tend to open if the head is firmly rotated dorsally (Fig. 2-1, B). In a dog, using a hand positioned on top of the muzzle, the examiner places the index finger (on one side) and the thumb (on the other side) just caudal to the upper canine teeth (Fig. 2-1, B) and rotates the head dorsally (Fig. 2-1, C). In a cat, the examiner places the index finger and thumb on the zygomatic arches to rotate the head dorsally (Fig. 2-1, D).

The gingival margins are examined. Viewing the area under the tongue can be facilitated by depressing the lower incisor area while pushing the thumb of the same hand into the intermandibular area, thus bringing the sublingual furrow into view (Fig. 2-1, E and F). The tongue is depressed to examine the pharynx (Fig. 2-1, G). The examiner inspects and palpates the hard palate and extends a finger onto the soft palate (Fig. 2-1, H). In a normal dog and cat, the hamular processes of the pterygoid bones can be palpated as two parallel bony ridges lying either side of the midline; inability to palpate these structures indicates the presence of a soft palate or nasopharyngeal mass. As the finger is extended further into the pharynx, a gag reflex should be obvious (soft palate contraction to close the nasopharynx, tongue contraction to attempt to expel the stimulating object from the pharynx).

The color, size, location, and symmetry of oral lesions should be noted because these findings are of major importance in developing a differential diagnosis list (described further in Chapter 3).

In a dog or cat that is unable or unwilling to open its mouth, it is important to note whether occlusion is normal and whether the animal opens its mouth when the examiner no longer is palpating or holding the head. The owner should be asked if the animal yawns and can manage food normally, play with or catch its ball, and other related questions. Some animals fiercely guard their mouths even under normal conditions. Other animals can have a painful oral lesion that may be aggravated by injudicious handling. If gentleness and patience do not permit eventual opening and inspection of the mouth, sedation or anesthesia may be necessary. In some circumstances (for example, severe atrophic myositis, coronoid process mass lesion, craniomandibular osteopathy) even with the animal under general anesthesia it still is impossible to open the mouth significantly. In that case the examiner should be prepared to perform a tracheotomy to permit continuation of the anesthesia without risk of aspiration during further diagnostic or therapeutic procedures.

In a dog or cat that is unable to close its mouth, the examiner determines whether the jaw is locked in an open position, such as in TMJ dysplasia or luxation, or can be closed by gentle digital pressure as, for example, with mandibular fracture or mandibular neuropraxia. Occlusion should be observed inasmuch as TMJ dysplasia and luxation cause the jaw to be

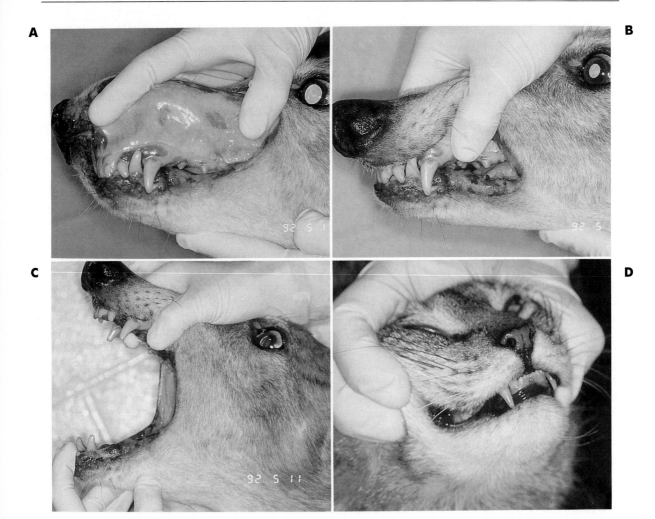

FIGURE 2-1

A, Physical examination of the oral cavity. The lip is lifted without attempting to open the jaws. The buccal alveolar mucosa is inspected and palpated. **B,** In a dog the index finger and the thumb are placed on the maxilla inside the lips, just caudal to the upper canine tooth. **C,** The head is moved dorsally by rotating the wrist, causing the mouth to open. **D,** In a cat the index finger and thumb are positioned just ventral to the zygomatic arch, and the head is rotated. **E,** The index finger of the other hand is used to depress the lower incisor teeth to open the mouth further. **F,** By pushing the thumb of the second hand into the intermandibular area as the lower jaw is depressed, the tongue is raised to permit inspection of the sublingual furrows. **G,** While the head is still rotated upwards by one hand, the index finger of the other hand is used to depress the dorsum of the tongue to permit inspection of the pharynx. **H,** With the tip of the finger pointing dorsally, the index finger is advanced gently but rapidly over the surface of the hard palate, advancing to the soft palate.

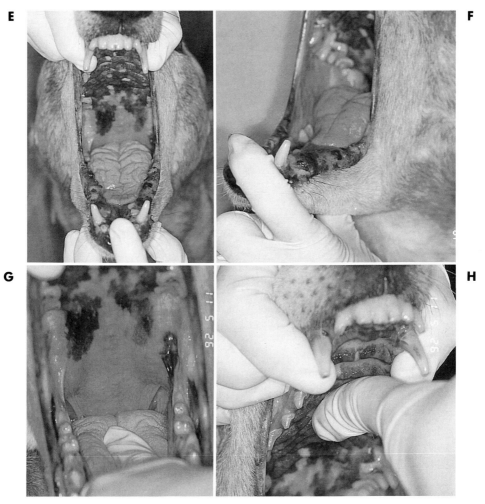

FIGURE 2-1, cont'd
For legend see opposite page.

pulled to one side unless the luxation is bilateral, and mandibular fracture often results in significant malocclusion.

The sense of smell can be a useful diagnostic tool in examining the animal's mouth. Because of their rapid growth, some malignant melanomas have large necrotic areas that produce a distinct, overpowering odor that is immediately detected. The mouth of a uremic dog has an ammoniac smell that is different from the typical odor of extensive periodontal disease. In spaniels with lip-fold dermatitis, *Proteus* or *Pseudomonas* organisms cause a classic seborrheic pyoderma smell.

Detailed examination of the periodontium by means of a periodontal probe is described in Chapter 4; examination of individual teeth is discussed in Chapter 6 and occlusal examination in Chapter 8.

Because the most common major oral diseases are chronic progressive diseases, recording the information obtained during a thorough oral examination is important. Examples of charts used to record this information are shown in Fig. 2-2.

If information about eating and drinking is not clear from the owner's description, the examiner should watch the animal eat or drink.

Text continued on p. 29.

A

MESA VETERINARY DENTAL SERVICE

858 NORTH COUNTRY CLUB DRIVE
MESA, ARIZONA 85201
(602) 833-7330

KENNETH F. LYON, D.V.M.
FELLOW, ACADEMY OF VETERINARY DENTISTRY

ASSOCIATED WITH
MESA VETERINARY HOSPITAL LTD.

CANINE DENTAL RECORD

Case Number: ____________

Patient: ______________________ Owner: ______________________
Breed: ______________________ Phone No.: ______________________
Age/Sex: ______________________ Date initiated: ______________________
Chief complaint: ____
____
Past dental history: ____
____
Existing home dental care: Brushing Oral Rinse Medication
Diet/Oral habits: ____

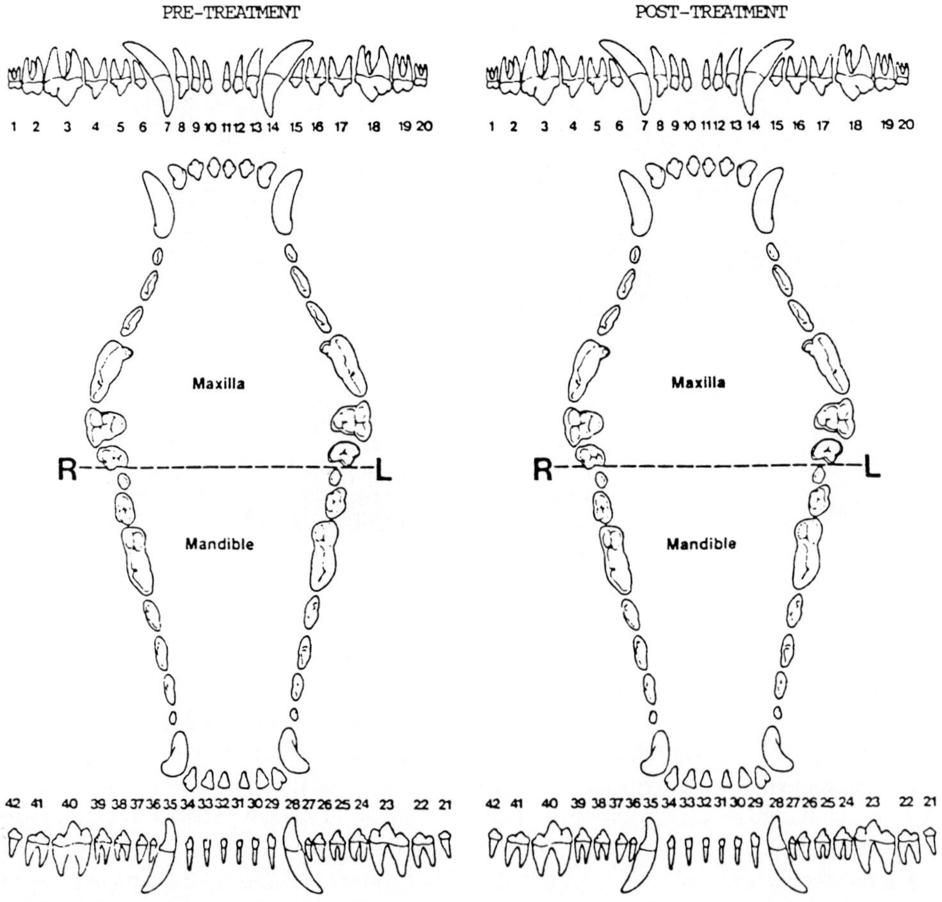

FIGURE 2-2
Examples of dental examination forms used by veterinary dentists. **A** and **B,** Courtesy of and copyright by Dr. K.F. Lyon.

CLINICAL EXAMINATION

General Assessment
mucosal color and contours:_____
_____
trauma:_____
caries:_____
salivary flow: dry   normal   excessive
lymphadenopathy:_____
tonsils/pharynx:_____
extraoral facial structures:_____
fistula:_____

Periodontal Evaluation
dental plaque: mild   moderate   severe   supragingival/subgingival
dental calculus: mild   moderate   severe   supragingival/subgingival
gingivitis: mild   moderate   severe   generalized/localized
periodontitis: mild   moderate   severe   generalized/localized
halitosis:_____
periodontal pockets:_____
gingival recession/root exposure:_____
mobile teeth:_____
periodontal abscess:_____

Endodontic Evaluation
fractured teeth:_____
carious teeth:_____
pulp exposure:_____
dental fistula:_____
radiographic evidence of periapical abscess:_____

RADIOGRAPHIC EXAMINATION_____
_____
_____

TREATMENT PLAN
Type of treatment
Oral Surgery   Treatment Sequence
  Extractions:_____
  soft tissue:_____
  jaw fracture:_____
Periodontal Treatment   Treatment Sequence
  dental prophylaxis:_____
  polishing:_____
  topical fluoride:_____
  subgingival curettage/root planing:_____
  gingivectomy:_____
  home care: brushing   oral rinses   diet
  follow up:_____
Endodontic Treatment   Treatment Sequence
  single root canal filling:_____
  multiple root canal filling:_____
  apicoectomy/retrograde filling:_____
  pulpotomy-direct pulp capping:_____
Dental Restorations   Treatment Sequence
  amalgam:_____
  composite resin:_____
  glass ionomer:_____
  light cure   chemical cure
Orthodontic Treatment_____
_____
_____
Bite evaluation:_____
TREATMENT
  Date   Procedure
  _____   _____

FIGURE 2-2, cont'd
Examples of dental examination forms used by veterinary dentists. **A** and **B**, Courtesy of
and copyright by Dr. K.F. Lyon.   *Continued.*

C

BEN H. COLMERY III, D.V.M.
DIP. American Veterinary Dental College
6011 Jackson Rd.
Ann Arbor, MI 48103

Owner Name _____

Patient Name _____ Age _____ M F A

Breed _____ Color _____

Referred by _____

CANINE DENTAL TREATMENT

Date _____

HISTORY:

Chief Complaint: _____ Diet: _____

Previous Dental Treatment: _____

Dental Home Care: _____

Other Pertinent History: _____

EXAMINATION:

WEIGHT: _____ lbs.

GEN. CONDITION: _____

HEART: _____/min.

Character: _____

FEM. PULSE: _____/min.

Character: _____

OCCLUSION:
a. Scissors
b. Brachygnatahic
c. Even
d. Anterior Crossbite
e. Posterior Crossbite
f. Prognathic
g. Wry
h. Other _____

SKULL TYPE:
a. Brachycephalic
b. Mesaticephalic
c. Dolicocephalic

TEMPOROMANDIBULAR PALPATION
a. Normal
b. Pain
c. Crepitus
d. Clicking
e. Inhibited Movement

SALIVARY FLOW:
a. Decreased
b. Normal
c. Increased

ANESTHETIC PROTOCOL:

INDUCTION
Valium _____ ml
Ketamine _____ ml
Biotal _____ ml
☐ Isoflurane/02

MAINTENANCE
☐ Oxygen
☐ Isoflurane
☐ Halothane

PROPHYLAXIS:
CROWN SCALING
a. Hand
b. Ultrasonic
c. Roto-pro
d. Other

SUBGINGIVAL
a. Exploration
b. Subgingival curettage
c. Root planing
d. Other _____

POLISHING
a. Fluoride Pumice
b. Tooth Varnish (Sealing)
c. Stannous Fluoride
d. Acidulated Fluoride

PERIODONTAL SURGERY:
a. Gingivectomy/Gingivoplasty
b. Open Curettage
c. Reverse bevel/Reposition flap
d. Lateral sliding flap
Other _____
_____
e. Free gingival graft
f. Periodontal splinting
g. Osseous implant
h. Biopsy
  ☐ Histo
  ☐ IFA
i. Culture/Sens

EXODONTIA:
a. Routine extraction
b. Sectioning
c. Buccal Cortical Bone RemovaL
d. Alveoloplasty
e. Suturing
  ☐ Absorbable
  ☐ Non-Absorb _____

ENDODONTICS:
a. Pulp cap
b. Root Canal
  ☐ ZOE
  ☐ Calcium Hydroxide
  ☐ Gutta Percha
  ☐ Other _____
c. Retrograde

ORTHODONTICS:
a. Impressions
b. Cheek elastic
c. Upper expansion
d. Lower Retainer
e. Maryland Bridge
f. Incline Plane
Other _____

RESTORATIONS:
a. Fillings
  ☐ Composite
  ☐ Light Bond
  ☐ Amalgam
  ☐ Glass Ionomer
  ☐ Other _____
b. Contouring
c. Bridge
d. Implant
e. Transplant
☐ Other _____
f. Build up
  ☐ Post
  ☐ Pins
g. Crown
  ☐ Impressions
  ☐ Cap
  ☐ Post and Core

RIGHT   PALATAL / LINGUAL   LEFT

R   L

CODE KEY

AF – Amalgam Filling	EP – Exposed Pulp	H – Gingival Hyperplasia	PH – Pulpal Hemorrhage
C – Calculus	F – Furcation Exposed	L – Loose Tooth	R – Rotated Tooth
CA – Caries/Cavity	Fx – Fractured Tooth	N – Neck Lesion	RC – Root Canal
CF – Composite Filling	G – Gingivitis	O – Missing Tooth	RD – Retained Deciduous
CR – Crown Restoration	GR – Gum Recession	P – Periodontal Pocket	WF – Worn Facets
E – Enamel Lesion	GV – Gingivectomy	PC – Pulp Cap	X – Extracted

X-ray Results: _____

Assessment: _____

Medications: _____

Feeding Instructions: _____

Special Instructions: _____

Re-Checks: _____

FIGURE 2-2, cont'd

Examples of dental examination forms used by veterinary dentists. **C,** Courtesy of and copyright by Dr. Ben Colmery.

GOODWOOD ANIMAL HOSPITAL, INC.
8778 Goodwood Blvd.
Baton Rouge, LA 70806
(504) 927-9940

GARY B. BEARD, DVM, Charter Diplomate
American Veterinary Dental College
ASHLEY B. OAKES, DVM, Dental Resident
DEBRA M. BEARD, DVM

Owner Name _____

Patient Name _____ Age _____ M F A

Breed _____ Color _____

Referred by _____

DATE _____

FELINE DENTAL RECORD

HISTORY

Chief Complaint _____ Weight _____

Known Medical Problems _____ Temp. _____

Previous Dental Treatments _____ Dental Homecare _____

EXAMINATION

SKULL TYPE:
Brachycephalic
Mesaticephalic
Dolichocephalic

OCCLUSION:
Scissors (normal)
Brachygnathic (overshot)
Even
Anterior Crossbite
Prognathic (undershot)
Wry

SOFT TISSUE ULCERATIONS:
None
Oropharynx
Tongue
Floor of Mouth
Buccal Lip (Cheeks)

TEMPOROMANDIBULAR PALPATION:
Normal
Painful
Clicking
Inhibited Movement

TOOTH MOBILITY
Class I
Class II
Class III

CALCULUS:
None
Mild
Moderate
Severe

CERVICAL LINE EROSION
Class I   Class IV
Class II   Class V
Class III

GINGIVITIS:
None
Mild
Moderate
Severe

PERIODONTAL DISEASE:
a. Grade I   - Marginal Gingivitis
b. Grade II - Gingivitis, Edema, Bleeds on probing
c. Grade III - Pocketing, Receded gums
d. Grade IV - Deep Pockets, Pus formation, Loose teeth
e. Grade V   - Abscessed teeth, Very mobile

BUCCAL VIEW

UPPER
R   L
LOWER

L

R

KEY
AR - Alveolar Bone Recession
C   - Calculus - I, II, III
CA - Cavity - Class 1 - 5
CLE - Cervical Line Erosion
EH - Enamel Hypoplasia
FE - Furcation Exposed - I, II, III
FX - Fractured Tooth
G   - Gingivitis
GH - Gingival Hyperplasia
GR - Gingival Recession
K   - Kissing Ulcer
MT - Mobile Tooth - Class I, II or III
M   - Missing Tooth
ONF - Oronasal Fistula
PE - Pulp Exposed
PP - Periodontal Pocket
R   - Rotated Tooth
RD - Retained Deciduous Tooth
RE - Root Exposed
SN - Supernumary Tooth
WF - Worn Facets

Diagnosis: _____

Plan: _____

Notes: _____

RECOMMENDED TREATMENT	EST.		EST.		EST		EST.
☐ Alveoloplasty		☐ Extraction		☐ Hemisection		☐ Restoration	
☐ Anesthesia/Sedation		☐ Feline Cervical Line Erosion		☐ Impression/Model		☐ Root Amputation	
☐ Apicoectomy		☐ Filling		☐ Lab Fee Estimate		☐ Root Canal	
☐ Bridge		☐ Flap Surgery (Periodontal)		☐ Odontoplasty		☐ Splinting (Acrylic/Wire)	
☐ Crown		☐ Fractured Tooth Repair		☐ Orthodontics		☐ Surgery (Oral)	
☐ Crown Build-Up - I, II, III		☐ Fracture Repair		☐ Pulp Capping		☐ Prophy - 1, 2, 3	
☐ Disarming		☐ Gingivectomy		☐ Pulpotomy (Vital)		☐ Curettege/Root Planing	
☐ Electrosurgery		☐ Gingivoplasty		☐ Radiography		☐ Wiring	

ORIGINAL

FIGURE 2-2, cont'd

Examples of dental examination forms used by veterinary dentists. **D,** Courtesy of and copyright by Dr. Gary B. Beard.

Continued.

E

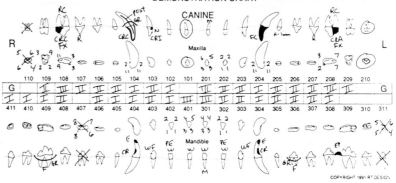

DEMONSTRATION CHART

COPYRIGHT 1991 RT DESIGN

DentaLabels CODE KEY

C	Calculus	FX	Fractured Tooth	PP	Periodontal Pocket
CA	Carious Lesion	G	Gingivitis	PU	Pulpitis
CR	Crowded Tooth	GR	Gum Recession	R	Rotated Tooth
CRA	Crown Restoration-Amalgam	H	Hyperplasia (Gingival)	RC	Root Canal
CRC	CR-Composite	I	Impacted Tooth	RD	Retained Deciduous Tooth
CRI	CR-Glass Ionomer	M	Mobile Tooth	RR	Root Resorption
D	Dehiscence	N	Neck Lesion	SD	Sulcus Depth
E	Enamel Lesion	O	Missing Tooth	V	Vital Pulpotomy
EP	Epulis	OD	Odontoplasty	W	Worn Tooth
F	Furcation Exposure	PD	Periodontitis	WF	Wear Facet
FC	Full Crown	PE	Pulp Exposure	X	Extracted Tooth

GINGIVITIS BOX SCORES:

Grade I = Thin red gingival line (subclinical gingivitis)
Grade II = Gingival edema (clinical gingivitis)
Grade III = Advanced gingivitis or early periodontitis

Copyright 1991 DentaLabels

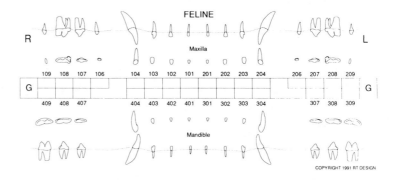

FELINE

COPYRIGHT 1991 RT DESIGN

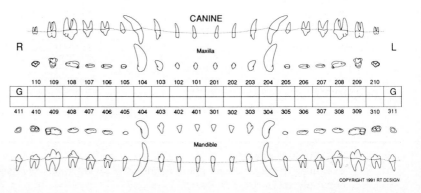

CANINE

COPYRIGHT 1991 RT DESIGN

FIGURE 2-2, cont'd
Examples of dental examination forms used by veterinary dentists. **E,** Summary forms for dogs and cats available as peel-off strips for insertion in existing hospital record. Copyright by and available from Denta-Labels, 19 Norwood Ave, Kensington CA 94707.

▶ RADIOGRAPHIC EXAMINATION

Oral radiography frequently is both essential, because the requisite information cannot be obtained in any other way, and rewarding, because of the contrasts among the teeth, bone, and intervening soft tissue (periodontal ligament). Excellent oral radiographs can be made only with use of correct technique. Anesthesia or sedation is essential to allow correct positioning of the x-ray beam and film because oral radiographs that are inadequately obtained rarely are of diagnostic value.

The five essential elements in good oral radiographic technique are the source of x-rays, the film itself, positioning, processing, and interpretation.

Source of X-Rays

A dental x-ray unit is ideal because the x-ray source is mounted on a universal joint that permits correct positioning with minimal need to adjust the position of the animal. Human dental x-ray units generally have a fixed milliampere (7 to 15 mA) and kilovolt peak (60 to 90 kVp) and are suitable for companion animal dentistry. The head is mounted on a long jointed arm that is attached to the wall or ceiling or supported on a wheeled base. For a small animal practice that intends to offer a full range of dental services, a dental x-ray machine is as valuable an investment as an air-driven high-speed dental handpiece system. The smaller the focal spot of the unit, the better will be the radiographic detail. The most up-to-date units have parallel-sided lead-lined collimator cylinders that reduce scatter. Reconditioned units often are available from dental supply houses at significant savings compared with new units, and veterinary supply houses are now offering units with a practical array of features (see Chapter 11).

Excellent oral radiographs can be made using standard veterinary radiography machines, which typically have 100 to 500 mA and therefore require a much shorter exposure time than do dental x-ray units (typical exposure factors are listed in Table 2-1). The major drawback to use of a unit with 100 mA or higher is that the head is less adaptable. In the hospital it is fixed in one location, and if an endodontic procedure is being performed, the x-ray machine will be unavailable for other uses for the duration of the pro-

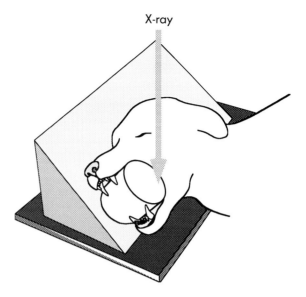

X-ray

FIGURE 2-3
Foam blocks used to obtain correct head position when using a fixed radiographic source for dental radiographs.

cedure. Units that have an x-ray source that can be raised or lowered and rotated or angled are preferable because it will be less necessary to contort the skull of the animal to achieve correct position. Foam blocks are useful for obtaining correct head positioning (Fig. 2-3). With nonscreen dental film (intraorally or extraorally), the x-ray source is brought much closer to the subject (the end of the collimator should just touch the most external part of the skull) so that the focus-film distance (FFD) is about 25 to 30 cm. With standard film in a screened cassette, the standard 75 cm (30-inch) FFD is maintained.

Radiographic Film

The most common technique used in oral radiography requires that the film be placed in the mouth during exposure. Therefore the film must be small enough to fit in the desired position without causing damage to adjacent tissues. Oral radiographic films are packaged in x-ray transparent but light-proof plastic holders that are flexible, and thus the film can be bent to conform to the shallow dental ledge without damaging the mouth or film. The sizes and types of

TABLE 2-1	Dental radiography

Dental Radiographic Film—Ultraspeed Type

4	Occlusal—DF50	5.7 × 7.6 cm
		(2¼ × 3 in)
2	Periapical—DF58	2.5 × 5.1 cm
		(1 × 2 in)
0	Periapical—DF54	2.2 × 3.5 cm
		(⅞ × 1⅜ in)

Technique Chart—Ultraspeed Film

Focal film distance: 30 cm (12 in)
Machine specifications (assumes dental x-ray unit with fixed mA and kVp): 10 mA to 70 kVp

	Weight of animal (kg)		
Exposure Time (seconds)	**<10**	**10-40**	**>40**
Occlusal view (incisors, canines)	0.15	0.2	0.3
Maxillary bisecting-angle view (premolars, molars)	0.2	0.25	0.4
Mandibular parallel view (premolars, molars)	0.2	0.25	0.3

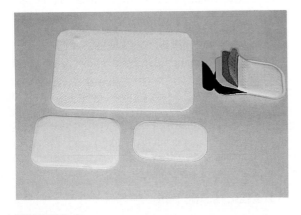

FIGURE 2-4
Dental radiographic film typically used in small animal dentistry. *Top left,* #4 film (DF50). *Top right,* An opened film, showing the film covered by paper and outer plastic wrapping. *Bottom left,* #2 film (DF58). *Bottom right,* #0 film (DF54).

film most commonly used in veterinary dentistry are described in Table 2-1 and shown in Fig. 2-4. These films are small, particularly the No. 0 (DF54) film commonly used in the mouth of cats. Handling and storing for easy identification are important. Peel-off radiodense markers are available so that each film during a procedure can be identified by number, with the exposure number, location, and purpose noted on a separate sheet for subsequent storage in a small envelope pack, or a dental film viewing and identification holder can be used (Fig. 2-5).

Dental films are identified with a small bump or button on one corner pointing toward the x-ray source (Fig. 2-6). Thus even when the radiographed side is not recorded at the time, it is simple to identify which side is which by orienting the bump. Given that the bump must have faced toward the x-ray source, there is only one way that the film can have been placed in the mouth. Some clinicians and technicians use a consistent system for film placement to make side identification even easier; for example, the film is always placed so that the bump is at the rostral end of the

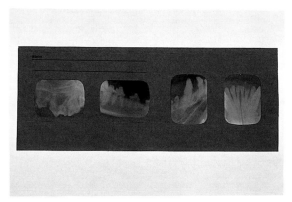

FIGURE 2-5
Dental film holder and identification card.

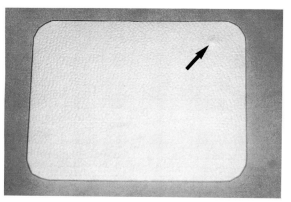

FIGURE 2-6
Dental radiographic film showing the dimple that is used to identify the side of the mouth that was radiographed.

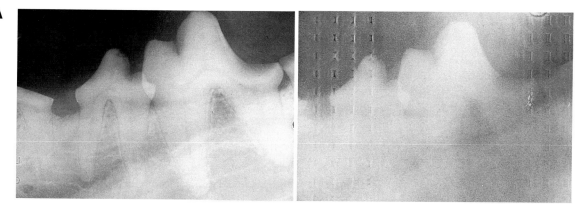

FIGURE 2-7
A, Dental radiograph taken with the correct side (dimple up) toward the radiographic source. **B,** Dental radiograph taken with wrong side toward the radiographic source. The image is blurred by the aluminum foil within the package.

film for the right side of the mouth, with the caudal end of the film on the left side of the mouth. If the film was exposed with the bump facing away from the x-ray source, the image will be blurred because of the aluminum foil layer that is placed behind the film within the film package (Fig. 2-7).

Position

The ideal oral radiograph is made in a parallel position; that is, the plane of the radiographic film is parallel to the long axis of the tooth and perpendicular to the plane of the x-ray beam (Fig. 2-8). The result is neither magnification nor foreshortening of the

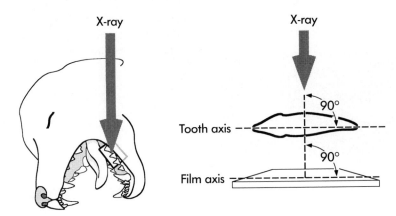

FIGURE 2-8
Parallel position technique for dental radiographs of the mandibular premolar teeth.

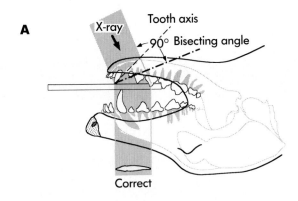

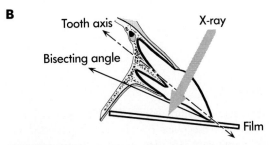

FIGURE 2-9
Bisecting angle technique for dental radiographs.
A, Lower canine tooth. **B,** Carnassial tooth.

tooth, and no superimposition of other structures obscures the radiographic detail. However, parallel-position oral radiographs of most teeth in dogs and cats are impossible to obtain because of the anatomy of the jaws. In human beings there is a distinct dental ledge in both the upper and lower jaws to accommodate the roots of the teeth, which permits placement of an intraoral radiograph parallel to the long axis of the tooth. The flat palate (for the upper jaw) and the shallow but caudally extending mandibular symphysis (for the lower jaw) in carnivores prevent achieving true parallel position for all teeth except the lower premolars and molars. For the teeth in the upper jaw, as well as the lower incisor and canine teeth (and the lower first premolar tooth in dogs), a compromise technique known as the bisecting angle technique must be used. The radiographic film is placed as close to parallel position as possible for the tooth to be examined; then an imaginary line is drawn bisecting the angle formed by the planes of the long axes of the tooth and the surface of the film. The x-ray beam is directed perpendicular to this bisecting angle line (Fig. 2-9). For the upper or lower incisor and canine teeth, this view is similar to be occlusal view used for intranasal radiographs. The bisecting angle line for the upper incisor and canine teeth corresponds to a line from the canine tooth tip to the medial canthus of the eye on that side. For the premolar and molar

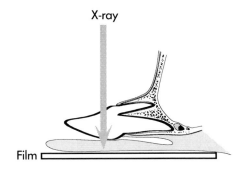

FIGURE 2-10
Parallel position technique for imaging upper premolar and molar teeth by using extraoral film position.

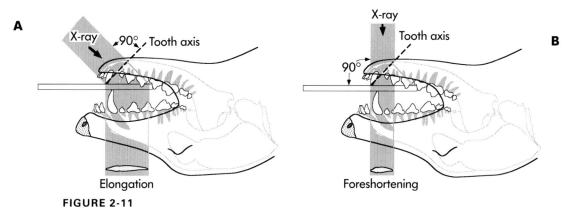

FIGURE 2-11
Effect of incorrect radiographic beam position. **A,** Beam perpendicular to tooth axis—tooth is elongated. **B,** Beam perpendicular to film axis—tooth is foreshortened.

teeth, oblique positioning of the head on an extraoral cassette or occlusal size No. 4 film will produce similar results (Figs. 2-3 and 2-10 to 2-16). If bisecting angle technique is not used, the image of the radiographed tooth will be lengthened or foreshortened (Fig. 2-11).

Processing

In most cases, dental radiographs are made during a dental examination or procedure, resulting in prolongation of the anesthesia while the radiograph is processed. Thus speed of processing is of considerable importance. Because of their small size, dental radiographs are physically awkward to process. They can be put through a standard automatic processor in a cycle that takes about 4 to 5 minutes, but they must be taped to a larger film to ensure that they work their way through the system correctly. Waterproof tape prevents caking of the processor rollers during drying. Automatic processors for dental films are available. Although they provide a correctly processed and dry film, they are slow (4 to 7 minutes, depending on model).

Standard wet-tank processing in a dark room is feasible but messy and time-consuming. The most rapid way to obtain a readable film is to use a high speed "chairside darkroom" kit (see Chapter 11). This kit consists of a box with two hand-entry portals. A safety light lid prevents passage of light, avoiding exposure of radiograph film, but permits the operator direct viewing of the wells and film. The box contains four wells: developer, water, fixer, and water. A metal single-radiograph clip is used to hold the film during processing. With use of the rapid-developer and fixative solutions, the film can be removed from the box for interpretation within 1 minute. However, the film is wet, and there is a tendency to underfix, which often results in processing artifacts. Nevertheless, consistent attention to correct fixing, rinsing, and drying after the initial inspection makes these units an excellent, cost-effective, timely way to process dental films. If a radiographic darkroom is readily available, a chairside developing box is not necessary; four beakers or glass jars are lined up, containing developer, water, fixer, and water.

A quick and clean alternative is the injectable developer-fixer system; after exposure the needle supplied with the system is used to inject the fluid though the injection point of the specifically packaged films that are used with this system. The film is massaged gently to spread the fluid; then 15 seconds later the package is opened and the film can be inspected. Additional fixing time is recommended after inspection of the wet film if it is to be retained as a permanent record.

Interpretation

Interpretation of oral films requires careful observation and excellent technique. A magnifying glass is helpful, particularly for cat oral radiographs or in circumstances that require discernment of fine details, such as in checking that a good apical seal has been achieved during a root canal procedure.

The oral structures consist of soft tissues, as well as hard tissues that are calcified to differing extents. These structures result in differing radiodensities that are in a specific pattern in normal animals. The most radiodense tissue is dental enamel covering the crowns of the teeth. Most of the tooth substance is made up of dentin, which is less radiodense than enamel but is readily seen because it is so even in density and specific in shape, forming the roots and the hard tissue of the crown beneath the enamel. Dentin is readily recognizable because it is surrounded by soft tissue: the pulpal tissues of the endodontic system and the periodontal ligament that attaches the tooth to adjacent bone. Normally the line between radiolucency and radiodensity can be followed entirely around and within the tooth (Fig. 2-12).

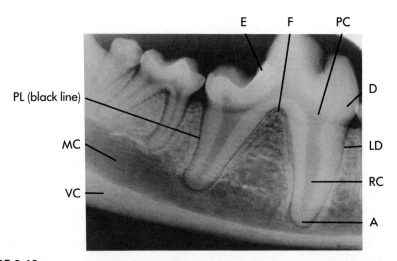

FIGURE 2-12
Normal radiographic dental and periodontal structures. *A,* apex of root in a mature dog; *E,* enamel; *D,* dentin; *F,* crestal bone in root furcation area; *LD,* lamina dura (cortex of alveolar bone); *PC,* pulp chamber in crown; *PL,* periodontal ligament; *RC,* root canal; *VC,* ventral cortex of mandible.

The bone surrounding the teeth is radiodense but much less evenly so compared with dentin. The thin cortical layer adjacent to the tooth (the alveolar wall) forms a white line known as the *lamina dura*. It is seen separated from the dentin of the root because of the radiolucent periodontal ligament between these structures (Fig. 2-12). The bone of the jaws adjacent to the lamina dura generally is trabecular in pattern, although many variations in pattern exist because of anatomic location and age. Figs. 2-13 to 2-16 show sets of oral radiographs from immature and mature cats and dogs. The mental foramina are the most obvious anatomic oddities that can cause misinterpretation (see Fig. 6-11). Details of radiographic interpretation of periodontal structures are described in Chapter 4, and endodontic radiographic features are described in Chapter 6.

▶ OTHER EXAMINATIONS
Culture

Indications for bacterial culture of oral lesions are rare because the flora of the normal oral cavity is so plentiful that pathogens (bacteria considered to be pathogenic when a culture is obtained from a normally sterile location) are common and multiple isolates are expected. Normal culture techniques will not identify flagellate organisms or the anaerobic flora that are considered to be the pathogens in periodontal disease. Fungal culture occasionally is useful to confirm the presence of *Candida albicans* and, rarely, for aspergillosis or systemic mycoses that may be affecting oral tissues.

Biopsy

Cytologic examination of oral tissues is useful if the sample is scraped from lesional tissue and the lesion is readily identifiable cytologically. The two most obvious examples of cytologically diagnosable lesions are squamous cell carcinoma and eosinophilic granuloma. For other lesions, surgical biopsy and microscopic examination of a formalin-fixed specimen are more accurate. Some oral neoplasms contain areas of necrotic tissue because of rapid growth; thus the location of the biopsy sample should include viable

tissue. It rarely is satisfactory to snip a small piece from the most protuberant area, even though it is tempting to do so in the consulting room as a way of avoiding anaesthesia and of expediting the diagnostic process. Because lesions such as fibrosarcoma may be hidden beneath a layer of normal tissue, the examiner should be prepared to extend the biopsy incision deeply. Open-ended skin biopsy punches are useful for obtaining deep samples.

For diagnosis of suspected autoimmune diseases by direct immunofluorescence, a specimen should be obtained from the freshest-looking area of disease, ideally with an intact epithelial bleb, and should include some adjacent grossly normal epithelium. The specimen should be placed in Michel's preservative instead of formalin.

For lesions that distort the hard or soft palate, or if there is a risk of creating an oronasal fistula, the biopsy procedure should be planned to avoid penetrating the lesion in full depth (keeping in mind the need to obtain lesional tissue). An alternative is to make a separate incision in a normal area and reflect an epithelial flap to gain entry to the biopsy site.

Additional Examinations

Examination for systemic disease is important, particularly in aging animals, to assess anesthetic risk or to determine the likelihood of oral lesions being secondary to a systemic condition. A complete blood cell count and standard serum chemistry panel are essential in many cases, and additional serum chemistry or clotting factor tests may be indicated (see Chapter 3). Urinalysis and cardiac examination are indicated when prognosis and management of urinary or cardiac diseases are essential factors in decision making for animals with chronic oral diseases. All cats with chronic oral inflammatory diseases should be tested for feline leukemia virus, feline immunodeficiency virus, and feline infectious peritonitis (see Chapter 5). Fluoroscopic examination of swallowing function may be useful for pharyngeal lesions but rarely adds information for oral cavity lesions. Electromyographic examination of tongue and pharyngeal tissues may be helpful but can be very confusing inasmuch as normal muscles in these areas may show changes that are considered indicative of disease in limb muscles.

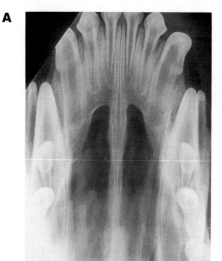

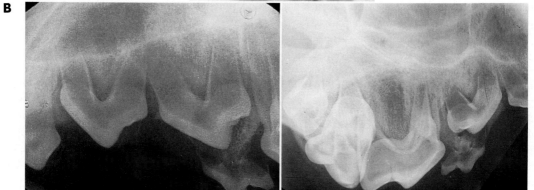

FIGURE 2-13
Oral-dental radiographic series from a clinically normal 5-month-old dog. The roots of the permanent teeth are incomplete. **A,** Occlusal view. Maxillary canine and incisor deciduous teeth are still in place. **B,** Bisecting angle view of maxillary PM1-3; a deciduous tooth is still in place. **C,** Bisecting angle view of maxillary PM3, 4, M1, 2; a deciduous tooth is still in place.

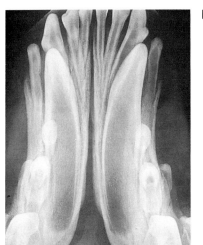

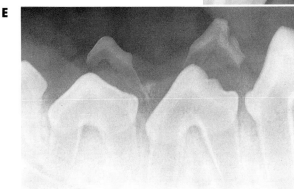

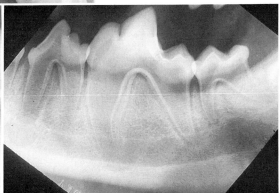

FIGURE 2-13, cont'd
Oral-dental radiographic series from a clinically normal 5-month-old dog. The roots of the permanent teeth are incomplete. **D,** Occlusal view of mandibular canine and incisor teeth; deciduous canine teeth are still in place. **E,** Parallel view of mandibular PM1-4; two deciduous teeth are still in place. **F,** Parallel view of mandibular P3-M3 (M3 is not yet erupted).

A

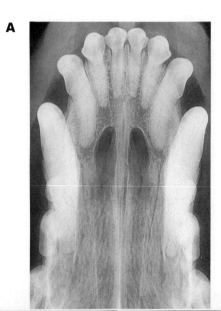

B 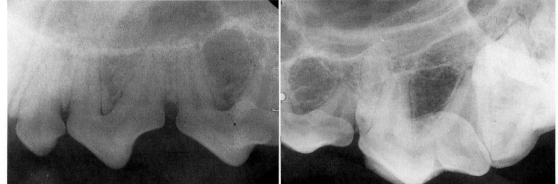 C

FIGURE 2-14
Oral-dental radiographic series from two clinically normal mature dogs. The apexes of the roots of the teeth are closed. The pulp chambers and root canals are wide in the younger dog (**B, C, E,** and **F**) and less wide in the older dog (**A** and **D**). **A,** Occlusal view of maxilla. **B,** Bisecting angle view of maxillary premolars. **C,** Bisecting angle view of maxillary PM3, 4, M1, M2.

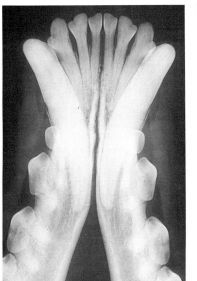

D

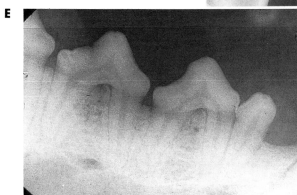

E

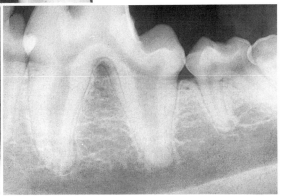

F

FIGURE 2-14, cont'd
Oral-dental radiographic series from two clinically normal mature dogs. The apexes of the roots of the teeth are closed. The pulp chambers and root canals are wide in the younger dog (**B, C, E,** and **F**) and less wide in the older dog (**A** and **D**). **D,** Occlusal view of mandible. **E,** Parallel view of mandibular PM1-3. **F,** Parallel view of mandibular PM4, M1, 2.

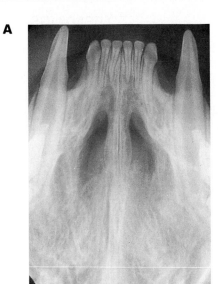

FIGURE 2-15
Oral-dental radiographic series from a clinically normal mature cat. **A,** Occlusal view of maxillary teeth. **B,** Bisecting angle view of maxillary premolar and molar teeth. **C,** Same view as **B,** with different vertical angulation showing superimposition of zygomatic arch over teeth. **D,** Mandibular occlusal view (from an older cat, showing a much narrower root canal). **E,** Mandibular parallel view of premolar and molar teeth.

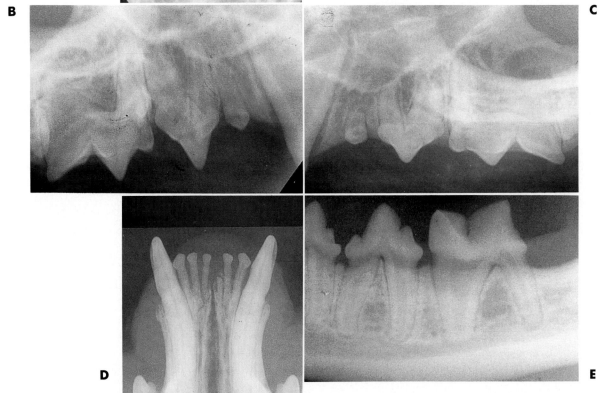

A

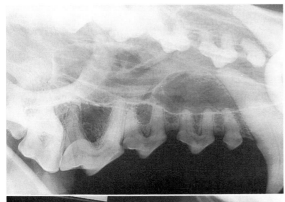

B

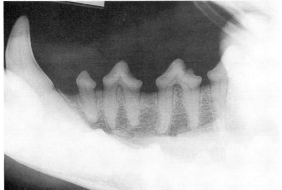

FIGURE 2-16
Radiographs taken from oblique position with extraoral film position. **A,** Maxilla. **B,** Mandible.

▶ SUGGESTED READINGS

Eisner ER: Problems associated with veterinary dental radiography, *Prob Vet Med* 2:46, 1990.

Emily P: Intraoral radiography, *Vet Clin North Am* 16:801, 1986.

Flamarens R, Franceschini G: Radiologie dentaire veterinaire, *Point Veterinaire* 10:19, 1980.

Harvey CE, Flax BM: Feline oral-dental radiographic examination and interpretation, *Vet Clin North Am, Small Anim Pract* 22:1279, 1992.

Hennet P, Poisson L, Paillasson P: Interet et limites de la radiologie en dentisterie veterinaire, *Point Vet* 23:295, 1991.

Morgan JP, Miyabayashi T: Dental radiography: aging changes in permanent teeth of beagle dogs, *J Small Anim Pract* 32:11, 1991.

Sager M, Bieniek KW: Verwendung von Zahnrontgenfilmen, *Prak Tierarzt* 11:51, 1988.

San Roman F, LLorens MP, Pena MT, Garcia FA, Prandi D: Dental radiography in the dog with a conventional x-ray device, *Vet Radiol* 31:235, 1990.

Zontine WJ: Dental radiographic technique and interpretation, *Vet Clin North Am* 4:741, 1974.

3

Oral Lesions of Soft Tissue and Bone: Differential Diagnosis

Oral lesions have many causes. Some primary lesions are common, others are rare, and some may be common or rare but are not a significant part of the wider clinical syndrome. Some result from a local cause and others from systemic abnormalities. Some have a characteristic appearance or location, whereas others vary widely in their appearance. This chapter describes this wide range, initially by appearance and location and then by etiology. The important primary oral diseases are described in detail in subsequent chapters (Chapter 4, Periodontal Disease; Chapter 5, Other Inflammatory Conditions; and Chapter 9, Neoplastic Conditions). Conditions that affect tooth substance are considered separately (Chapters 6 and 7). This three-step approach (appearance, location, and etiology) is used because it is confusing to consider all the lesions that occur in the mouth in a one-description system. In a few instances the appearance of the lesion is highly diagnostic. In other cases the combination of the appearance, location, and history leads to a reliable primary diagnosis. In some cases, however, several conditions will appear on the differential diagnosis list; either more specific diagnostic tests are required or response to therapy for the most common condition on the list is assessed. This chapter is not an exhaustive description of all oral conditions, although it mentions about 30 causes of oral ulcer-

ation, for instance. The challenge to the clinician is to use all the information available to make an informed clinical judgment and to follow the case to ensure that it is progressing as expected. If the result (of a diagnostic test or response to therapy) is not satisfactory, an alternative course of action is required.

The mouth consists of an epithelium of variable thickness, beneath which are connective tissue, muscle, and bone. The thinness of the buccal and sublingual epithelium permits subepithelial changes to be visible. The rich vasculature of oral structures means that lesions affecting vessels are likely to occur in oral structures. Because of the rapid turnover of oral tissues (particularly tongue epithelium), conditions that cause systemic or metabolic defects often result in oral lesions. As noted in Chapter 2, a good general history and physical examination are essential to avoid focusing on the oral lesion that may be only the most readily visible sign of body-wide disease.

▶ DISEASES THAT AFFECT ORAL EPITHELIAL SURFACES

Generalized Oral Lesions

The healthy oral mucosa has a glistening surface, pink or pigmented, with small vessels visible on the superficial buccal mucosa that can be blanched easily with finger pressure (see Fig. A-1).

Abnormalities that result from nonoral diseases but that are evident from inspection of the buccal oral mucosa include the following.*

Clinical dehydration

The oral mucosa is dull or tacky but otherwise intact. Clinical dehydration results in absence of the normal layer of oral fluid. This condition usually is not an oral problem, but a causative or coexisting oral or pharyngeal lesion can result in the inability to drink.

Hypotension, shock, or anemia

The oral mucosa is pale and may be dry but otherwise normal. These conditions usually do not reflect an oral problem. Pulse pressure and hematocrit levels should be checked.

Hypoxia

The oral mucosa is cyanotic (blue-gray). Hypoxia usually is not an oral problem. Respiration, pulse rate, and pressure should be checked.

Generalized oral hyperemia

The oral mucosa is bright red throughout the mouth but not ulcerated or asymmetric. If redness is uniform throughout the mouth but the mucosa is of normal thickness and glistens, a nonoral problem such as pyrexia secondary to infection most likely is present elsewhere. Other mucosal surfaces and body temperature should be checked.

If the color change is widespread in the mouth, but the mucosal surfaces are unevenly affected or are ulcerated, possible causes are chemical trauma, systemic diseases, or oral autoimmune or other immune-mediated diseases. Such lesions are described in greater detail in subsequent sections of this chapter.

Local or Irregular Oral Lesions
Inflammatory or ulcerated lesions

Lesions that are centered on the gingival margins but that are generalized or symmetric indicate *peri-*

---

*The Atlas, pp. 49-80, contains color plates of many oral lesions, arranged by location.

odontal diseases (including acute, severe conditions such as acute necrotizing gingivitis in dogs or gingivitis-stomatitis in cats). Periodontal diseases are described in Chapter 4 and other severe inflammation-associated diseases in Chapter 5 (see also Figs. A-60 and A-86 to A-91 in the Atlas).

Focal lesions located on the mucosa of the cheek, where the cheek is in contact with plaque-laden surfaces of major teeth when the lip is in a normal dependent position, are contact ulcers or "kissing" lesions of ulcerative stomatitis (see Figs. A-40 and A-41, p. 59).

Similar desquamative lesions sometimes are seen on the lateral margins of the tongue from contact with the lingual surface of the lower premolar and molar teeth (see Fig. A-20, p. 54) or as flattening and depigmentation of the palatal mucosa adjacent to the palatal surfaces of the upper premolar and molar teeth (see Fig. A-110, p. 78). Ulcerative stomatitis is described in greater detail in Chapter 5.

Lesions located primarily on the tongue, which cover much of its surface in irregular white patches partially covering a chronically inflamed or ulcerated epithelium, indicate candidiasis (see Fig. A-7, p. 51). If the dorsal surface of the tongue is generally but irregularly raised in areas of granulation tissue, vegetative foreign bodies are likely to be embedded (see Fig. A-12, p. 52).

Other conditions also cause lesions primarily on the tongue, but the lesions are less generalized (they may be irregular or symmetric), and adjacent areas of the tongue are normal. Examples are ulcerated lesions from chemical trauma (see Fig. A-10, p. 52) and, in cats, herpes and calicivirus lesions (see Fig. A-6, p. 51). Only rarely does calicivirus occur in dogs. Linear dorsal ulceration of the tongue without adjacent inflammation results from prolonged protein deprivation in an animal that continues to attempt to eat (see Fig. A-11, p. 52).

Petechia or frank hemorrhage without significant areas of inflammatory or ulcerative disease generally indicates local trauma or vascular lesions of systemic cause. The location and extent of the lesion should be assessed and the skin or other mucosal surfaces observed for similar lesions. Petechia may result from diseases that cause vasculitis, such as uremia (see

Figs. A-14, p. 53; and A-112, p. 79), leptospirosis (see Fig. A-9, p. 51), diabetes mellitus (see Fig. A-112, p. 79), or local immune-mediated phenomena such as epidermal necrolysis (see Fig. A-13, p. 52). The most common causes of frank hemorrhage are tooth eruption (associated with eruption gingivitis or pericoronitis in young animals), oral trauma (see Figs. A-16 and A-17, p. 53; and A-59, p. 63), periodontal disease (particularly during tooth loss or in association with ulcerative gingivitis or stomatitis), and oral neoplasms. Inflammatory diseases or minor trauma may cause intermittent hemorrhage in animals with coagulopathy.

Deeply ulcerative lesions are most likely to be neoplastic (see Fig. A-84, p. 71), particularly if they invade bone. Recent dental extraction or exfoliation sites may appear to be areas of bone ulceration, and chronic osteomyelitis associated with vascular damage during extraction or as a result of severe osteomyelitis may occur as an ulcerated lesion surrounded by a zone of firm, enlarged tissue (see Fig. A-58, p. 63).

Protuberant lesions also are most likely to be gingival hyperplasia (see Figs. A-81 and A-82, p. 70) or neoplastic.* With some neoplasms the epithelium characteristically is intact and in others is ulcerated (see Chapter 9). Small, symmetric protuberant lesions may be buccal or sublingual granulomatous hyperplasia ("gum chewer" lesions; see Fig. A-42, p. 59). Other causes of protuberant lesions are sublingual ranula (salivary mucocele) (see Figs. A-29 and A-30, p. 56); sublingual edema secondary to pharyngeal abscessation (see Fig. A-27, p. 56); craniomandibular osteopathy; chronic maxillary or mandibular osteomyelitis; endodontic, dentigerous, or bone cysts (see Fig. A-57, p. 63); isolated chronic inflammatory lesions such as eosinophilic granuloma (described in Chapter 5; see also Figs. A-5, p. 50; A-18, p. 54; A-36, p. 58; and A-106, p. 77).

Table 3-1 and the box on p. 47 list the common or major lesions by type of lesion and by primary location.

---

*See Figs. A-3, A-4, A-18, A-21, A-22, A-32 to A-35, A-48 to A-56, A-83, A-85, A-105, and A-106 in the Atlas, pp. 49-80.

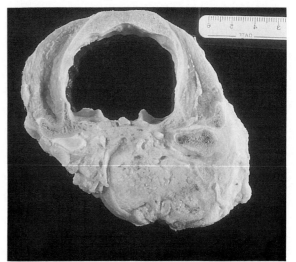

A

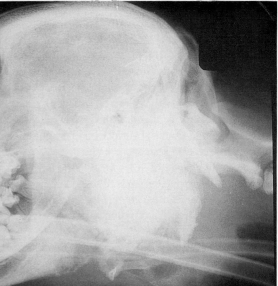

B

FIGURE 3-1
Craniomandibular osteopathy lesions in a West Highland white puppy. **A,** Section through skull at caudal end of mandible. **B,** Radiograph showing calcified tissue at caudal end of mandible.

TABLE 3-1	Major oral diseases by type of lesion
Type of lesion	**Likely diagnosis**
Generalized Mucosal Changes	
Dull, tacky surface, otherwise normal	Dehydration
Pale, otherwise normal	Shock, anemia
Cyanotic, otherwise normal	Hypoxemia
Hyperemic, otherwise normal	Pyrexia
Inflammation without Ulceration	
Centered on gingivae, symmetric	Periodontal disease
Spreading from gingivae; glossopalatine folds	Gingivostomatitis (cats)
Inflammation and Granulation, Hyperplasia	
Gingival (large dogs)	Gingival hyperplasia
Gingival, buccal glossopalatine folds, pharyngeal (cats)	Gingivostomatitis
Buccal fold, sublingual furrow, typically symmetric	Traumatic buccal or sublingual mucosal hyperplasia
Inflammation and Ulceration	
Mucocutaneous junction or scattered, generalized	Autoimmune mucosal diseases
Gingival margins	Periodontal disease
Gingival margins, spreading	Acute necrotizing ulcerative gingivitis
Centered on cheek opposite canine or carnassial teeth	Ulcerative stomatitis
Tongue, dorsal surface	Candidiasis, vegetative foreign body, caustic ingestion; FCV, FVR (cats)
Palate	Occlusal abnormality causing traumatic ulceration
Ulceration with Little or No Inflammation	
Dorsum of tongue	Protein deprivation
Anywhere, single lesion	Neoplastic
Anywhere, single or multiple	Chemotherapy, neutropenia of any cause
Vasculitis or Petechia	
Gingival or tongue most likely but could be anywhere	Uremia, leptospirosis, viral hepatitis, hypothyroidism
Fistulization	
On or close to MGJ	Endodontic disease, periodontal abscess
Edema	
Sublingual, lip	Pharyngeal abscess, electric cord injury
Necrosis	
Tongue	Electric cord injury, uremic vasculitis, leptospirosis
Palate	Electric cord injury

FCV, Feline calicivirus; *FVR,* feline viral rhinotracheitis; *MGJ,* mucogingival junction.   *Continued.*

TABLE 3-1	Major oral diseases by type of lesion—cont'd
Type of lesion	**Likely diagnosis**
Protuberant Mass	
Single mass, anywhere	Neoplasia
Single mass, tongue, palate, philtrum	Eosinophilic granuloma (cat)
Multiple masses, edge of tongue	Eosinophilic granuloma (dog)
Mucocutaneous junction, single or multiple, papillomatous	Viral papillomatosis
Symmetric, gingival	Gingival hyperplasia
Single, on tongue	Calcinosis circumscripta
Single, sublingual	Ranula
Symmetric, buccal or sublingual mucosa	Traumatic granulation hyperplasia
Frank Bleeding, No Gross Ulceration	
Any age, anywhere	Traumatic laceration
Young dog, gingival margin	Eruption
Gingival margin	Exfoliated tooth, uremic vasculitis, coagulopathy

▶ ETIOLOGY OF BACTERIAL, MYCOTIC, AND VIRAL DISEASES
Bacterial Oral Diseases
Periodontal disease

Periodontal disease, by far the most common oral disease in any species, results from accumulation and maturation of bacterial plaque. It is described in detail in Chapter 4.

Gingivostomatitis

Gingivostomatitis in cats is a severe and common oral inflammatory condition or group of conditions that may result from a hypersensitivity response or other abnormal reaction to gingival margin organisms (see Figs. A-88 to A-94, pp. 72 and 73). It is described in Chapter 5.

Ulceromembranous stomatitis

Ulceromembranous stomatitis (Vincent's stomatitis, trench mouth, acute necrotizing ulcerative gingivitis) is a severe but uncommon form of gingivitis or stomatitis associated with the presence of *Fusobacterium* and spirochete organisms though many other types of bacteria often are present. Severe acute gingivitis (pain, bleeding) is the major lesion, with ulceration of the interdental papilla as the classic initial lesion (see Fig. A-40, p. 59). It may progress to necrosis of soft tissues and exposure of bone. Diagnosis is by examination of a Wright-Giemsa–stained smear. This condition is described further in Chapter 5.

Other bacterial infections

Other primary bacterial infections are rare. *Actinomyces* spp. are gram-positive coccobacilli that are found in the mouths of dogs and cats. Gingivitis, ulceration of the lips, fetid odor, and drooling may occur. Pyogranulomatous periodontitis has been reported with sulfur granules (firm aggregates of bacterial material) in the actinomycotic exudate. *Feline leprosy* is caused by *Mycobacterium lepraemurium* and occasionally occurs with solitary or multiple raised, painless, plaquelike oral lesions (tongue and lips). Diagnosis is by Ziehl-Neelsen stain for acid-fast organisms or by biopsy. Oropharyngeal lesions occasionally develop in dogs or cats as a result of tularemia and infection with *Dermatophilus congolensis* and *Mycobacterium bovis*.

Major Intraoral Lesions by Common Locations

Dog

Generalized or randomly scattered

Neutropenia, chemotherapy or vasculitis ulcerations or petechia (uremia, leptospirosis, epidermal necrolysis)
Autoimmune blebs or ulcers (pemphigus vulgaris or bullous pemphigoid)

Tongue: dorsal surface

Candidiasis, vegetative glossitis, caustic chemical ulceration, nutritional ulceration, calcinosis circumscripta, neoplasia, electric cord injury, traumatic laceration

Tongue: lateral margin

Eosinophilic granuloma, neoplasia, ulcerative stomatitis (desquamation and ulceration), calcinosis circumscripta

Tongue: frenulum or sublingual

String foreign body, ranula, acute edema secondary to abscess, traumatic sublingual granulation-hyperplasia, calcinosis circumscripta

Lip

Autoimmune diseases (systemic or discoid lupus erythematosus), spaniel lip-fold dermatitis, schnauzer and Shar-pei conformational abnormalities, neoplasia, electric cord injury

Buccal mucosa

Traumatic buccal granulation-hyperplasia, ulcerative stomatitis, neoplasia

Gingiva

Periodontal disease, acute necrotizing ulcerative gingivitis, neoplasia

Palate

Neoplasia, electric cord injury, occlusal abnormality causing ulceration, congenital cleft

Cat

Generalized or randomly scattered

Autoimmune blebs or ulcers (pemphigus vulgaris)

Tongue

FVR or FCV ulceration, eosinophilic granuloma, caustic chemical ulceration, electric cord injury

Tongue: frenulum or sublingual

String foreign body, squamous cell carcinoma, edema secondary to pharyngeal abscess

Lip

Eosinophilic granuloma, neoplasia

Buccal mucosa

Gingivostomatitis, neoplasia

Gingiva

Periodontal disease, gingivostomatitis, neoplasia

Hard palate

Eosinophilic granuloma, neoplasia, electric cord injury, traumatic midline separation, congenital cleft

Glossopalatine fold

Gingivostomatitis

Saliva is bactericidal, and oral tissues heal rapidly. *Localized abscesses* usually result from foreign body penetration (see Figs. A-25 to A-28, pp. 55 and 56) and do not require treatment other than drainage and removal of the cause, although the foreign body itself may be gagged out before examination. The abscess pocket usually is sublingual or in the retropharynx or the orbit. If in the orbit, opening the mouth causes exophthalmos and severe pain as the coronoid process rotates forward to press on the orbital tissues. With pharyngeal abscesses, the neck and intermandibular tissues are firm, hot, and painful. In pharyngeal or sublingual abscesses, often a zone of severe edema involves the entire lip. In cats particularly, a pharyngeal infection or foreign body will cause sublingual edema that appears similar to a ranula (see Fig. A-27, p. 56), but no fluid can be aspirated and the pitting edema is obvious on squeezing the tissue.

Mycotic Oral Diseases

Mycotic stomatitis caused by *Candida albicans* is uncommon. It is associated with immunopathy or with prolonged antibiotic use. Lesions appear as white plaques with an ulcerated bleeding surface beneath, usually on the tongue and lips (see Fig. A-7, p. 51). Lesions also may be seen on other mucocutaneous junction areas. Diagnosis is by India ink–stained smear or culture of the plaque material. For description of treatment, see Chapter 5.

Nasal aspergillosis or penicilliosis occasionally penetrates the nasopalatine ducts and occurs with ulceration or hyperemia around the incisive papilla (see Fig. A-108, p. 78). Very rarely, lesions of one of the systemic mycoses, such as blastomycosis or histoplasmosis, may be present in oral tissues such as the tongue (see Fig. A-8, p. 51).

Viral Oral Diseases

Primary viral diseases of the oral cavity are rare. Exceptions to this rule are the herpes virus (FVR) and calicivirus (FCV), which cause viral respiratory disease in cats, and viral papillomatosis in dogs. FVR and calicivirus infection in cats may occur with tongue or pharyngeal ulceration in addition to (but only rarely without) sneezing and nasal discharge (see Fig. A-6,

p. 51). A similar acutely ulcerated glossitis, which is caused by calicivirus in dogs, is rare. FCV also causes severe glossopalatine-fold stomatitis (faucitis).

Diseases that result in immunosuppresion, such as feline leukemia virus (FeLV), feline immunodeficiency virus (FIV), and feline infectious peritonitis (FIP) infection, will predispose the animal to oral lesions. The possible association among FCV, FeLV, FIV, and FIP infection and gingivostomatitis in cats is discussed in Chapter 5.

Viral papillomatosis in dogs is a self-limiting condition typically seen in puppies. It produces warts, often in multiple clusters on the buccal mucosa and mucocutaneous junction area of the lips (see Figs. A-31, p. 57; and A-56, p. 63); treatment rarely is necessary for this self-limiting disease (see Chapter 9).

Distemper (in dogs) and panleukopenia (in cats) also may cause oral ulceration or inflammation, but clinical signs resulting from lesions in other areas are much more obvious.

▶ TRAUMATIC DISEASES
Fractures of Jaws

Fractures of jaws are described in Chapter 10, and fractures and avulsions of teeth in Chapter 6; falls from a height can cause a longitudinal split in the hard palate of cats (see Chapter 10). These conditions generally are obvious from inspection. Nondisplaced mandibular fracture may produce a swelling at the fracture site without malocclusion or mucosal damage.

Lacerations

Lacerations may result from external trauma or from ingested foreign bodies (see Fig. A-17, p. 53). Hemorrhage from the oral mucosa may be profuse.

Foreign Bodies

Foreign bodies may be recognized immediately because of rapid jaw or tongue movements and dysphagia (see Figs. A-24 to A-28, pp. 55 and 56). The most common areas of penetration are the root of the tongue and pharyngeal walls or floor. The sublingual area

Text continued on p. 81

Atlas of Oral Pathology of the Dog and Cat

This section includes clinical slides of many of the conditions described in the text, illustrating the range of abnormalities and the similarity of the gross appearance of many of the lesions. They are arranged by location.

▶ NORMAL

A 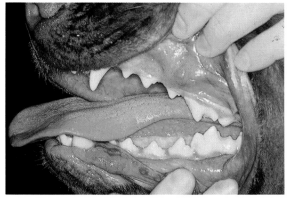 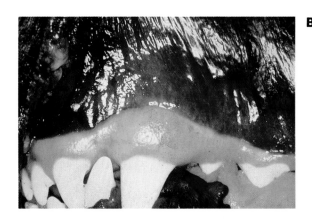 B

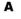

FIGURE A-1
A, Dog with the lip lifted to show the normal buccal and lingual mucosa, buccal gingivae, and teeth. **B,** Gingiva (unpigmented) and alveolar mucosa (pigmented) of a dog, showing the mucogingival junction and variation in gingival height.

▶ TONGUE AND SUBLINGUAL LESIONS

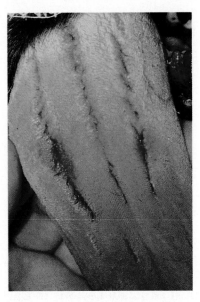

FIGURE A-2
Tongue of a dog with hairs growing from two lateral and one midline row of follicles on the dorsal surface.

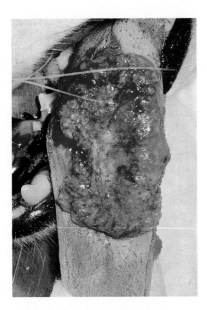

FIGURE A-3
Squamous cell carcinoma of the dorsal tongue of a dog.

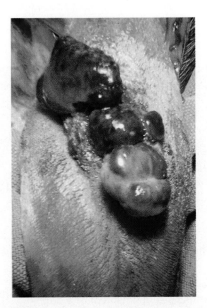

FIGURE A-4
Malignant melanoma of the dorsal tongue of a dog.

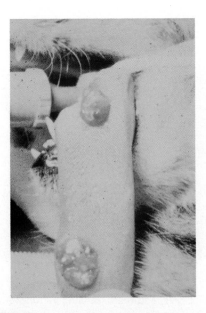

FIGURE A-5
Two eosinophilic granuloma lesions on the dorsum of the tongue of a cat.

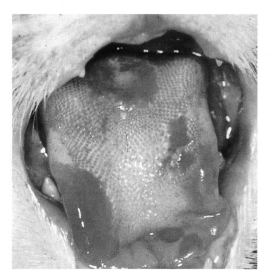

FIGURE A-6
Ulcers of the dorsum of the tongue caused by Feline viral rhinotracheitis in a cat.

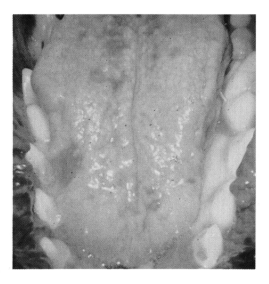

FIGURE A-7
Candida infection of the dorsal tongue of a dog; note extensive whitish plaques.

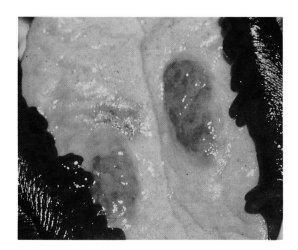

FIGURE A-8
Blastomycosis granulomas on the dorsal tongue of a dog.

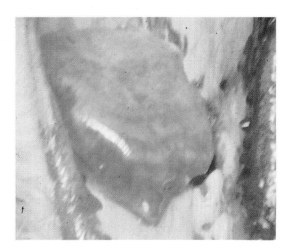

FIGURE A-9
Necrotic glossitis caused by leptospirosis in a dog.

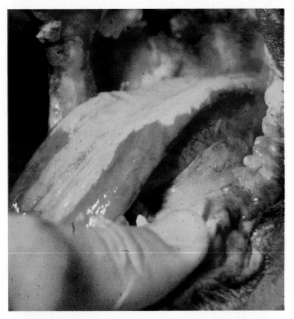

FIGURE A-10
Ulcerations of the lateral margins of the tongue of a dog caused by ingestion of caustic lye.

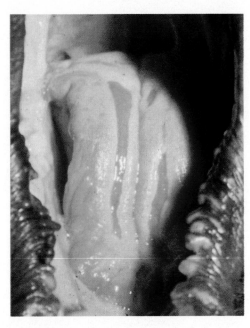

FIGURE A-11
Linear ulcerations on the dorsal tongue of a dog caused by malnutrition.

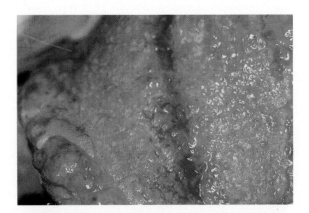

FIGURE A-12
Granulomas of the entire dorsal tongue of a dog caused by penetration of fragments of plant material.

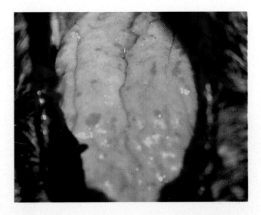

FIGURE A-13
Acute epidermal necrolysis (drug eruption following gold salt therapy), seen as spotting on the tongue surface of a dog.

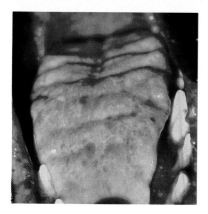

FIGURE A-14
Ulceration of the dorsal tongue of a dog caused by severe uremia.

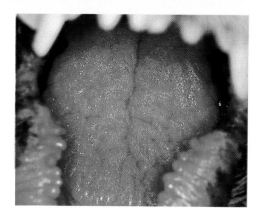

FIGURE A-15
Xerostomia and irregular thickening of the tongue and lips (cause unknown) of a dog.

A   B   C

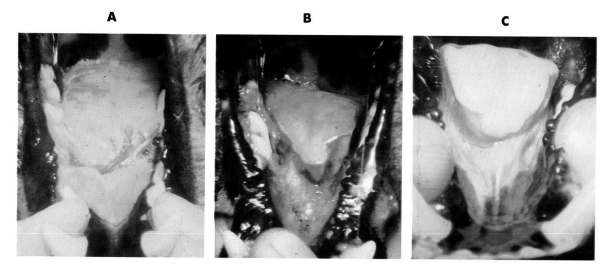

FIGURE A-16A
Necrosis of the free end of the tongue of a dog caused by chewing on electrical cord. **B,** Several days after the injury the necrotic section has sloughed. **C,** The tongue has healed 18 days after the injury.

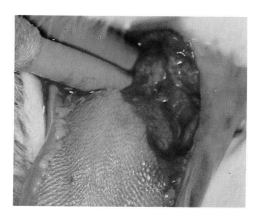

FIGURE A-17
Deep traumatic laceration of the root of the tongue of a cat.

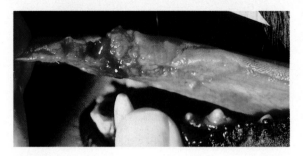

FIGURE A-18
Squamous cell carcinoma of the lateral margin of
the tongue of a dog.

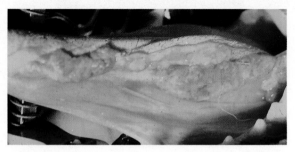

FIGURE A-19
Eosinophilic granuloma of the lateral margin of a Siberian Husky.

FIGURE A-20
Ulceration of the lateral margin of the tongue in a
dog with ulcerative stomatitis.

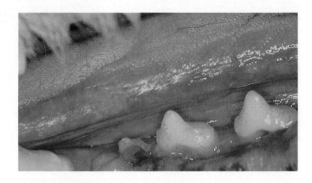

FIGURE A-21
Squamous cell carcinoma of the root of the tongue
of a cat.

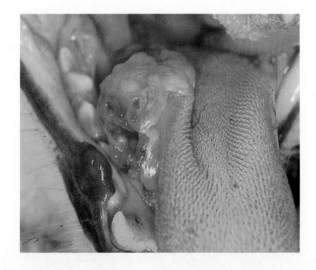

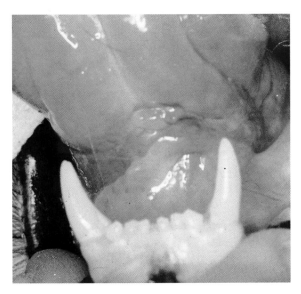

FIGURE A-22
Squamous cell carcinoma of the root of the tongue
of a cat causing edema of the sublingual frenulum.

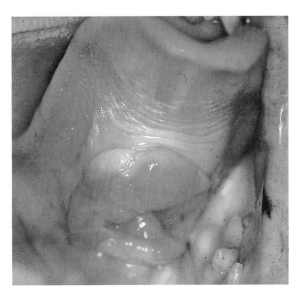

FIGURE A-23
Granuloma of unknown cause of the frenulum of the
tongue of a cat.

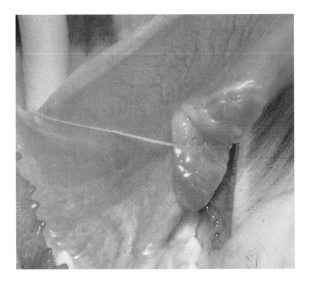

FIGURE A-24
Granuloma of the frenulum of the tongue of a dog
caused by a foreign body trapped beneath the
tongue.

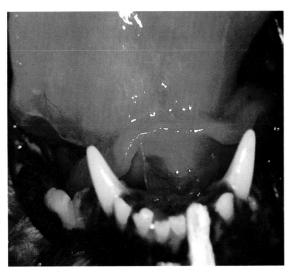

FIGURE A-25
Edema and granulation of the frenulum of the
tongue of a dog caused by an intermandibular foreign body abscess.

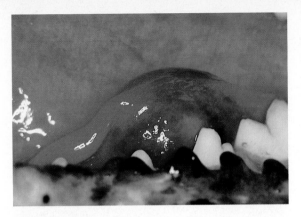

FIGURE A-26
Sublingual foreign body abscess in the tongue of
a dog.

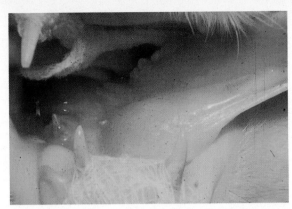

FIGURE A-27
Sublingual edema of the tongue of a cat caused by a
pharyngeal foreign body.

FIGURE A-28
Sublingual and lingual edge granulomas in a dog
caused by chewing on plant material.

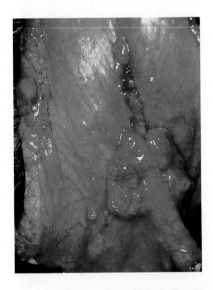

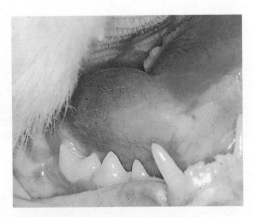

FIGURE A-29
Ranula (sublingual sialocele) in a cat.

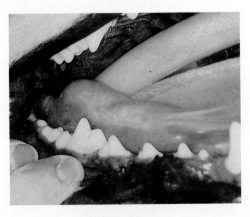

FIGURE A-30
Ranula in a dog.

▶ LIP AND BUCCAL VESTIBULE LESIONS

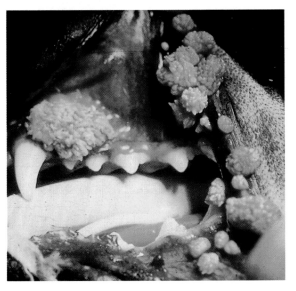

FIGURE A-31
Viral papillomatosis lesions in a young dog.

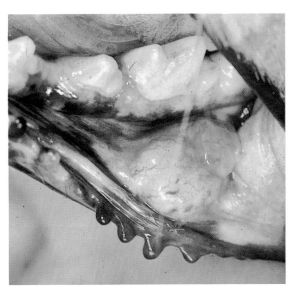

FIGURE A-32
Adenocarcinoma of the salivary tissue of the buccal fold in an old dog.

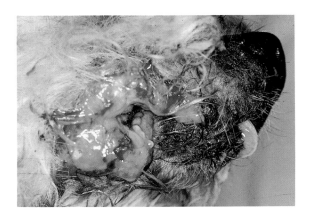

FIGURE A-33
Extensive squamous cell carcinoma of the lip of a dog.

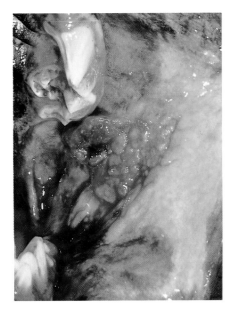

FIGURE A-34
Squamous cell carcinoma of the vestibule of a dog.

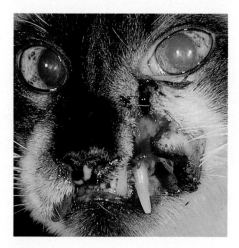

FIGURE A-35
Squamous cell carcinoma of the lip of a cat.

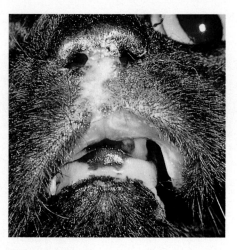

FIGURE A-36
Eosinophilic granuloma of the upper lip of a cat.

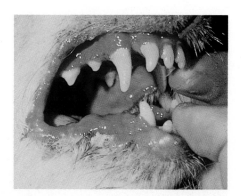

FIGURE A-37
Mucocutaneous junction lesions caused by systemic lupus erythematosus in a dog.

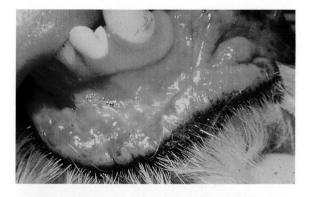

FIGURE A-38
Discoid lupus erythematosus lesion of the lip of a dog.

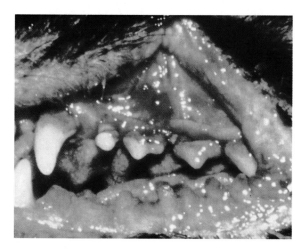

FIGURE A-39
Generalized inflammation and ulceration of the gingiva and buccal mucosa of a dog.

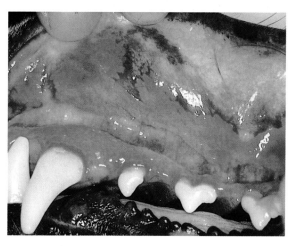

FIGURE A-40
Severe acute ulcerative gingivitis and stomatitis in a dog.

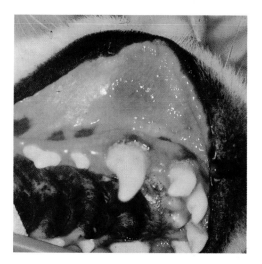

FIGURE A-41
Localized ulceration of the upper lip mucosa that contacts the upper canine tooth of a dog.

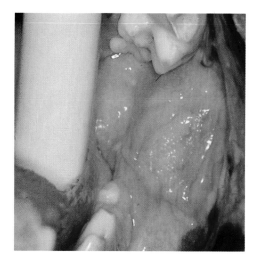

FIGURE A-42
Traumatic buccal granulation and hyperplasia ("cheek-chewers" lesion) in a dog.

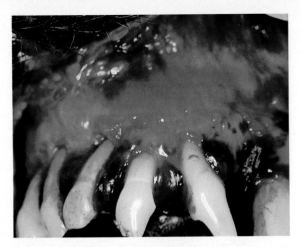

FIGURE A-43
Ulceration and granulation of the incisive gingiva and labial mucosa caused by penetration of chewed plant material in a dog.

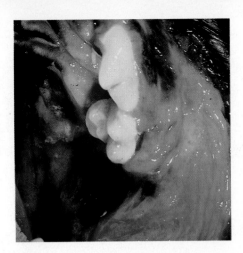

FIGURE A-44
Bullous autoimmune disease of the buccal mucosa of a dog.

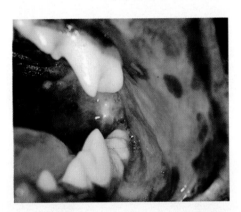

FIGURE A-45
Severe ulcerative stomatitis in areas of the buccal mucosa in contact with the premolar and molar teeth of a dog.

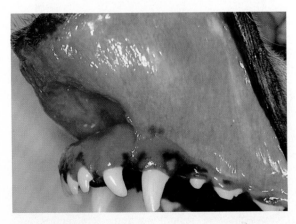

FIGURE A-46
Traumatic avulsion of the upper lip and nasal cartilages from the premaxilla in a dog.

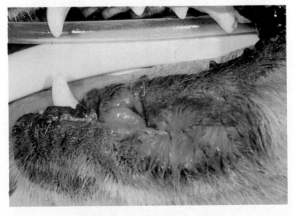

FIGURE A-47
Lip-fold dermatitis in a dog.

▶ GINGIVAL AND JAW LESIONS IN DOGS

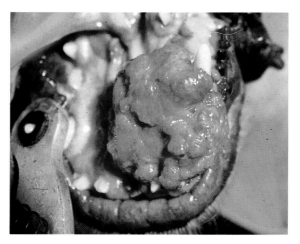

FIGURE A-48
Acanthomatous epulis of the lower incisor and canine area.

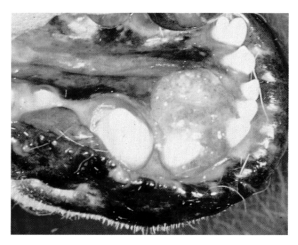

FIGURE A-49
Squamous cell carcinoma of the incisive gingiva.

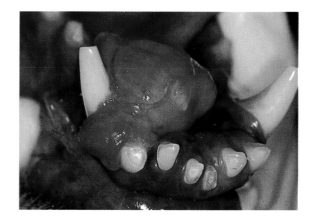

FIGURE A-50
Partially melanotic melanoma of the rostral end of the mandible.

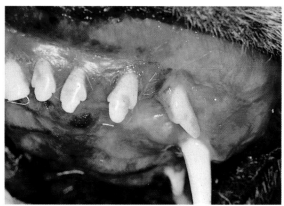

FIGURE A-51
Fibrosarcoma of the premaxilla and maxilla that has deprived teeth of their apical blood supply, as shown by the coronal discoloration.

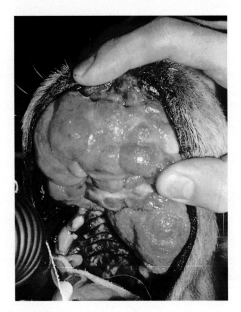

FIGURE A-52
Huge fibrosarcoma of the upper jaw.

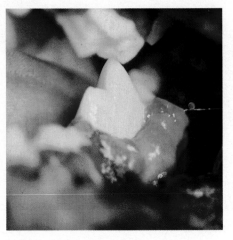

FIGURE A-53
Gingival swelling resulting from a mandibular osteosarcoma.

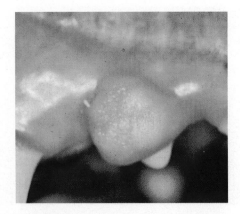

FIGURE A-54
Fibrous epulis lesion arising from the gingiva of the first premolar tooth.

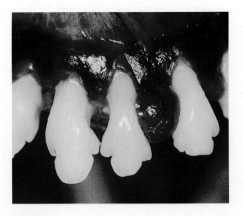

FIGURE A-55
Pigmented fibrous epulis lesion lying between two incisor teeth.

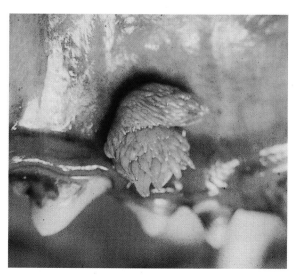

FIGURE A-56
Single viral papilloma lesion at the gingival margin.

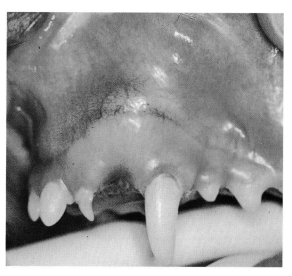

FIGURE A-57
Dentigerous cyst in the premaxilla.

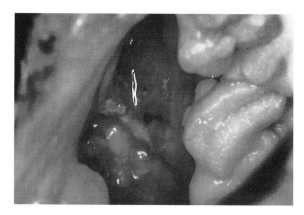

FIGURE A-58
Chronic maxillary osteomyelitis of unknown cause that has resulted in a huge oronasal fistula following several attempts at surgical treatment.

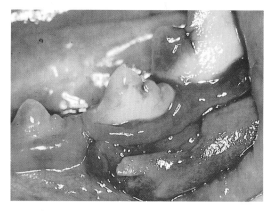

FIGURE A-59
Bone foreign body wedged into the buccal fold.

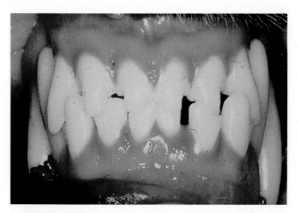

FIGURE A-60
Early gingivitis. There is increased vascularity to the marginal gingiva.

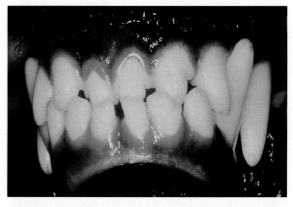

FIGURE A-61
Gingival inflammation has caused edema and swelling of the marginal gingiva of the upper central incisor teeth.

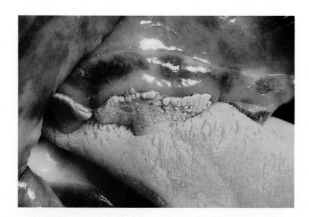

FIGURE A-62
Extensive rough-surfaced calculus on the buccal surface of the upper fourth premolar and first molar teeth with moderate gingival edema or hyperplasia.

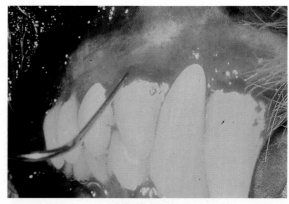

FIGURE A-63
Acute gingivitis.

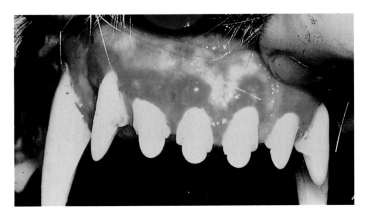

FIGURE A-64
Severe chronic gingivitis and early periodontitis.

A

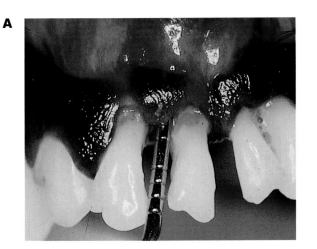

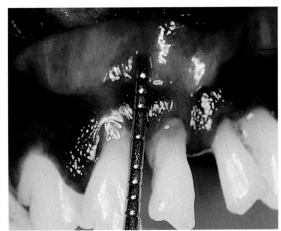

B

FIGURE A-65
A, and **B,** Moderate periodontitis—2 mm of gingival recession and a 4 mm pocket on the distal surface of a central incisor.

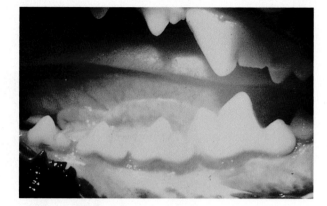

FIGURE A-66
Generalized gingival recession.

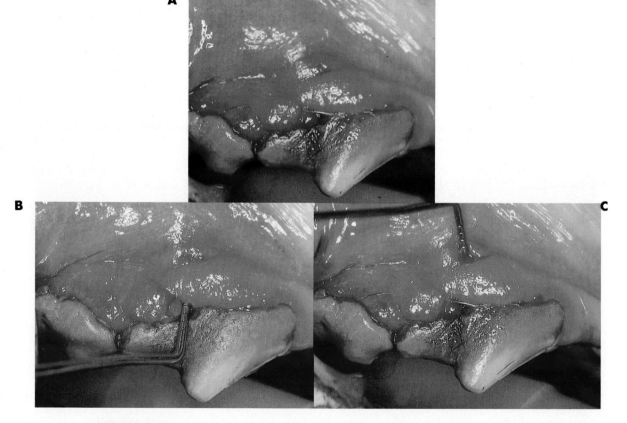

FIGURE A-67
A-C, Plaque and calculus accumulation, gingival inflammation, periodontitis (7 mm pocket) and fistula at the mucogingival junction of an upper fourth premolar tooth.

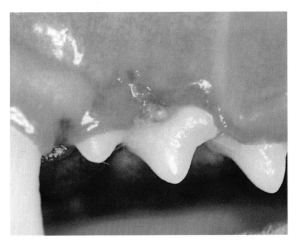

FIGURE A-68
Rotation of the upper second premolar tooth with loss of all attached gingiva and furcation exposure at the location of attachment of the upper lip frenulum.

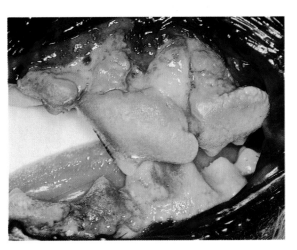

FIGURE A-69
Very extensive generalized plaque and calculus accumulation and periodontitis.

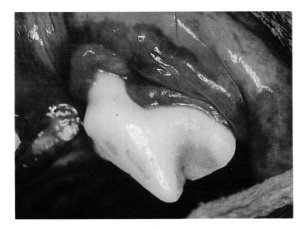

FIGURE A-70
Loss of all attached gingiva over the buccal surface of the mesial root of the upper fourth premolar tooth with ulceration of the exposed buccal mucosa.

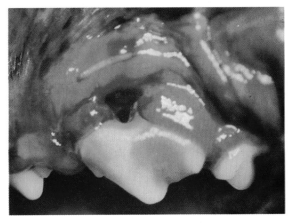

FIGURE A-71
Complete furcation involvement of the upper fourth premolar tooth with moderate gingival hyperplasia around other teeth.

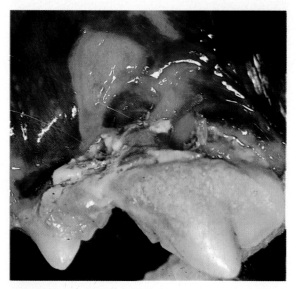

FIGURE A-72
Extensive buccal ulceration following periodontal abscessation over the mesial root of the upper fourth premolar tooth.

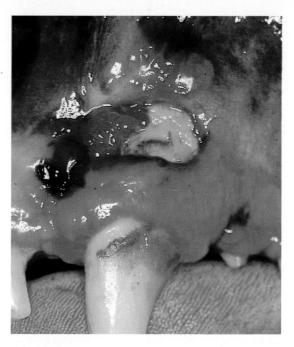

FIGURE A-73
Periodontal abscessation has resulted in a fenestration at the mucogingival junction of this canine tooth. Another possible cause of this lesion is endodontic disease, although the crown is intact.

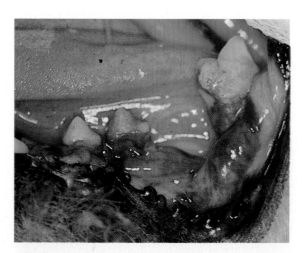

FIGURE A-74
Pathologic fracture of the mandible caused by periodontal disease. The jaw was unstable.

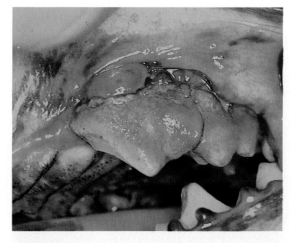

FIGURE A-75
The upper fourth premolar and first molar teeth are still present; however the first, second, and third premolar teeth have been lost, with healing of the gingival tissues.

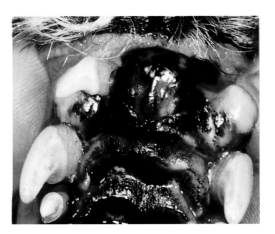

FIGURE A-76
Five incisor teeth have been lost, and there is extensive loss of attachment around the remaining incisor and canine teeth.

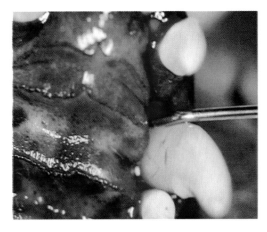

FIGURE A-77
Twelve-millimeter pocket on the palatal surface of an upper canine tooth in a narrow-nosed dog.

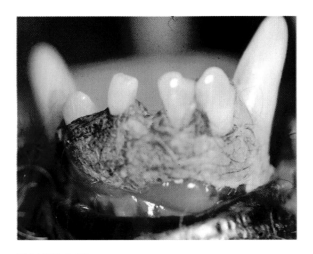

FIGURE A-78
Extensive entanglement of matted hair around the incisor teeth of a dog with dermatologic disease.

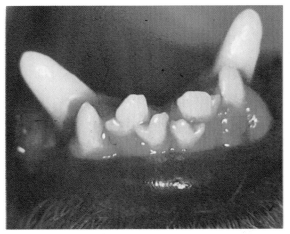

FIGURE A-79
Crowding of the incisor teeth and gingival inflammation.

A
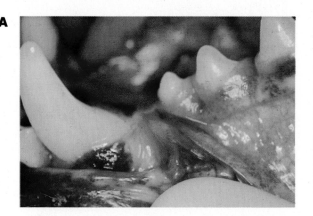
B
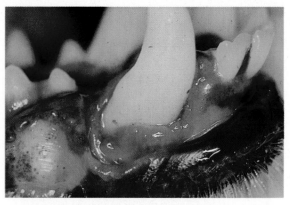

FIGURE A-80
A, Normal lower lip frenulum attachment. **B,** Periodontitis and gingival recession is most severe where the lip frenulum normally is attached.

FIGURE A-81
Moderate generalized gingival hyperplasia.

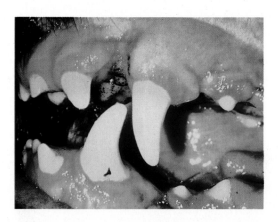

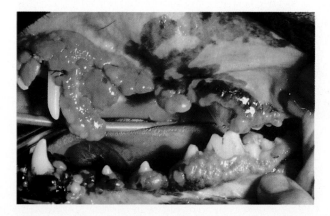

FIGURE A-82
Generalized severe gingival hyperplasia that has covered the crowns of several teeth.

▶ GINGIVAL AND JAW LESIONS IN CATS

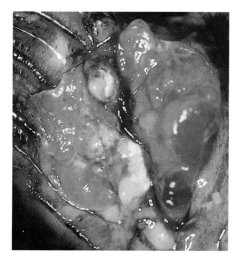

FIGURE A-83
Squamous cell carcinoma of the maxilla.

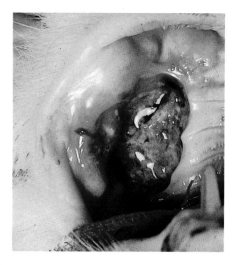

FIGURE A-84
Squamous cell carcinoma of the maxilla that is
mainly destructive rather than protuberant.

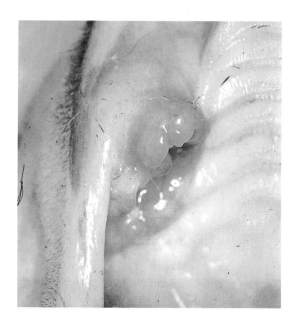

FIGURE A-85
Fibrosarcoma of the maxilla.

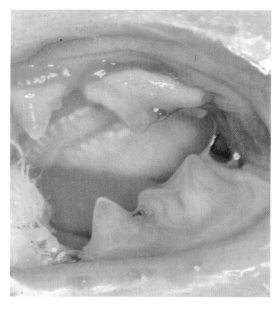

FIGURE A-86
Moderate calculus deposition with minimal visible
gingival tissue inflammation or loss.

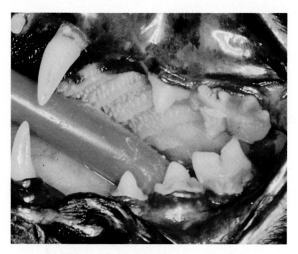

FIGURE A-87
Calculus deposition, periodontitis, and gingival recession with minimal externally visible inflammation.

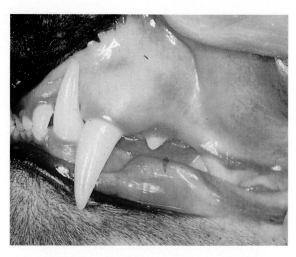

FIGURE A-88
Acute gingivitis. The inflammation affects only the marginal gingiva of the canine tooth but most or all of the attached gingiva of the premolar teeth.

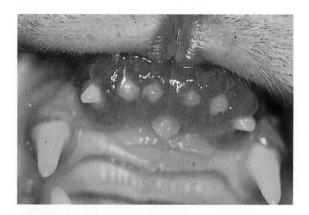

FIGURE A-89
Extensive acute gingivitis of the incisor teeth.

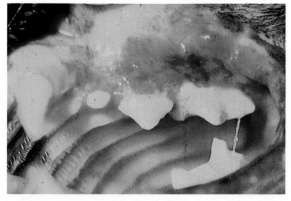

FIGURE A-90
Gingivitis and buccal stomatitis affecting the premolar area.

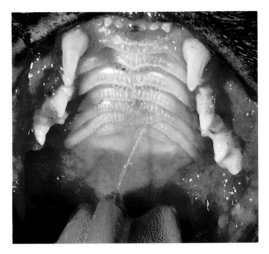

FIGURE A-91
Severe generalized gingivitis and buccal stomatitis.

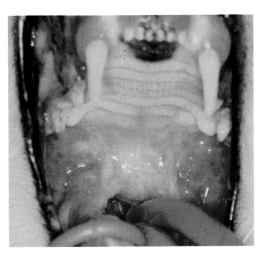

FIGURE A-92
Inflammation of the glossopalatine folds (faucitis).

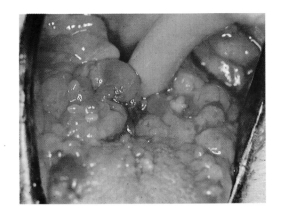

FIGURE A-93
Severe glossopalatine fold and pharyngeal inflammation and granulation.

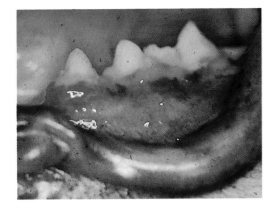

FIGURE A-94
Acute gingival inflammation affecting the mesial root and the distal root (to a lesser degree) of the lower third premolar tooth.

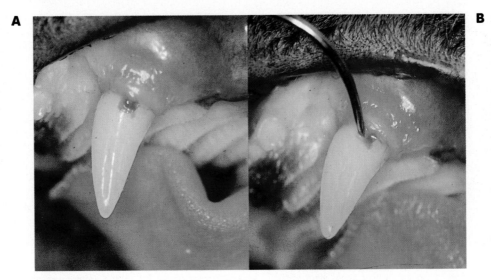

FIGURE A-95
A, External odontoclastic resorptive lesion affecting the upper canine tooth. **B,** A dental explorer assessing the extent of the lesion.

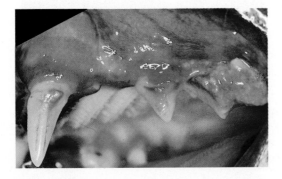

FIGURE A-96
Generalized periodontal inflammation that is more severe around the distal root of the third premolar tooth indicating the presence of an external resorptive lesion at that location.

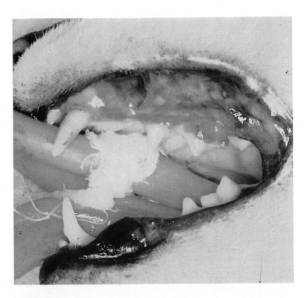

FIGURE A-97
Hyperplastic granulation that is covering the distal root of the upper fourth premolar tooth indicating the presence of an external resorptive lesion.

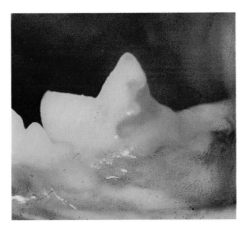

FIGURE A-98
Cavitation and granulation of the distal crown of the lower first molar tooth.

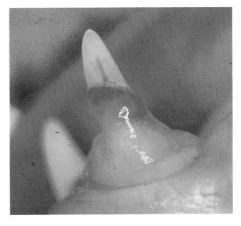

FIGURE A-99
Extensive hyperplasia and granulation growing over a large external resorptive lesion on the canine tooth.

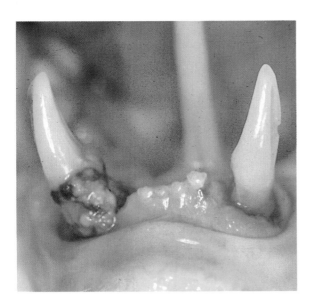

FIGURE A-100
Extensive resorptive changes around the roots of the lower canine teeth.

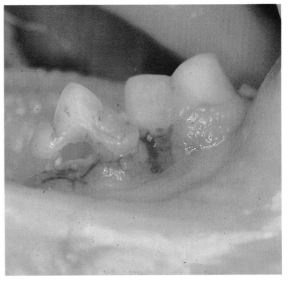

FIGURE A-101
External resorptive lesion that has eaten its way completely through the mesial root of the lower fourth premolar tooth.

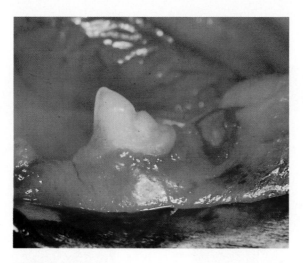

FIGURE A-102
A fragment of the mesial root of the lower first molar tooth is visible, although no crown of this tooth
remains. The acute inflammation around the mesial
root of the third premolar tooth indicates the presence of another resorptive lesion.

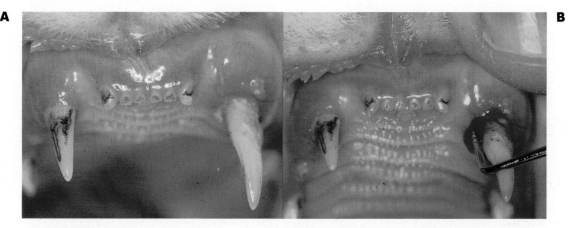

FIGURE A-103
A, Extrusion of the left upper canine tooth. The tooth was not mobile, but a deep pocket
was present palatally **(B).**

▶ PALATAL LESIONS

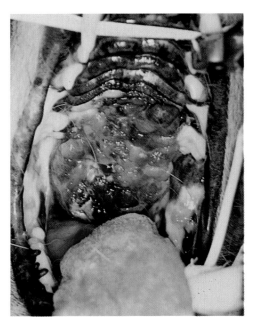

FIGURE A-104
Extensive malignant melanoma of the palate of
a dog.

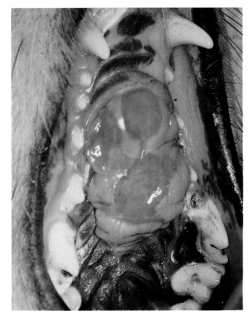

FIGURE A-105
Palatal fibrosarcoma of a 2-year-old dog.

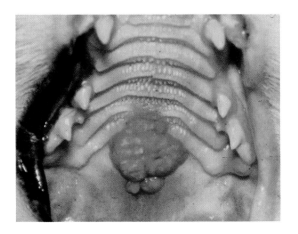

FIGURE A-106
Extensive eosinophilic granuloma of the palate of
a cat.

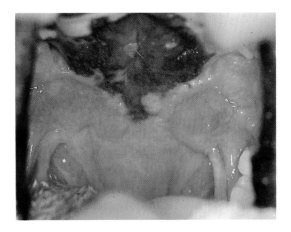

FIGURE A-107
Multiple granulomas of unknown cause in the
pharynx of a dog.

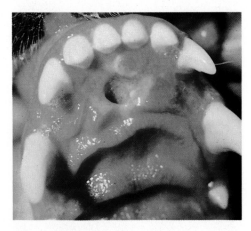

FIGURE A-108
Inflammation and ulceration of the incisive area, with fistulation through the masopalatine duct in a dog with nasal aspergillosis/penicilliosis.

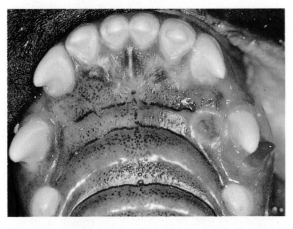

FIGURE A-109
Ulceration of the palate adjacent to the upper canine tooth caused by occlusal trauma from a base-narrow canine tooth.

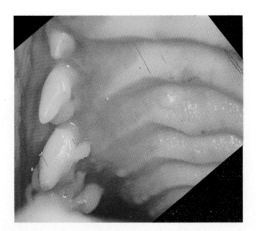

FIGURE A-110
Ulceration of the palatal gingival margins in a dog with buccal ulcerative stomatitis.

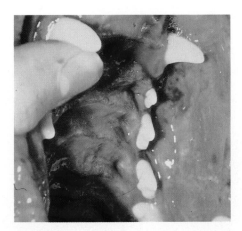

FIGURE A-111
Palatal and buccal ulceration in a dog with bullous autoimmune disease.

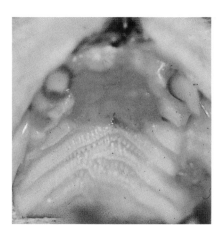

FIGURE A-112
Palatal ulceration in a cat with diabetes and uremia. The cat was FeLV and FIV positive.

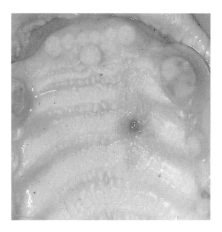

FIGURE A-113
Palatal sinus of undiagnosed cause that caused severe hemorrhage in a cat.

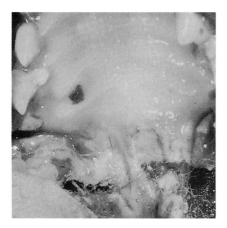

FIGURE A-114
Severe pharyngeal chemical burns in the soft palate of a cat (necropsy specimen).

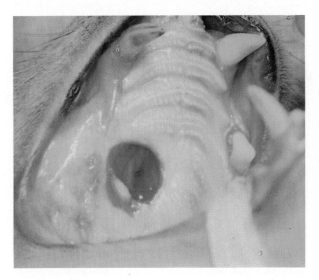

FIGURE A-115
Palatal defect in a cat caused by an electrical cord injury.

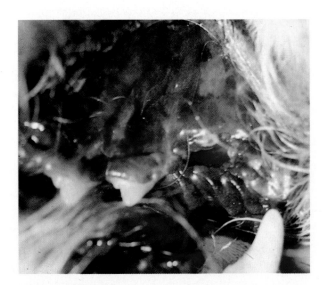

FIGURE A-116
Oronasal fistula caused by periodontal disease in a dog.

must be examined to locate strings caught around the tongue (see Fig. A-24, p. 55).

Small plant burs such as burdock *(Arctium lappa)* may penetrate deeply into the tongue or lip. The lesions initially appear as small papules; the necrotic center sloughs to form a discrete ulcer with a granular center. The surrounding tissue is normal, or the entire surface of the tongue may be affected (see Figs. A-12, p. 52; and A-28, p. 56).

Chemical Burns

Chemical burns are rare. Corrosive chemicals or gastric reflux are possible causes. Dysphagia or inability to eat is the most obvious sign. The lesions are acute-onset ulcers covered by necrotic debris (see Figs. A-10, p. 52; and A-114, p. 79).

Electric Cord Injury

Electric cord injury occurs most often in young dogs and cats. The effects may be local or systemic. Immediately after injury, pulmonary edema may be life-threatening. It may take several days before the extent of local injury is clearly defined. Necrosis of parts of the tongue and lips is common (see Fig. A-16, p. 53), and more extensive electrical burns can cause necrosis of dental pulp tissue and maxillary, palatal, or mandibular bone (see Fig. A-115, p. 80).

Radiation Therapy Sequelae

Radiation directed at normal tissue included in the radiation portal can cause erythema, mucositis, and superficial desquamation. On a long-term basis, radiotherapy may lead to radioosteonecrosis, although this condition rarely is recognized in dogs or cats.

Exposure to Sunlight

Acute and chronic glossitis can occur in working dogs exposed to sunlight in areas with high humidity and temperature. Principal signs are salivation, drooling, inappetence, and awkward, dipping drinking style. Variable redness and loss of papillae appear on the rostrodorsal portion of the tongue. Ultraviolet light–sensitizing agents may have contributed to development of severe lesions of this sort in military dogs in Vietnam.

Snakebites

Progressive and extensive local edema with petechiae, ecchymotic hemorrhage, or hematoma can result from snakebites. The bite wound may not always be visible.

Traumatic Buccal or Sublingual Hyperplasia

Proliferative, cauliflower-like lesions result from self-induced oral trauma to buccal mucosa along the bite plane or on the sublingual mucosa ("cheek chewer" lesion; see Fig. A-42, p. 59). A sublingual ranula can be traumatized or ruptured by teeth.

Management of traumatic diseases is described in Chapter 10.

▶ DISEASES RELATED TO NUTRITION

Structures with a rapid cell turnover that are continually exposed to chemical, mechanical, thermal, and microbial insults are particularly susceptible to injury when compromised by deficient nutrition. The tongue has the highest rate of cell turnover in the mouth and is the structure most likely to show nutritional deficiency lesions.

Protein-Calorie Malnutrition

Oral lesions have been described in the malnourished animal with depressed cell-mediated immunity, with an underlying protein-losing enteropathy or nephropathy, or subsequent to stress resulting in diminished IgA secretion and concomitant increased susceptibility to pathogens. The typical lesion is a linear ulceration of the dorsum of the tongue (see Fig. A-11, p. 52).

Hypervitaminosis A

A diet high in raw liver, with resultant hypervitaminosis A, causes proliferative gingivitis and retarded development or early loss of incisor teeth in young cats.

Mineral and Vitamin Deficiencies

Vitamin and mineral deficiencies are now rare in the companion animal population. A calcium-poor diet leading to hyperparathyroidism results in demineralization of the alveolar cortical bone. In young dogs this can result in gingival recession; however, it is not a major factor in periodontal bone loss and exfoliation of teeth associated with periodontal disease (see Chapter 4).

Severe niacin deficiency causes black tongue (hyperemia and ulceration of the tongue and other areas of the oral mucosa) in dogs. Severe biotin deficiency can cause salivation and scaling of the skin of the lips.

▶ IMMUNE-MEDIATED DISEASE

Many immune-mediated conditions cause oral lesions. Their appearance is briefly described here. Immune-mediated or inflammatory lesions primarily centered in oral or adjacent tissues are described in more detail in Chapter 5.

Hypersensitivity Diseases

Drug eruptions, including toxic epidermal necrolysis and swelling from insect stings, are rare oral conditions caused by a hypersensitivity response. There is no particular pattern to location of these lesions. Scattered oral ulceration is the most common presentation for drug eruption and toxic epidermal necrolysis. Insect stings cause swelling that generally is short-lived and without ulceration. These conditions are described in Chapter 5.

Autoimmune Diseases

Any of the autoimmune diseases known to cause skin lesions can occur in oral epithelium. They occur most often at the mucocutaneous junction margins, particularly of the oral cavity (see Figs. A-37 and A-38, p. 58; A-44, p. 60; and A-111, p. 78). Less often, the lesions may be wholly contained within the oral cavity (pemphigus vulgaris and bulbous pemphigoid). In the early stage, the lesions have a typical bleb— a superficial epithelial layer raised by a localized area of fluid. The blebs soon burst, and a more generalized or irregular epithelial ulceration or granulation of tissue is seen. The mucocutaneous junction lesions cause halitosis, bleeding from the lips, and discomfort in eating, drinking, and grooming. For further detail, including treatment, see Chapter 5.

Immunosuppressive Diseases

Conditions that suppress immune system function result in opportunistic infections, particularly in areas constantly subject to the presence of bacteria and other microflora. The lesions generally are centered on the gingival margins or adjacent tissue; they are ulcerated and surrounded by a zone of acutely inflamed tissue (although if neutrophil function is suppressed, ulceration may occur with little or no inflammation).

▶ NEOPLASTIC DISEASES

Benign and malignant tumors are common and important causes of oral disease; they are described in detail in Chapter 9.* In general, single asymmetric protuberant or ulcerative lesions in or on oral structures should be assumed to be neoplastic until proved otherwise by biopsy.

▶ GENETIC AND DEVELOPMENTAL CONDITIONS
Cleft Lip and Palate

Congenital or inherited clefts may involve the primary palate (incisive bone) or the secondary palate, or both. Congenital cleft of hard palate usually is on the midline and almost always is associated with a midline soft palate defect. Soft palate defects may be midline or unilateral. These conditions are described further in Chapter 10.

Gray Collie Syndrome—Cyclic Neutropenia

The gray collie syndrome is inherited as a simple recessive autosomal disease. Clinical signs result from infection during neutropenic periods. The most common signs include fever, stomatitis, pharyngitis (often severe and recurrent), and skin infections. Oral lesions may be the major clinical disease manifestation, with severe periodontal disease and large, deep, recurrent ulcers.

---

*See also Figs. A-3, A-4, A-18, A-21, A-22, A-32 to A-35, A-48 to A-56, A-83 to A-85, A-104, and A-105 in the Atlas, pp. 49-80.

von Willebrand's Disease

Hemorrhagic bleeding diathesis is caused by a deficiency of von Willebrand's factor (vWF). This condition is particularly common in the Doberman breed. Oral lesions include spontaneous gingival bleeding or excessive bleeding after tooth extraction or oral surgery. Diagnosis is by vWF antigen assay, platelet aggregation and platelet agglutination assays for vWF, and indirect assay for vWF-activated partial thromboplastin time and bleeding time.

Cheilitis

In schnauzers, microcheilia predisposes the lips to trauma and accumulation of food in lip folds, with subsequent infection and inflammation. In spaniels, prominent lateral lip furrows allow for trapping of food and moist dermatitis in association with seborrhea (see Fig. A-47, p. 60). In Shar-peis, excessive lip folds result in inflammation and infection (see Chapter 10). In giant-breed dogs, excessive lower lip length results in channeling of saliva and severe drooling, often with moist dermatitis of the lower lip (see Chapter 10).

"Bird Tongue"

This lethal glossopharyngeal defect is inherited as a simple, recessive autosomal gene condition, with upward and inward curling of the fimbriated margins of the tongue that gives the tongue a narrow and pointed appearance. The tongue normally has fimbriated edges in very young dogs and cats.

▶ METABOLIC AND MISCELLANEOUS CONDITIONS

Oral mucosal ulceration and increased susceptibility to endogenous infection and trauma may be a manifestation of many systemic diseases. Compromise of tissue metabolism may complicate diseases such as acute renal failure, septicemia, and liver disease.

Uremia

Uremia (renal or postrenal) results in increased ammonia production from urea in saliva, interfering with the normal mucosal protective systems. Uremia also causes vascular damage; ammonia irritation, dehydration, and uremia-related clotting abnormalities result in vasculitis. This combination predisposes the oral mucosa to ulceration and hemorrhage, with brownish discoloration of the dorsal surface of the tongue; there may be necrosis and sloughing of the tongue, xerostomia, and hemorrhage from the gingivae (see Figs. A-14, p. 53; and A-112, p. 79). Uremic patients are immunocompromised as a result of uremic intoxication and protein and calorie malnutrition. Halitosis (a sharp ammoniacal smell) may be easily detected. Preoperative creatinine testing is mandatory in any older animal with halitosis and periodontal disease.

Leptospirosis

Leptospirosis causes severe inflammation and ulceration of oral mucosa, leading to necrosis if there is concurrent uremia (see Fig. A-9, p. 51). Oral manifestations vary depending on the bacterial species. *Leptospira canicola* causes severe congestion of oral mucous membranes, and there may be uremia-related oral ulceration, hemorrhage, glossitis, and necrosis especially of the tip of the tongue. *L. icterohaemorrhagiae* can cause severe oral mucous membrane congestion and thrombocytopenia-related petechiae and hemorrhage. Primary signs of liver or kidney disease usually are obvious.

Viral Infectious Canine Hepatitis

Viral infectious canine hepatitis may cause extreme hyperemia and petechiae in the oral mucosa, in addition to the more obvious signs associated with liver disease.

Feline Panleukopenia

Feline panleukopenia may cause oral ulceration, particularly in the milder nongastroenteritis form of the disease. Other signs are depression, anorexia, and fever.

Diabetes Mellitus

Diabetes mellitus may cause severe or more rapidly progressive periodontal disease in diabetic animals, as has been shown in humans, although this has yet to be documented in dogs or cats. Diabetes in humans causes dryness (xerostomia) of the mouth. Diabetic vasculitis may cause oral lesions (see Fig. A-112, p. 79).

Hypoparathyroidism and Hyperparathyroidism

Hypoparathyroidism is a deficiency in parathyroid hormone production. Oral manifestations are infrequent and poorly understood sequelae to hypoparathyroidism and hypocalcemia. Enamel hypoplasia and abnormal dentin formation may be an outcome of disease occurring while deciduous and permanent teeth are calcifying. Ulceration and necrosis of the margin of the tongue and mucocutaneous junctions, halitosis, and salivation are seen occasionally in mature animals.

Hyperparathyroidism causes decalcification of the jaws.

Hypothyroidism

Hypothyroidism is caused by a deficiency of thyroid hormone, most commonly a result of a primary thryoid abnormality or an acquired autoimmune problem. The progressive slowing of metabolic function causes insidious disease that affects multiple organ systems. The interference with normal development and eruption of the teeth, macroglossia, puffy and thickened lips, retarded condylar growth, and delayed apexification of the permanent dentition seen in children with hypothyroid cretinism have not been observed to date in dogs or cats.

Most primary thyroid abnormalities in the dog have an inherited autoimmune basis. Oral lesions in the hypothyroid animal result from underlying immune-mediated processes and bleeding tendency. Periodontal disease is extensive in breeds with low thyroid hormone concentrations, such as Dobermans, and oral mucosal bleeding may occur.

Aplastic Anemia

Aplastic anemia (normocytic normochromic non-regenerative anemia) usually is due to bone marrow failure. Oral manifestations are attributed to pancytopenia. Pallor of the mucous membranes is consistent with anemia. Gingival bleeding is the most common oral manifestation; petechiae and purpura of oral and pharyngeal tissues also occur; and ulcers without surrounding erythema may be present.

Toxicity

Warfarin and indanedione may cause the appearance of petechiae on the oral mucosa, as well as gingival hemorrhage. Evidence of bleeding from other body systems usually is present. Thallium poisoning causes erythema, exudative inflammation, and finally necrosis of oral epithelium, lips, conjunctiva, and feet. Systemic signs also are present.

Chemotherapy

Chemotherapy may cause large, irregular, and foul-smelling ulcers that are surrounded by pale mucosa as a result of concurrent anemia. The ulcers lack the usual zone of inflammatory response surrounding ulcers of other cause. Ulcers generally occur about 1 week after the start of therapy. Bacterial invasion secondary to severe neutropenia may play a role in ulcer formation. Ulcers may be infected with organisms not commonly associated with oral infection, such as gram-negative enteric bacilli.

Chrysotherapy

Chrysotherapy (aurothioglucose therapy) often causes stomatitis, a common toxic side effect. Toxicity most frequently develops during the initial course of therapy and is related to the total body content of gold.

Neutropenia

Neutropenia commonly manifests as ulceration of the oral mucosa, with large, deep, painful, irregular ulcers and necrosis. The lack of surrounding inflammatory response is characteristic. Neutropenia or pancytopenia can result from high-dose whole body radiation, drug therapy (for example, cyclophosphamide and doxorubicin), exogenous estrogen toxicity, chloramphenicol toxicity in cats, phenylbutazone toxicity in dogs, as a side effect of cephalosporin treatment, and from viral diseases such as panleukopenia, parvovirus, and FeLV infection.

Calcinosis Circumscripta

Calcinosis circumscripta is an idiopathic deposition of amorphous calcified material in the skin and subcutis, most typically in young, large-breed dogs, causing chalky, gritty nodules embedded in the tongue and buccal mucosa.

Ranula

Ranula is a unilateral soft fluctuant swelling in the sublingual furrow from accumulation of extravasated saliva. The mass may become large enough to be traumatized by the teeth (see Figs. A-29 and A-30, p. 56).

Sublingual Edema

Sublingual edema may appear as a unilateral or bilateral edematous mass in the sublingual furrow secondary to pharyngeal venous obstruction caused by a foreign body abscess or surgery (see Figs. A-25 and A-27, pp. 55 and 56).

Lingual Myositis–Granuloma

Lingual myositis–granuloma occasionally causes progressive dysphagia in dogs. The tongue is symmetrically enlarged and firm. External lesions may occur because of traumatic ulceration secondary to gross enlargement. Biopsy and cultures have failed to reveal a specific etiologic agent.

▶ DISEASES THAT AFFECT THE BONE OF THE JAWS AND THE MASTICATORY APPARATUS

Osteomyelitis

Severe proliferative osteomyelitis secondary to periodontal disease, occlusive trauma, or poorly performed extraction procedures is seen only rarely (see Fig. A-58, p. 63). There may be considerable necrosis and new bone formation. Management is described in Chapter 10.

Craniomandibular Osteopathy

Excessive periosteal new bone is formed on the base of the skull and caudal end of the mandible, typically in immature West Highland White dogs but occasionally in other breeds. There may be enough abnormal bone to prevent the mouth from opening (Fig. 3-1). The condition does not develop further once the dog is skeletally mature, which may be too late if the dog is unable to open its mouth.

Temporomandibular Joint Dysplasia

Temporomandibular joint dysplasia is seen in Irish setters, bassets, spaniels, and other breeds. The coronoid process of the mandible becomes locked outside the zygoma, and the dog is unable to close its mouth. The open-jaw locking may correct spontaneously, or the coronoid process may need to be manipulated back into place. Long-term treatment of this condition is described in Chapter 10.

Mandibular Neuropraxia

Mandibular neuropraxia is caused by stretching of the branches of the masticatory muscle–motor nerves when the animal attempts to open its mouth too far or to carry heavy weights (rocks or branches) in the mouth. The mandible hangs and can be closed to the maxilla with little effort by the veterinarian, but it drops open once the hand is removed. Recovery occurs without treatment over a 2- to 4-week period.

Tetanus

Toxins produced by *Clostridium tetani* cause muscle spasms, particularly of the masticatory and facial muscles, even though the site of infection may be anywhere in the animal. The animal may be unable to open its mouth and the lips may be pulled back (Fig. 3-2). Generalized weakness or inability to use limb muscles also may be present.

Masticatory Muscle Myositis of Dogs

Masticatory muscle myositis includes the conditions known as eosinophilic myositis and atrophic myositis of masticatory muscles. It is an autoimmune disease that affects the masticatory muscles supplied by the trigeminal nerve. It is limited to these muscles because they contain a unique group of myosin components in the type 2M myofibers. The autoimmune response causes necrosis, phagocytosis, and fibrosis.

The condition occurs in adult, large-breed dogs, particularly German shepherds and related breeds. Swelling of the temporal and masseter areas may be noted by the owner, but the primary clinical sign is trismus, which can progress to a total inability to open the jaws even 1 mm (see Fig. 5-1). Standard laboratory tests rarely are helpful; eosinophilia is found occasionally, and creatine kinase (CK) concentration usually is normal. Biopsy of affected muscle shows ne-

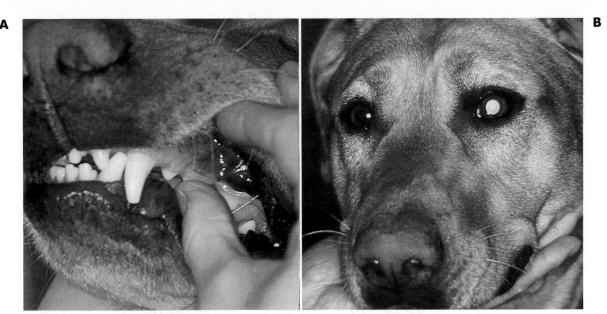

FIGURE 3-2
Tetanus-induced trismus (**A**) and facial distortion (**B**) in a dog.

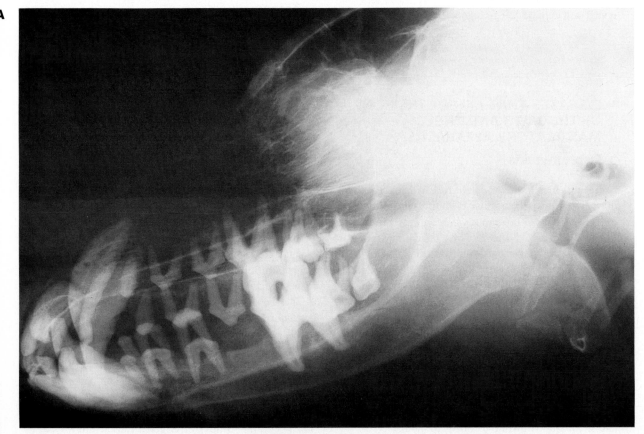

FIGURE 3-3
For legend see opposite page.

B

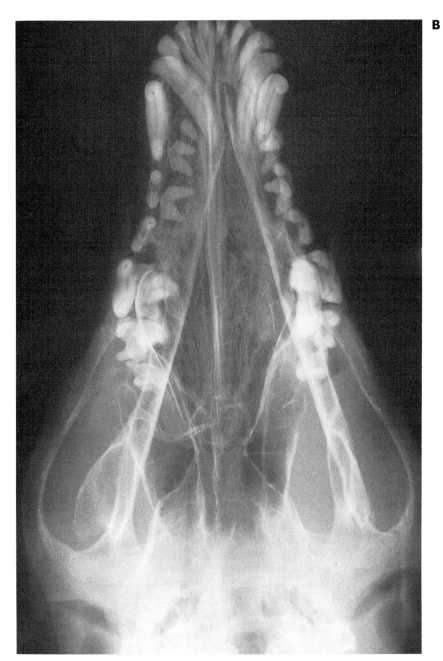

FIGURE 3-3
A and **B,** Radiographs of a dog with renal secondary hyperparathyroidism ("rubber jaw"). The laminae durae are no longer visible, and the overall density of the bone is poor.

crosis, phagocytosis, atrophy with fibrosis, and, in occasional cases, eosinophilic infiltration. A specific diagnostic test to examine for autoantibodies to type 2M myosin in muscle and serum is more helpful.* Treatment is described in Chapter 5.

Carnassial Abscess

Carnassial abscess (facial abscess, dental fistula) is seen as a swelling or draining tract below the medial canthus of the eye, typically in middle-aged or older dogs, usually mongrels. This is most often an endodontic disease (discussed in Chapter 6).

Hyperparathyroidism

Hyperparathyroidism results in resorption of calcium from bone as the body attempts to maintain calcium homeostasis. The common causes of hyperparathyroidism are nutritional deficiency (prolonged feeding of a diet with an abnormally low ratio of calcium to phosphorus as, for example, in meat without bone) and chronic kidney disease (secondary renal hyperparathyroidism). The condition is progressive, with a distinct and consistent pattern of affected bones. The first bone affected is the mandible, followed by the maxilla, then the other bones of the skull, the axial skeleton, and finally the long bones of the limbs. Before the rest of the skeleton is affected, the bones of the jaws may be severely demineralized, which is evident clinically as softening, commonly referred to as "rubber jaw." The first radiographic sign is loss of the lamina dura (cortical plate of the alveolus surrounding the roots of teeth), followed by loss of density of mandibular trabecular and cortical bone (Fig. 3-3). The bone will remineralize if the nutritional deficiency is corrected or the kidney disease is successfully treated. This condition does not cause periodontitis unless plaque accumulation is permitted; however, it will exacerbate bone loss and exfoliation of teeth in animals with plaque-induced periodontitis (see Chapter 4).

---

*Available through Comparative Neuromuscular Laboratory, Office of Veterinary Services, Room B200, Basic Science Building, University of California–San Diego, La Jolla, CA 92093.

▶ SUGGESTED READINGS

Baker MK: Ulcerative glossitis—a facet of feline panleukopenia, *J S Afr Vet Assoc* 46:295, 1975.

Bennet D, Prymak C: Excision arthroplasty as a treatment for temporomandibular dysplasia, *J Small Anim Pract* 27:361, 1986.

Bradley WA: Gingivitis in maltese terriers, *Vet Rec* 110:618, 1982.

Chastain CB et al: Actinomycotic periodontitis in a cat, *JAAHA* 13:65, 1977.

DeMonbreun WA, Goodpasture EW: Infectious oral papillomatosis of dogs, *Am J Pathol* 8:43, 1932.

Douglas SW, Kelley DF: Calcinosis circumscripta of the tongue, *J Small Anim Pract* 7:441, 1966.

Dubielzig RR: Proliferative dental and gingival diseases of dogs and cats, *JAAHA* 18:577, 1982.

Fox MW: Abnormalities of the canine skull, *Can J Comp Med Vet Sci* 9:219, 1963.

Humphreys GU: Dropped jaw in dogs, *Vet Rec* 95:222, 1974.

Jennings PD et al: Glossitis of military working dogs in Vietnam: experimental production of tongue lesions, *Am J Vet Res* 35:1295, 1974.

Kolata RJ, Burrows CF: The clinical features of injury by chewing electrical cords in dogs and cats, *JAAHA* 17:219, 1981.

Madewell BR et al: Oral eosinophilic granuloma in Siberian husky dogs, *JAVMA* 177:701, 1980.

McKeever PJ, Klausner JS: Plant awn, candidal, nocardial, and necrotizing ulcerative stomatitis in the dog, *JAAHA* 22:17, 1986.

Padgett GA, Mostosky UV: Animal model: the mode of inheritance of craniomandibular osteopathy in west highland white terrier dogs. *Am J Med Genet* 25:9, 1986.

Pool RR, Leighton RL: Craniomandibular osteopathy in a dog, *JAVMA* 154:657, 1969.

Potter KA et al: Oral eosinophilic granuloma of Siberian huskies, *JAAHA* 16:595, 1980.

Riser WH et al: Canine craniomandibular osteopathy, *J Am Vet Radiol Soc* 8:2331, 1967.

Robins GM, Grandage J: Temporomandibular joint dysplasia and open mouth jaw locking in the dog, *JAVMA* 171:1072, 1977.

Robins GM: Dropped jaw—mandibular neuropraxia in the dog, *J Small Anim Pract* 17:753, 1976.

Rowland GN, Fetter AW: Nutritional secondary hyperparathyroidism. In Bojrab MJ, editor: *Pathophysiology in small animal surgery,* Philadelphia, 1981, Lea & Febiger.

Stedham MA et al: Glossitis of military dogs in South Vietnam, *JAVMA* 163:272, 1973.

Stewart WC et al: Temporomandibular subluxation in the dog: a case report, *J Small Anim Pract* 16:345, 1975.

Thivierge G: Granular stomatitis in dogs due to burdock, *Can Vet J* 14(4):96, 1973.

Watson ADJ, Huxtable CRR, Farrow BRH: Craniomandibular osteopathy in Doberman pinschers, *J Small Anim Pract* 16:11, 1975.

4

Periodontal Disease

Etiology and Pathogenesis

Periodontal disease is caused by accumulation of bacterial plaque on the teeth and their supporting structures. Periodontal disease includes gingivitis (inflammation confined to the gingival soft tissues) and periodontitis (the more severe form in which bone supporting the tooth is lost, with eventual loss of the tooth). It is a progressive, usually nonregenerative and incurable disease if plaque is not controlled, but it is preventable and manageable with proper treatment techniques.

Periodontal disease is the most common disease occurring in dogs and cats. Age, body weight, head shape, diet, and chewing behaviors affect prevalence. There is general agreement that more than half the companion-animal dog population has some measurable disease, which increases with age to 80% or more by 5 years of age. The epidemiology of periodontal disease is detailed later in this chapter.

Maintenance of a healthy periodontium requires good oral hygiene, correct tooth alignment and occlusal forces, systemic health, and a nutritionally and abrasively adequate diet.

▶ PERIODONTAL ANATOMY

The periodontal tissues (*periodontium* or *attachment apparatus*) consist of cementum, gingivae, al-

veolar bone, and the periodontal ligament (Fig. 4-1).

The tooth-gingiva interface is a unique area in the body. The enamel surface of the crown of the tooth is incapable of healing after eruption because it lacks viable connective tissue or epithelial cover. Enamel is very hard and cannot respond to occlusal forces by deforming. After eruption to full crown height, the enamel surface cannot be altered by any bodily process except loss of substance by abrasion or chemical erosion. At the point of attachment in a normal healthy tooth, the enamel meets the cementum, also a dense structure but with connective tissue components that permit laying down of new tissue and inorganic matrix. The cementum is penetrated by collagen fibers of the periodontal ligament that retain the root of the tooth in the alveolus. The epithelial attachment also is focused at the cementoenamel junction (CEJ). In the 1- to 2-mm space of the CEJ–soft tissue junction, there is a need to accommodate the mechanical stress resulting from use of the jaws and teeth, yet maintain the attachment. The result is a papilla of soft tissue whose inner (sulcular) lining is protected. Additional protection is provided by the enamel bulge, the thickened area of the crown of the tooth that lies immediately coronal to the CEJ. Thus a concave area is formed (the "neck" of the tooth) that accommodates the gingival attachment in a protected position. A disadvantage of this protected environment is that plaque can be retained rather than removed by dietary

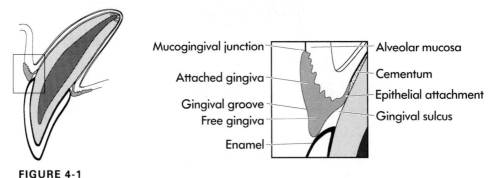

FIGURE 4-1
Diagram of a cross section of a tooth showing the periodontal tissues. Inset shows enlarged detail of the gingival area.

abrasion. The gingival sulcus is thus the focus of periodontal disease for understanding cause and implementing management.

Cementum

Cementum contains the collagenous fibers of the periodontal ligament that anchor teeth to alveolar bone. It is an avascular, mineralized connective tissue that covers the roots of teeth. The inorganic content of cementum is lower than that of enamel, dentin, and bone, and it is softer than these other tissues. Cementum resorption and deposition continue throughout life. Cementum is thickest toward the tooth apex and thinnest at the CEJ.

Gingiva

The gingiva overlies the bony alveolar processes of the maxilla and mandible and surrounds the tooth itself. The gingiva consists of parakeratotic stratified squamous epithelium, with prominent rete pegs overlying the lamina propria (connective tissue) on its external surface. Anatomically, the gingiva is divided into the attached gingiva and the marginal (unattached or "free") gingiva.

The attached gingiva is the part of the oral mucosa that covers and is bound to the alveolar processes of the jaw and surrounds the necks of the teeth. The gingival sulcus is the shallow crevice or space around the tooth bounded by the surface of the tooth on one side and the marginal epithelium lining the free margin of the gingiva on the other (Figs. 4-1 and 4-2).

The gingiva is the first line of defense against periodontal disease, protecting the subjacent bone and supporting tissues. Without an adequate zone of attached gingiva (approximate minimum is 2 mm) the crestal and alveolar bone will be lost to disease. The height of the attached gingiva is an important clinical parameter, defined as the distance between the mucogingival junction and the projection on the external surface of the bottom of the gingival sulcus, or the periodontal pocket. The attached gingiva is coral-pink or pigmented, stippled, firm, resilient, and tightly bound to the underlying periosteum of alveolar bone. At its crest the marginal gingiva normally is shaped like the edge of a knife.

The attached gingiva meets the relatively loose and movable alveolar mucosa at the MGJ, which is recognizable clinically as a distinct furrow. There is a change in pigmentation in some animals; the buccogingival height varies considerably, being greatest over the canine teeth (Fig. 4-1, *inset*). The alveolar mucosa apical to the MGJ is smooth, shiny, and pink or pigmented. On the lingual aspect of the mandibular teeth, the attached gingiva changes abruptly into the mucous membrane lining the sublingual sulcus. On the palatal aspect of maxillary teeth, the attached gingiva merges into ridges of masticatory mucosa (rugae), which cover the hard palate.

The MGJ remains stationary throughout adult life. Changes in the height of the attached gingiva are due to loss of attachment or recession.

The gingival sulcus is the (normally) shallow space

that is coronal to the attachment of the junctional epithelium and is bounded by the tooth on one side and the sulcular epithelium on the other.

The crest and facial surfaces of the marginal gingiva are keratinized. The surface of the marginal gingiva adjacent to the tooth is the sulcular epithelium. It is nonkeratinized stratified squamous epithelium (usually three to four cells thick) without rete pegs, but with large intercellular spaces. It acts as a semipermeable membrane that permits passage of tissue fluid from the gingival connective tissue; thus bacteria and injurious bacterial by-products from the sulcus can enter the tissue. Neutrophils and other inflammatory cells can readily pass into the sulcular space. The lamina propria (the connective tissue of the gingiva) is rich in blood vessels, lymphatics, nerves, and collagen fiber bundles that extend from the cementum of the tooth into the marginal or attached gingiva. Also present are plasma cells, lymphocytes, neutrophils, and some mast cells; these cells are a chronic inflammatory response to sulcular bacteria.

At the apical extent of the sulcular epithelium is the epithelial attachment. This is a strip of stratified squamous epithelium attached to the CEJ by hemidesmosomes and a basement membrane. The level of the epithelial attachment is an indicator of the crest of existing alveolar bone. Normal sulcus depths are 1 to 2 mm in the dog (occasionally 3 to 4 mm around canine teeth of giant-breed dogs) and up to 1 mm in the cat. Pocket depth may be increased because of regression of the epithelial attachment apically or enlargement of marginal gingiva as a result of inflam-

mation or hyperplasia, or a combination of these processes.

Alveolar Bone

The alveolar processes are ridges of the jaw bones that contain tooth sockets (the alveoli). Alveolar bone consists of dense compact bone; the cribriform plate, which lines the sockets; dense compact bone of the facial and lingual plates; and supporting alveolar bone consisting of cancellous trabeculae. Radiographically, the cribriform plate is a radiopaque line called the *lamina dura,* adjacent to and paralleling the radiolucent periodontal ligament (discussed in the next section). Blood and lymphatic vessels and nerves penetrate the cribriform plate, extending from underlying cancellous bone into the periodontal ligament. Alveolar bone responds readily to external and systemic influences, generally by resorption and, under specific circumstances, by remodeling.

Where collagenous fibers of the periodontal ligament are embedded in alveolar bone, the fibers, referred to as *Sharpey's fibers,* are continuous with those embedded in cementum.

Periodontal Ligament

The periodontal ligament is a connective tissue structure that attaches and supports the tooth in the alveolus. It is located between the tooth root and cribriform plate of the alveolus. Consisting primarily of collagenous fibers, it also contains cells of several types, blood vessels, nerves, lymphatics, ground substance, and a few elastic fibers. Collagen fibers of the

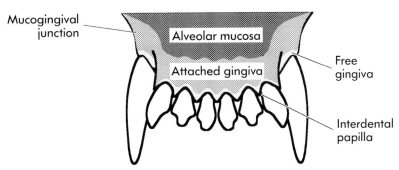

FIGURE 4-2
Landmarks of normal gingiva of the upper canine and incisor teeth.

periodontal ligament are arranged in bundles that run between the cementum of a tooth to the cementum of an adjacent tooth, or to the alveolar bone. These principal fibers of the periodontal ligament serve as attachment for the tooth to the alveolar bone and cushion the tooth and bone from occlusal forces.

The synthesis and resorption functions of the periodontal ligament are performed by cementoblasts, fibroblasts, and osteoblasts, as well as cementoclasts, fibroclasts, and osteoclasts. The periodontal ligament is in a constant state of repair and remodeling in response to local, functional, and systemic factors. Within limits the number and size of principal fiber bundles will increase with increased masticatory forces. Excessive occlusal forces, however, will result in necrosis of the periodontal ligament, and a decrease or cessation of mastication results in atrophy of the periodontal ligament. Progenitor cells in the periodontal ligament can give rise to any of the cellular elements.

The blood supply to periodontal structures is very rich. The major arteries are branches of the maxillary artery, particularly the sphenopalatine, palatine, and mandibular arteries. Venous drainage occurs via the pharyngeal, lingual, and facial veins. The sensory nerve supply to the teeth and jaws is via the trigeminal cranial nerve (V).

▶ PLAQUE

In a healthy dog or cat fed a "natural" diet that requires tearing and separation of swallowable pieces, the teeth and gingival tissues are largely self-cleaning; that is, plaque is wiped off before it has time to mature to a pathogenic thickness and bacterial mix. When circumstances change so that plaque accumulates, the disease process starts.

A clean crown surface (such exists after teeth scaling and polishing) is smooth and dry. This condition lasts a very short time inasmuch as a glycoprotein layer is laid down on the tooth surface as soon as there is contact with oral fluids. This glycoprotein layer, the pellicle, is invisible; however, it forms a surface that permits adhesion of bacteria that are constantly present in oral fluids. Initially the bacteria that adhere are largely aerobic gram-positive organisms, generally

actinomyces and streptococci in dogs and cats. Within 24 hours there is a smooth layer of bacterial plaque over the entire tooth surface, except for those areas that are cleansed naturally by dietary abrasion. Over the next several days the growth of the initial plaque population provides a rough, adhesive, but still largely invisible surface that favors the retention and growth of other organisms. As the plaque thickens, matures, and extends further down the gingival sulcus, the environment becomes more hospitable for growth of anaerobic organisms, motile rods, and spirochetes. It is the anaerobes that generally are considered to be organisms responsible for the pathologic changes that lead to periodontal tissue destruction and loss of periodontal attachment.

Koch's postulate states that, to prove an infectious cause of a disease, the organism must be harvested from diseased tissues, cultured in a pure state, produce the disease when inoculated into the target tissue, and be recultured from the artificially produced diseased tissues. Although it is impossible to fulfill Koch's postulate because of the complexity of oral flora and related conditions in the mouth, the research conducted to date indicates that the primary cause of periodontal disease is the accumulation of anaerobic bacterial plaque on the tooth surfaces. Thus the ultimate object of all periodontal therapy is control of plaque. Evidence of the cause-and-effect hypothesis between the accumulation of plaque and initiation of periodontal disease is based on several observations: gingival inflammation and subsequent tissue loss do not develop at the same rate in gnotobiotic animals as in animals with a "normal" periodontal flora, even though calculus accumulates; frequent mechanical removal of all plaque completely prevents the start of periodontal inflammation; and chemical control of plaque accumulation also effectively prevents development of the disease.

Periodontal tissue destruction occurs markedly less rapidly in rodents maintained on a calculus-inducing diet that contains an antibiotic. The rate of tissue destruction can be increased considerably in animals with a "normal" periodontal flora by placing a ligature of porous material (silk or cotton) around the tooth at the gingival margin; however, placement of the ligature in germ-free rats does not result in an increased rate of tissue destruction. Periodontal disease in germ-free rats and hamsters can be greatly accelerated by inoculating either specific flora from affected non–germ-free animals or pure cultures of oral organisms from a human source. The effect of bacteria is not limited to tissue inflammation and subsequent destruction; the rate of calculus deposition in rats bred to produce little calculus can be increased by caging them with rats that have been bred to form large amounts of calculus. Conclusions based on observations from one group of animals such as rodents must be applied to other animal groups (such as carnivores) with some caution. In rodents, even germ-free animals maintained in "ideal" circumstances, a very slowly progressive form of periodontal disease develops, perhaps because of the gingival attachment changes associated with a continually erupting dentition. However, parallel studies conducted in dogs, as well as clinical studies in humans, lead to the same basic conclusion: bacterial plaque causes periodontal disease.

In the dog, frequent (daily or twice daily) and thorough mechanical removal of plaque prevents development of periodontal inflammation and tissue loss. In one study, plaque was identified by disclosing solution and removed daily by brushing and polishing the teeth on one side only; the other side of the mouth was not touched. At the end of 4 years the brushed-polished side was clinically normal; no accumulation of calculus, inflammation, or loss of periodontal ligament attachment occurred, whereas the untreated side showed extensive calculus deposition and pocket formation or recession, and mobility or loss of teeth was common.

Plaque is a soft, cream-gray amorphous deposit. Thin layers of plaque may not be visible unless stained with a disclosing solution or scraped from the teeth with a periodontal probe. Plaque consists of bacteria in a matrix of salivary glycoproteins and extracellular polysaccharides mixed with epithelial cells, leukocytes, macrophages, lipids, carbohydrates, inorganic substances, and water. It is impossible to rinse plaque away with water; it must be removed by the diet or mechanically by means of hand instruments, toothbrush, or other oral hygiene aids.

The flora of the oral cavity is rich both in total number of organisms and in the range of organisms present. There are several relatively distinct ecologic niches in the mouth. Supragingival plaque and subgingival plaque are two distinct morphologic and microbiologic entities (Tables 4-1 to 4-3). Supragingival plaque is seen above the free gingival margin, and subgingival plaque is found below the free gingival margin. Because it is so difficult to determine where in the pocket a particular sample is taken from, "subgingival" plaque generally is lumped together into one category in studies of bacterial culture, although it has been shown by electron microscopy in a dog with mild gingivitis that subgingival plaque has distinct "layers." A dense mixed population was seen at the orifice of the gingival sulcus: gram-positive and gram-negative coccal and rod forms with little intermicrobial matrix. Next was a more loosely arranged mix, predominantly of filamentous organisms. Deeper within the sulcus, gram-negative filamentous organisms were again predominant. Deeper still was a layer of spirochetes associated with other gram-negative organisms. The most apical space was filled with closely packed spirochetes, arranged parallel to each other and perpendicular to the root surface. At the epithelial junction the spirochetes were more loosely arranged and occasionally were seen in the intercellular spaces of the junctional epithelium. Because of the difficulties associated with culturing and quantifying spirochetes, the pathologic or etiologic significance of this observation is not known.

It is easy to accept the idea that organisms found more commonly in deep pockets somehow are involved as causative agents. This, however, is a simplistic conclusion. First, deep periodontal pockets are unique ecologic niches—anaerobic but with an abundance of organic debris. The organisms present simply may be those best adapted to this environment rather than playing a causative role. This is hypothesized to be particularly true of spirochetes. Second, it is known that periodontitis is a disease with periods of active tissue destruction followed by longer periods of quiescence. Unless acute inflammatory or tissue-destructive activity can be shown at the time of sampling, bacterial culture as a means of elucidating the cause of periodontal disease is a flawed technique. Clinical criteria, such as gingival bleeding index or more definitive criteria such as histologic examination or biochemical analysis of pocket fluid for products of active tissue destruction, can be used. Even these criteria, however, are only poorly correlated with presence or absence of subsequent bone loss in humans.

Although no one now doubts that plaque bacteria are essential for development of periodontal disease, the emphasis is shifting to investigation of the factors that influence the host-plaque bacteria interaction (see later discussion of pathogenesis).

TABLE 4-1	Change of aerobic flora in periodontal disease				
		Gingivitis		Periodontitis	
	Healthy	Supragingival	Subgingival	Supragingival	Subgingival
Colony-forming unit	1.3×10^3	3×10^6	2.1×10^4	0.76×10^6	4.8×10^4
Total flora (%)	36.5	14	13	2.3	1.5

Data from Hennet P, Harvey CE: *J Vet Dent* 8:9, 1991.

TABLE 4-2	Streptococci and actinomyces in periodontal disease in the dog				
	Gingivitis (% of total CFU)		Periodontitis (% of total CFU)		
	Supragingival	Subgingival	Supragingival	Subgingival	
Streptococcal esculin negative plus *Streptococcus faecalis* (enterococci and nonenterococcus group D)	4.5	1.3	1.8	1.4	
Streptococcal esculin *(S. mitis)**	3.9-4.4	2.2-2.4	12.3	10.9	
Total actinomyces	24.1	17.8	10.9	2.1	
Actinomyces (aerobes and facultative)	6.1	8.4	2.0	0.95	

Data from Hennet P, Harvey CE: *J Vet Dent* 8:9, 1991.
*Includes facultative and anaerobic bacteria.

TABLE 4-3	Predominant subgingival anaerobic flora		
	Healthy gingiva (%)	Gingivitis (%)	Periodontitis (%)
Anaerobes (%)	25-48	70	74-95
Gram-positive cocci	3	7	5-12
Nonpigmented bacteroides	16	ND	19
Black-pigmented bacteroides (mainly *Porphyromonas gingivalis*)	6	15	20-34
Fusobacterium	7	25	10-40
Other gram-positive rods	5	10	6-25
Microaerophilic bacteria	17-30	ND	7-15
Spirochetes	+	+ +	+ + +

Data from Hennet P, Harvey CE: *J Vet Dent* 8:18, 1991.
ND, No data.

Plaque Bacteria in Dogs and Cats

Findings of supragingival and subgingival plaque on culture or direct smear from dogs and cats whose gingiva appear clinically healthy or have gingivitis and periodontitis are shown in Tables 4-4 and 4-5.

In dogs, the principal pathogens in subgingival flora are believed to be bacteroides (now divided into *Bacteroides* sp., *Prevotella* sp., and *Porphyromonas* sp.) and *Fusobacterium* spp.; aerobic organisms are uncommon in subgingival flora from dogs with periodontitis.

TABLE 4-4	Relationship of gingival index scores to percentage composition of subgingival plaque flora in cats

	Mean percentage of cultivable flora ± SE in sites with gingival index scores of:			
	0-1	**1.5-2**	**2.5-3**	**Significance***
Total anaerobes	53.4 ± 11.6	78.0 ± 3.8	89.7 ± 4.6	$p < 0.02$
Gram-Negative Rods				
Anaerobic	50.0 ± 10.8	66.6 ± 4.7	76.0 ± 6.2	NS
Fac/aerobic	12.5 ± 2.9	7.5 ± 2.5	3.4 ± 2.0	NS
Gram-Positive Rods				
Anaerobic	3.4 ± 2.0	9.7 ± 2.9	8.7 ± 3.0	NS
Fac/aerobic	18.8 ± 9.8	11.4 ± 3.3	1.2 ± 0.7	$p < 0.02$
Gram-Negative Cocci				
Anaerobic	0.0 ± 0.0	0.6 ± 0.4	0.0 ± 0.0	NS
Fac/aerobic	0.8 ± 0.5	0.7 ± 0.4	0.4 ± 0.3	NS
Gram-Positive Cocci				
Anaerobic	0.0 ± 0.0	1.2 ± 0.6	5.1 ± 2.2	$p < 0.02$
Fac/aerobic	14.5 ± 7.8	2.5 ± 1.3	5.4 ± 4.4	NS
Black-pigmented *Bacteroides*	25.0 ± 9.5	32.8 ± 6.3	41.6 ± 8.6	NS
Anaerobic fusiform bacilli	4.8 ± 2.8	5.2 ± 1.9	7.9 ± 3.9	NS
F. nucleatum	3.1 ± 2.6	1.5 ± 0.6	1.6 ± 1.1	NS
W. recta	0.0 ± 0.0	0.1 ± 0.08	0.0 ± 0.0	NS
A. actinomycetemcomitans	0.0 ± 0.0	0.0 ± 0.0	0.0 ± 0.0	NS
Capnocytophaga spp.	0.7 ± 0.7	0.2 ± 0.1	0.0 ± 0.0	NS
E. corrodens	0.0 ± 0.0	0.2 ± 0.1	1.1 ± 1.1	NS
P. multocida	5.2 ± 3.1	5.2 ± 2.1	0.5 ± 0.4	$p < 0.05$
Actinomyces spp.	0.02 ± 0.02	0.3 ± 0.2	0.1 ± 0.1	NS
Peptostreptococcus anaerobius	0.0 ± 0.0	1.2 ± 0.6	5.1 ± 2.2	$p < 0.02$
Mean gingival index	0.7	1.9	2.6	—
Mean total count × 10^5 CFU	9.9 ± 5.7	8.1 ± 2.6	11.1 ± 4.4	NS
Number of samples	6	17	7	—

From Mallonee DH, Harvey CE, Venner M, Hammond BF: *Arch Oral Biol* 33:677, 1988.
NS, not significant.
*Probability that all population means in row are equal (Kruskal-Wallis).

TABLE 4-5	Relationship of gingival index scores to frequency of detection of bacterial groups in cats		
	Frequency of detection (%) in sites with gingival index scores of:		
	0-1	1.5-2	2.5-3
Gram-Negative Rods			
Anaerobic	100	100	100
Fac/aerobic	100	82	71
Gram-Positive Rods			
Anaerobic	67	94	100
Fac/aerobic	100	94	57
Gram-Negative Cocci			
Anaerobic	0	12	0
Fac/aerobic	50	41	43
Gram-Positive Cocci			
Anaerobic	0	29	71
Fac/aerobic	83	53	29
Black-pigmented *Bacteroides*	100	100	100
Anaerobic fusiform bacilli	50	71	57
F. nucleatum	33	59	29
W. recta	0	12	0
A. actinomycetemcomitans	0	0	0
Capnocytophaga spp.	17	12	0
E. corrodens	0	12	14
P. multocida	100	76	43
Actinomyces spp.	17	18	14
Peptostreptococcus anaerobius	0	29	71

From Mallonee DH, Harvey CE, Venner M, Hammond BF: *Arch Oral Biol* 33:677, 1988.

In cats, black-pigmented bacteriodes (Porphyromonas) are found in all healthy and diseased samples, and *Peptostreptococcus* sp. are common in diseased samples. *Actinomyces* sp. also are common in both types of samples. One study showed an increase in detection of *Fusobacterium nucleatum* in gingivitis samples, but another larger study did not. *Actinobacillus actinomycetemocomitans* (the cause of juvenile periodontitis in humans) has not been found in culture studies, but circulating antibodies to *A. actinomycetemcomitans* were significantly higher in cats with gingivitis than they were in cats with clinically normal gingiva (however, there is cross-reactivity between *A. actinomycetemcomitans* and *Pasteurella* spp., which are very common in the mouth of cats).

Pasteurella spp. are common in the mouth and pharynx of both dogs and cats. Isolates from cats are more likely to be the human pathogens, *Pasteurella multocida* and *P. septica*. These organisms are more significant as the cause of abscess and cellulitis after cat bite wounds than as a cause of oral disease.

▶ CALCULUS

Dental plaque undergoes mineralization to form calculus, which can form above the gingival crest (supragingival calculus) or below the crest on the tooth root (subgingival calculus). Saliva provides the minerals for supragingival calculus (commonly known as "tartar"). The heaviest supragingival calculus depositions are found on the buccal surfaces of maxillary fourth premolars and first molar teeth in dogs and fourth premolar teeth in cats, adjacent to the parotid and zygomatic salivary ducts. Supragingival calculus is gray-brown, bulky, fairly brittle, and easy to remove (see Fig. A-62, p. 64).

Two studies of the chemical composition of dental calculus in carnivores have been reported. One study (10 days, 20 sample sites) showed that the principal component is calcium carbonate (calcite form) mixed with small amounts of calcium phosphate apatite. Variation occurred between samples in the calcite/apatite ratio, as well as the calcite/apatite ratio between the inner and outer layers of single samples. The investigators of these studies also examined precipitable calcium salts in mandibular and parotid saliva, which was found to be principally calcium carbonate calcite, compared with calcium phosphate apatite in human saliva. The addition of a calcium solution to canine saliva caused the precipitation of calcium salts, whereas addition of a phosphate solution did not result in any visible precipitation. The second study included 87 dogs and 17 cats. The principal component of calculus was calcium carbonate apatite (65% of dog samples, 76% of cat samples); a combination of carbonate apatite and calcium carbonate was the primary component in 17% of dog samples and 24% of cat samples.

Calculus promotes gingivitis because it provides a rough surface for accumulation of additional plaque. It is the bacteria-laden surface plaque that is the main irritant to the periodontium.

Subgingival calculus, particularly calculus attached to the roots of severely affected teeth, differs from supragingival calculus in color. Typically it is very dark or even black because of incorporation of iron pigments from degraded hemoglobin and production of pigments by subgingival bacteria. Subgingival calculus can be detected by running a dental curet or explorer along a root surface or by visual inspection during gingival flap surgery or gingivectomy. A roughened root surface may be due to the presence of calculus, or it may be due to demineralization of cementum (root caries) or external odontoclastic resorption.

The pattern of development of calculus accumulation is described in Prevalence and Patterns of Periodontal Disease.

Mouth breathing leads to dehydration of the oral cavity, which renders the plaque tougher and stickier and increases the rate of deposition of calculus in humans. Anecdotal comments suggest that the same may be true of dogs, although physiologic panting and nasopharyngeal airway obstruction do not cause xerostomia in dogs.

▶ DIET AND PERIODONTAL DISEASE

The natural diet of the wild carnivore has a plaque-retarding effect. In rigidly controlling and optimizing the nutritional content, palatability to the pet, and acceptance of commercially available dog foods by the pet-owning public, we have created materials that in gross form do not closely resemble the natural diet of wild carnivores. By selective breeding for specific body size, head shape, and occlusive pattern, we have created dogs that would not manage well even with a diet that closely resembles that of wild carnivores. By either route, plaque formation is enhanced, inflammatory periodontal disease is more common, and long-term health hazards secondary to intermittent bacteremia are more likely to occur in an aging pet population.

Several studies have shown that the form of the diet is much more important in controlling plaque build-up and gingival inflammation than is the nutritional content of the diet in dogs. Gross changes in carbohydrate and protein content have no effect on rate of plaque build-up. Gross distortion of the dietary calcium-phosphorus ratio leads to demineralization of periodontal bone but does not cause more rapid periodontal tissue breakdown. The general conclusion from reported studies is that a fibrous or dry food diet is more beneficial than a soft food diet. Even if dry food is somewhat better at retarding plaque formation than is canned food, it is far from optimal. From published studies to date, the diet that promotes optimal oral health in dogs contains large pieces, each of which contains calcified material and softer but fibrous material (for example, whole oxtail or whole tracheoesophagus).

The known differences in severity of periodontal disease among ages and types (body weights) of dogs (see p. 106) may be due in part to differences in specific anatomic factors such as tooth size relative to jaw bone height or thickness and gingival sulcus depth or to a tendency for owners of small-breed dogs to be more likely to feed a soft food diet. Both factors may be involved, each exacerbating the other.

In a Japanese study of the calculus found in 2649 companion animal dogs, the prevalence of calculus ("present" or "abundant") was significantly lower in dogs fed dry food or leftovers compared with canned, soft-moist, and home-cooked food.

Several products are now available that are designed to improve oral health by encouraging chewing action (described under in the section on home care under Treatment).

► PATHOGENESIS OF PERIODONTAL DISEASE IN DOGS

Supragingival plaque strongly influences the growth, accumulation, and pathogenic potential of subgingival plaque, especially in the early stages of gingivitis and periodontitis. Once the disease has progressed and periodontal pocket formation has taken place, the influence of supragingival plaque on all but the most coronally located subgingival plaque is minimal.

Gram-negative organisms can result in rapid tissue destruction because of their elaboration and release of endotoxins and their ability to invade the adjacent gingival tissue.

Periodontal disease begins as an infiltrate subjacent to the epithelium of the gingival margin and rapidly extends throughout the marginal gingiva to affect the connective tissue underlying both the oral and the sulcular epithelium (Fig. 4-3, *A* and *B*). In addition, there are pathologic alterations of both the sulcular and the oral epithelium of the marginal gingiva. Initially, the marginal gingiva becomes swollen, edematous, and friable, and it encroaches on the crown of the tooth (see Figs. A-60 to A-62, p. 64). Periodontal pocket depth increases as a result of enlargement of the gingiva (pseudopocket; Fig. 4-3, *C*). Later, sulcular epithelium begins to lose integrity and becomes

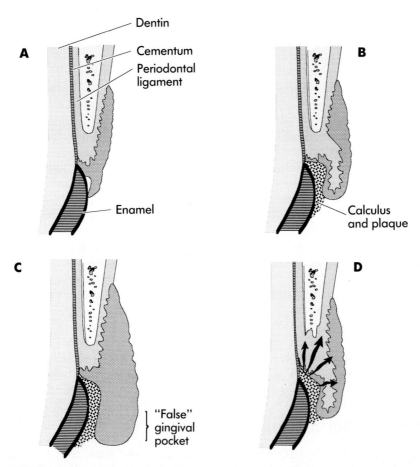

FIGURE 4-3
Pathogenesis of periodontal disease. **A,** Normal gingival-tooth relationship. **B,** Plaque accumulation and marginal gingivitis. **C,** Formation of a pseudopocket by gingival edema or hyperplasia. **D,** Pathways of invasion of sulcular bacteria.

more porous, allowing bacteria and their by-products to gain access to deeper periodontal structures, and the inflammatory lesion is found throughout the entire thickness of the marginal gingival tissue (Fig. 4-3, *D*). Spontaneous gingival bleeding or bleeding on exploration of the pocket with a periodontal probe may occur (see Fig. A-63, p. 64).

The predominant histologic features in early gingivitis are vasculitis, loss of perivascular collagen, and neutrophil migration. There is a significant correlation between extent of plaque and pocket depth, and between extent of plaque and hyperplastic tissues, with the additional factor of infection by periodontal pathogens.

The cellular and biochemical events that result initially in stimulation of an inflammatory response and that can lead to destructive change are now being elucidated. Data from one species, however, cannot reliably be applied to another species, particularly with regard to cats compared with dogs and humans. Events that are normally considered to be protective, such as the inflammatory response secondary to bacterial contamination or bacterial antigen stimulation of lymphocytes to produce immunoglobulins, may ultimately be harmful because of overstimulation. Thus neutrophils that die after bacterial engulfment may burst, littering the site with biochemical by-products that stimulate prostaglandin release and initiate tissue-destructive effects such as osteoclast stimulation.

The division between gingivitis and periodontitis is not absolute because methods of determining bone loss are relatively crude, and early signs of bone loss may be missed. Uncontrolled gingivitis leads to periodontitis, in which the bone and supporting connective tissues are gradually (and sometimes rapidly) destroyed. Periodontitis usually is considered to be permanent. Because of the bone loss, periodontitis can cause a significant increase in depth of the pocket where plaque can accumulate (see Fig. A-67, p. 66) and continue its destructive process unless gingival recession occurs at a rate similar to that of bone loss (see Fig. A-66, p. 66). Typically in dogs, uncontrolled periodontitis leads eventually to tooth loss (see Figs. A-75 and A-76, p. 69) although often without clinically obvious pain or other disabling side effects. Severe periodontal disease in cats often is more painful.

Periodontal disease progresses from the marginal gingiva to the gingival sulcus, with subsequent reduction and loss of the epithelial attachment. Without the epithelial attachment the underlying alveolar bone and periodontal ligament are exposed and subsequently destroyed (Fig. 4-4). The epithelial attachment is not in fact destroyed; the sequence is infiltration of inflammatory cells loaded with bacteria into the sub-

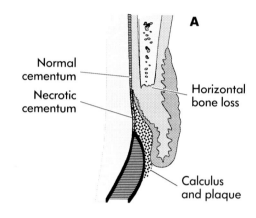

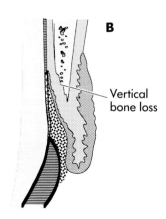

FIGURE 4-4

Types of periodontal pocket. **A,** Suprabony pocket: the entire thickness of crestal bone is lost. **B,** Infrabony pocket: loss of bone on the alveolar cortex only, leaving part of the outer cortical plate intact.

epithelial spaces, loss of integrity of the subepithelial connective tissue attachment, and downward growth of the epithelial attachment on the cemental surface. With periodontitis in dogs, the acutely inflamed, highly vascular, collagen-poor granulation tissue of gingivitis becomes more chronic, featuring dense inflammatory infiltrates that consist predominantly of plasma cells and lymphocytes. This change in predominant type of inflammatory cell is accompanied by a change in predominant lymphocyte type from T cell to B cell. Both cellular and humoral responses are present in periodontitis. The soft tissues behave in one of two ways. Either the hyperplastic granulation tissue remains located near the CEJ (see Figs. A-65 and A-67, pp. 65 and 66) and a deep periodontal pocket forms comparable to that usually seen around human teeth or the soft tissue retreats along the root surface as the bone resorbs (gingival recession; see Fig. A-66, p. 66). In the latter case the disease may progress to the point of tooth exfoliation without significant pocket formation.

Whether associated with gingival hyperplasia or gingival recession, the loss of supporting bone results in loosening and eventual loss of the tooth. The pattern of tissue loss varies, although there are general patterns in dogs of particular body weight and jaw conformation (see Figs. A-75 and A-76, p. 68 and 69). Beagles have been studied most extensively. In this breed, bone loss begins at the furcation of the upper fourth premolar and the interdental space between the upper fourth premolar and first molar teeth, then progresses to the third and second premolars and around the first premolars. Bone resorption appears sooner and more severely in the furcation regions than interproximally but is most severe buccally. The incisors and first and second premolars are the teeth most frequently lost from periodontitis, usually exhibiting bilateral symmetry. The patterns of periodontal disease in dogs are described in more detail later in the chapter.

Local factors, such as impaction of hair into pockets (see Fig. A-78, p. 69) as a result of excessive grooming associated with skin disease, crowding of teeth (see Figs. A-68, p. 67; and A-79, p. 69), and proximity to the frenulums of the lips (see Figs. A-68, p. 67; and A-80, p. 70) have an effect that is described further on pp. 108-110.

▶ CLINICAL FEATURES
Examination of Periodontal Tissues
Inspection

The examiner assesses for the normal number of teeth, noting that first and second premolar teeth in dogs and incisors and premolar teeth in cats may be completely covered by hyperplastic or inflamed gingiva.

The extent of plaque and calculus on the crowns or exposed roots of the teeth is evaluated. In many cats and dogs, there is so much accumulated calculus that the normality of the shape and size of some teeth cannot be determined. The contour of the MGJ is followed to ascertain if adequate gingiva surrounds each tooth. Is the gingiva inflamed, granulomatous, or ulcerated? Is there bleeding or purulent debris visible at the gingival sulcus? The adjacent buccal, lingual, and palatal mucosa are examined for areas of inflammation or ulceration. The examiner notes if the periodontal tissues are symmetric; one of the hallmarks of inflammatory periodontal disease is that the extent of disease often varies considerably from rostral to caudal, but it generally is symmetric. If a tooth has been lost as a result of periodontal disease, the contralateral tooth may be present but is likely to be severely diseased.

Palpation

The examiner presses each of the teeth to determine mobility. The incisor teeth may move in response to firm pressure, particularly in cats or small dogs. The other teeth normally cannot be moved, even with very firm pressure. A tooth that moves freely in response to light pressure or that can be depressed into the alveolus is unlikely to be salvageable.

The gingiva is palpated. This may induce pain in an awake animal with periodontal inflammation, and the periodontal tissues may feel less firm and resilient than normal. When deep pockets are present, pressing the gingiva often causes purulent or bloody fluid to exude from the periodontal pocket.

Probing

The depth and contour of the gingival sulcus and periodontal pockets are determined with a blunt-ended periodontal probe, marked to permit easy identification of depth in millimeters (see Fig. A-65, p. 65). Various types of probes are available (see Fig. 11-17).

The extent of attachment loss from periodontal disease is determined by measuring the distance between the CEJ of the tooth and the apical extent of the pocket (the epithelial attachment, beyond which the periodontal probe will not penetrate). The periodontal pocket depth is determined by measuring the distance from the height of the marginal gingiva (gingival crest) to the epithelial attachment.

The periodontal probe is inserted gently, parallel to the long axis of the tooth root, until it can be advanced no further. Then it is moved gently horizontally, walking along the floor of the sulcus to determine the area of deepest loss of attachment (Fig. 4-5). Bleeding after gentle probing indicates gingival inflammation (see Fig. A-63, p. 64). For multirooted teeth the normally bone-filled space between the roots (the furcation) is probed.

Pocket depth varies around the circumference of the tooth in many instances, and roots of multirooted teeth may be affected to very different extents. The area of deepest pocket measurement generally is considered to be the most severely affected area; however, the recession of gingival tissue and bone, the presence of an infrabony pocket, and furcation involvement complicate the circumstances.

An infrabony (intrabony) pocket consists of loss of attachment without bone resorption in the area of the pocket; that is, the pocket extends apically beyond the existing bone level (Fig. 4-4, *B*). The probe meets the firm resistance of the bone when angled away from the tooth. Infrabony pockets are described by depth and by the extent of the bony circumference involved. The surrounding alveolar bone is thought of as forming four "walls" (buccal, mesial, lingual/palatal, and distal). When bone is present around the entire circumference of the lesion, a "four-wall" (or "cup") lesion is present. When bone is missing on one face, a three-wall defect is present. Two- and one-wall pockets have two and three faces of the tooth root without bony support, respectively. In general, the prognosis for reattachment after scaling, root planing, and pocket curettage increases with the number of walls still present. Because of the shallow dental ledge

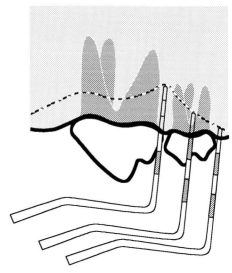

FIGURE 4-5
A blunt-tipped periodontal probe is "walked" around the sulcus, or pocket, to determine depth.

for maxillary teeth in dogs and cats, the presence or absence of the palatal wall can be difficult to determine; the root may be exposed to the nasal cavity or maxillary sinus recess if the palatal wall is absent, which may not be clinically obvious even if the pocket is probed (see Fig. A-77, p. 69). This condition can progress to formation of an oronasal fistula (see Fig. A-116, p. 80).

Pocket depth is not necessarily correlated with the severity of attachment loss. Protuberant hyperplastic gingival tissue may contribute to a deep pocket (or pseudopocket if there is no true attachment loss) (see Figs. A-81 and A-82, p. 70). Shallow is not necessarily good; gingival recession may keep pace with attachment loss, resulting in the absence of a "pocket" but also minimal remaining attachment (see Figs. A-66, p. 66; and A-70, p. 67).

Furcation involvement refers to the situation in which the bone between the roots in multirooted teeth (where the roots bifurcate or trifurcate) is resorbed as a result of periodontal disease. The furcation involvement may be incomplete (a periodontal probe can enter the furcation but not pass completely through) or com-

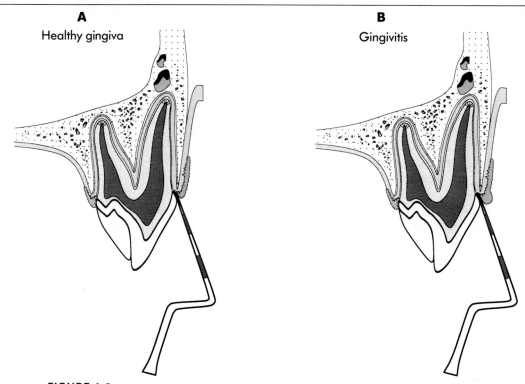

FIGURE 4-6

Clinical stages of periodontal disease. **A,** Healthy gingiva. **B,** Gingivitis. **C,** Early periodontitis. **D,** Moderate periodontitis. **E,** Advanced periodontitis.

plete (see Figs. A-68 and A-71, p. 67). Furcation involvement can be present in association with deep pockets or with little or no pocketing if accompanied by gingival recession. Furcation involvements are clinically significant because they permit food debris and plaque to accumulate in areas that are difficult to cleanse.

Stages of Periodontal Disease

Periodontal disease is an ongoing process with active and inactive phases. The following stages are presented sequentially.

1. *Health* (see Figs. 4-6, *A,* and A-1, *A* and *B*, p. 49). Gingival tissues are coral pink or pigmented in color, with good topography. The gingival tissue is firm and resilient, with defined stippling and minimal sulcular depth. There may be evidence of tissue loss as a result of previous disease.

2. *Gingivitis* (see Figs. 4-6, *B*, A-60, A-61, and A-63, p. 64). Gingival inflammation, erythema, gingival bleeding on probing in more advanced cases, and loss of stippling occur. No deterioration of bone supporting the tooth structure is seen.

3. *Early periodontitis* (see Figs. 4-6, *C*, and A-64, p. 64). Gingival topography is normal or may show hyperplasia, inflammation of periodontal ligament, and minor loss of attachment with minimal pocket development, crestal bone loss, or lack of tooth mobility (except for incisor teeth in small-breed dogs).

4. *Moderate periodontitis* (see Figs. 4-6, *D*, and A-65, p. 65). There may be moderate loss of attachment, with moderate to deep-pocket formation. Hyperplasia may mask pocket depth or gingival recession may reduce pocket depth; 30% to 50% loss of bone support may occur,

C
Early
periodontitis

D
Moderate
periodontitis

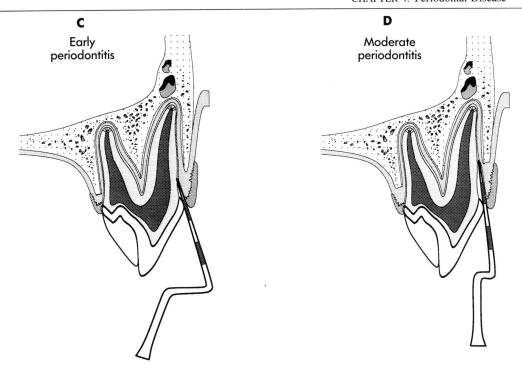

FIGURE 4-6, cont'd
For legend see opposite page.

gingival topography no longer is normal, and only slight tooth mobility is seen (moderate tooth mobility for incisors).

5. *Advanced periodontitis* (see Figs. 4-6, *E*, and A-67 to A-74, pp. 66-68). Advanced breakdown of supporting periodontal tissues, severe pocket depth or significant gingival recession, severe loss of attachment, more than 50% loss of bone support, and advanced tooth mobility (less so for multirooted teeth) occur.

6. *Exfoliation of teeth* (see Figs. 4-6, *F*, A-75, and A-76, pp. 68 and 69). After healing of the empty alveolus, inflammation recedes, the dental ledge may atrophy, and a smooth epithelium-covered jaw surface is present. The result of healing may be an oronasal fistula (see Fig. A-116, p. 80).

E
Advanced
periodontitis

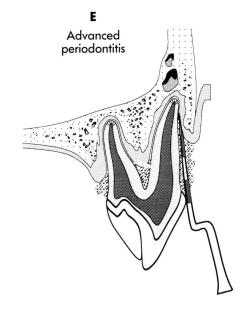

Hyperplastic Gingivitis

Gingival hyperplasia, which often occurs in association with plaque-induced periodontal disease, results in pseudopockets (see Figs. 4-3, A-81, and A-82, p. 70).

An apparently separate clinical condition occurs in some dogs, with gradual development of firm, raised gingival margins, often not associated with grossly obvious gingival inflammation and calculus deposition. This is particularly common in boxer dogs, in whom an inherited cause has been hypothesized, but also is recognized as a specific entity in other—usually large- and giant-breed dogs,—typically collies, standard poodles, retrievers of various sorts, and mastiffs. The gingival margin may be symmetrically enlarged, particularly in the incisor tooth area, or may reveal protuberant masses that can be mistaken for neoplasms. Chronic administration of drugs (diphenylhydantoin, nitrendipine, nifedipine, and cyclosporine) causes gingival hyperplasia in cats, dogs, and humans; plaque accumulation is necessary for this effect to occur.

▶ RADIOGRAPHIC FEATURES OF PERIODONTAL DISEASE

Radiographic evaluation of periodontal disease requires excellent radiographic technique because many of the signs are subtle. Interpretation depends on changes in the normally readily visible sequence of radiodensity and radiolucency in the dental and bony tissues. The earliest change is a slight loss of sharpness and density of the crestal bone (Fig. 4-7, *B*). This is followed by progressive loss of mineralization of the lamina dura from the crestal bone apically (Fig. 4-7, *C*). In multirooted teeth, this also is seen as a progressively lengthening furcation radiolucency (Fig. 4-7, *D*).

Radiographs are particularly useful for determining whether periodontal bone loss has reached the apex

FIGURE 4-7
For legend see opposite page.

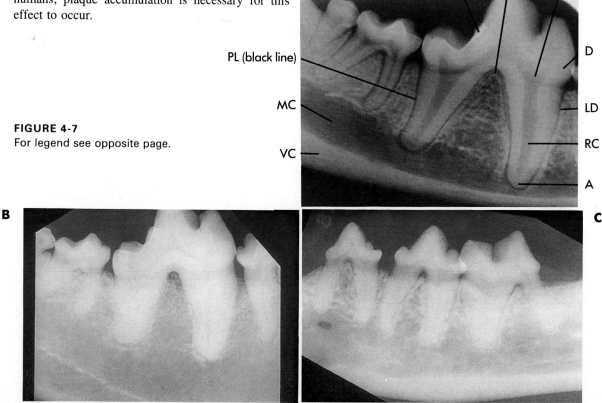

D

FIGURE 4-7

Radiographic features of periodontal disease. **A,** Radiographically healthy periodontium. (For identification of specific structures see Fig. 2-12.) **B,** Early periodontitis—loss of crestal bone density. **C,** Moderate periodontitis—loss of crestal bone height and deeper loss of lamina dura density, with early furcation involvement. **D,** Moderate periodontitis—loss of furcation bone of PM2. **E,** Severe periodontitis (distal root) extending to the apex of the root of the first molar. Also loss of bone around the entire mesial root of the second molar, with radiolucencies present in both roots. **F,** Severe periodontitis. The third premolar tooth is missing. There is a small area of radiodense lamina dura on the mesial side of the mesial root of the fourth premolar. Irregular root surface densities (calculus) on the distal root of the fourth premolar and root resorption or caries on the distal surface of the mesial root of the same tooth. A pathologic fracture extends through the ventral mandibular cortex directly beneath the distal root of the fourth premolar. **G,** Tooth with cavitation. **H,** Severe vertical bone loss close to the apex of the distal root of the first molar tooth. Also oblique bone loss of the distal root of the fourth premolar tooth; this root has an oblique fracture midway along its length and apparent resorption coronally.

E

F

G

H

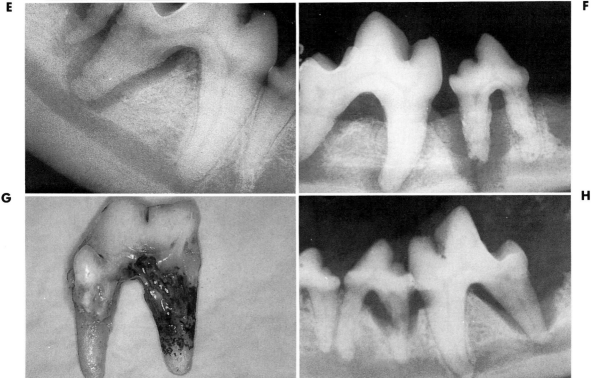

of the root and whether root caries or external odontoclastic resorption (neck lesions) exists (Fig. 4-7, *E* to *H*), inasmuch as these lesions will alter the prognosis or treatment plan, or both, for that tooth. Radiographs also are a timely reminder that there may be little healthy tissue left holding the jaw intact (Fig. 4-7, *F*)!

Staged radiographic signs of periodontitis have correlated with clinical measures of plaque, calculus, mobility, pocket depth, and furcation exposure in dogs and cats, but no such correlation could be shown with gingivitis without periodontitis.

Periodontal bone loss usually is termed *horizontal* or *vertical:* horizontal bone loss describes an even loss of bone around several adjacent roots, so that a horizontal line connecting the radiographic limit of bone can be drawn parallel to the long axis of the jaw (Fig. 4-7, *C* and *D*). This is the most common pattern found, particularly around teeth in which the roots are 5 mm or less apart, because the osteoclastic stimulation resulting from periodontal pocket disease affects approximately 2.5 mm of the tissue surrounding the pocket itself. In larger dogs, or for canine teeth in cats, which have greater interdental distance, vertical bone loss is more common. In this condition the bone loss occurs parallel to the long axis of the root, and adjacent roots may have a normal attachment (Fig. 4-7, *E*, *G*, and *H*). In many cases the radiographic bone loss pattern is not strictly horizontal or vertical but is oblique (Fig. 4-7, *H*), reflecting the profile of the inflamed and infiltrated tissue adjacent to the pocket.

▶ PREVALENCE AND PATTERNS OF PERIODONTAL DISEASE

Dogs

Because the teeth vary greatly in size and function, as well as degree of regular dietary abrasion of the crown surface and gingival margin area, there is wide variation in the extent of disease affecting particular animals, groups of animals, and areas of the mouth.

Incisor teeth, having relatively small single roots compared with the adjacent canine teeth, tend to be lost earlier than other teeth, particularly in small-breed dogs that have relatively less bone supporting each tooth (see Fig. A-76, p. 69). The leverage effect on

a single root magnifies the mobility resulting from bone loss and further weakens periodontal fibers.

Canine teeth have massive roots, and thus even though the root is single, the area of periodontal attachment is so large that mobility does not become clinically apparent until massive tissue destruction has occurred. The resultant pockets may be pus-filled and may contribute to formation of periodontal abscesses or gingival clefts (see Fig. A-73, p. 68), often causing oronasal fistulae in small-breed dogs (see Figs. A-77, p. 69; and A-116, p. 80).

Premolar teeth develop periodontal lesions unevenly. The accumulation of plaque and calculus worsens in a caudal direction. However, because of differences in the height of the gingiva (free gingival margin and MGJ), the rostral (mesial) teeth may be more severely affected. This is particularly true of the second premolar tooth, in which the frenulum attaching the upper lip to the maxilla is predisposed to pull away the attached gingiva from the bone overlying this tooth (see Fig. A-80, p. 70).

The upper fourth premolar (carnassial) tooth is the tooth most severely affected with plaque and calculus accumulation, most of which attaches to the buccal (lateral) aspect of the crown (see Figs. A-67, A-69, and A-70, p. 67). This area is not subjected to routine dietary abrasion because the lower carnassial teeth occlude lingual to the upper carnassial teeth. Pocket formation often is much more severe on the buccal or distal aspects (see Figs. A-69 and 72, pp. 67 and 68), although the tooth remains in the mouth because the buccal roots are large and the palatal root often is much less affected.

Several studies of the prevalence of periodontal disease in dogs have been reported. They differ in criteria used to define the extent of disease, population included (such as large, small, client-owned, laboratory housed), extent to which diet is considered, country of origin, and other factors. Thus considerable differences are reported in the results, but some general conclusions can be drawn.

In a British survey of oral-dental diseases in 600 dogs of unstated source, periodontal disease accounted for 73% of cases. On detailed examination of 63 dogs anesthetized for nonoral reasons at a North American veterinary hospital, virtually all had at least incipient gingival inflammation, and mobility was common in incisor teeth; 53% of the dogs had one or more pockets deeper than 3 mm, and 39% showed gingival hyperplasia (most commonly in the premolar area). In a similar study of 62 mongrel dogs anesthetized at a veterinary hospital in Denmark (the report does not mention whether the dogs were seen because of oral disease), only 2 of the 62 dogs had clinically healthy

gingiva—both were less than 6 months old. Plaque was found in 60 of 62 dogs and calculus in 50. Plaque index, calculus index, and gingival index increase with increasing age (Fig. 4-8). Both plaque and calculus are significantly but independently correlated with gingival index. No differences between sexes could be shown.

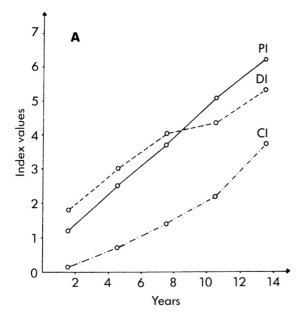

FIGURE 4-8

A, Graph indicating increasing calculus deposition *(CI),* plaque deposition *(DI,* debris index) and periodontal inflammation *(PI)* with age in the teeth of 62 dogs. **B,** Graph indicating increasing frequency and severity of periodontitis with age in dogs and increased extent of disease in upper teeth *(top data set)* compared with lower teeth *(bottom data set).* Data from teeth from canine *(C)* to third molar *(M3)* are shown for each age group. *Open portion of bar,* mild to moderate periodontitis; *cross-hatched portion of bar,* severe periodontitis; *black portion of bar,* tooth lost. *(A from Gad T:* J Periodont Res *3:268, 1968.* **B** *from Hamp SE et al:* Vet Radiol *25:86, 1984.)*

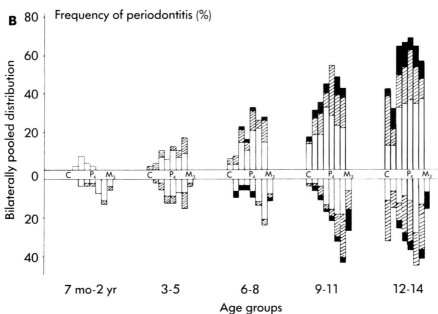

In another study from Scandinavia 162 randomly selected dogs were examined by necropsy; 50 breeds, classified as small, medium, or large, were represented. The overall frequency of calculus deposits was 83%; 52% had one or more teeth missing, and 64% had periodontitis. Plaque and gingival inflammation were not recorded, but each head was sectioned and radiographed in lateral position. As with the previous study, periodontitis increased significantly with age (Fig. 4-8, *B*). Calculus was first seen on the upper molar, carnassial, and canine teeth. Periodontitis was more evident in the upper teeth than in the lower teeth and was more severe around carnassial and molar teeth than around canine and noncarnassial premolar teeth (periodontitis in incisor teeth was not recorded). Periodontitis and lost teeth were more common in small dogs than in large dogs (Table 4-6). Poodles were particularly severely affected, although the prevalence in dachshunds and boxers—breeds of dissimilar weight but similar jaw length—was comparable. Individual variation among dogs of the same breed was very wide.

A study conducted in Germany examined 281 dogs of which 218 (77.5%) had periodontitis, which was more common in older dogs, in smaller dogs, and in the upper jaw.

A study from Switzerland of 200 dogs is the exception to this general pattern of high prevalence of some measurable periodontal disease; 125 of the 200 dogs had no obvious gingival disease. The prevalence and severity increased with age.

In the largest survey reported to date, 2649 ran-

TABLE 4-6	Dogs of breeds represented by 10 dogs or more and all other dogs classified as small, medium, or large; mean age, number of teeth with slight or advanced periodontitis, and number of teeth lost due to periodontitis

Group/breed	No. of dogs	Mean age (yr)	Slight periodontitis		Advanced periodontitis		Lost teeth	
			No.	x̄*	No.	x̄	No.	x̄
Small								
Poodle	26	8.8	123	4.6	111	4.3	45	1.7
Dachshund	16	8.2	70	4.4	41	2.6	8	0.5
Others	35	7.2	108	3.1	80	2.3	32†	0.9
Total	77	8.0	301	3.9	232	3.0	85	1.1
Medium								
Others	18	4.9	26	1.4	9	0.5	1	0.1
Large								
German shepherd	17	5.9	16	1.0	8	0.5	1	0.1
Boxer	10	8.9	53	5.3	24	2.4	5	0.5
Others	28	7.1	87	3.1	19	0.7	11	0.4
Total	55	7.1	160	2.9	51	0.9	17	0.3
Varia								
Mongrels	12	6.5	30	2.5	9	0.8	0	0.0

From Hamp SE et al: *Vet Radiol* 25:86, 1984.
*x̄, Mean number of affected or lost teeth per dog.
†Includes 22 premolars of two chihuahuas.

domly selected dogs were examined by veterinarians in Japan, who recorded the presence of calculus, missing teeth, and halitosis. Calculus was classified as absent, present, or significant and was found to be increasingly frequent with increasing age and with increased prevalence in small-breed dogs. This study also examined the relationship between calculus and type of food fed; these findings are described earlier in Diet and Periodontal Disease.

Several studies examined beagle dogs kept under laboratory conditions, including the only detailed longitudinal studies in dogs reported to date. In 12 dogs (6 male, 6 female) that were fed dry dog food over a period of several years, the sequence of development of calculus was followed. By 9 months of age, deposition started on the buccal surface of the upper fourth premolar tooth, the mesial surface of the upper first molar tooth, and the distobuccal surfaces of the second and third premolar teeth. Gingival inflammation was limited to the free gingival margin and was most noticeable in the areas where calculus had deposited. By 15 months of age, calculus was moderately thick on the upper carnassial and first molar tooth, particularly buccodistally (carnassial) and buccomesially (first molar) where the two teeth are in contact. Calculus was now evident buccally on the upper canine tooth and buccally on the lower third and fourth premolar and first molar teeth. There was no calculus at this stage lingually, although slight plaque build-up and mild gingival inflammation occurred. Gingival inflammation was most evident buccally over the upper carnassial and first molar teeth. By 20 months, calculus covering the upper carnassial and first molar tooth was extensive and was accompanied by severe gingival inflammation and pocket formation. Calculus, accompanied by gingival inflammation, was clearly evident on buccal surfaces of other teeth. Lingual calculus had not yet formed although several premolar teeth showed linguogingival inflammation. Although the general pattern was clear, there was considerable variation among dogs in the rate of deposition of calculus and extent of gingival inflammation. At about 20 months of age the teeth were scaled on one side, with rapid recovery to clinical gingival health on that side. By 6 weeks after scaling, plaque and calculus accumulation patterns were sim-

ilar to those seen in the dogs at 9 months. At about 6 months after scaling, no differences could be seen between the treated and untreated sides. No differences between male and female dogs were discernible. The same study briefly describes observations on calculus formation in a larger group of 125 dogs.

A similar rate of development was seen in 39 beagles in another study, although gingival inflammation scores were higher in the mandible than in the maxilla. Calculus scores, as well as pocket depth and recession, were greater for the maxillary teeth. Again, no differences between sexes were seen. As in the previous study the site of most extensive calculus deposition was on the upper carnassial and the first molar teeth.

A study of 40 beagles aged 1 to 8 years included clinical and histologic examinations; gingivitis was observed in younger animals, periodontitis in older dogs.

The teeth of another group of 20 beagles were scaled at 10 months of age and allowed to accumulate plaque and calculus in a soft food diet. Mean plaque index rose rapidly by 1 month and then stayed stable. The calculus index continued to increase for 2 years, then stayed stable. Gingival inflammation was evident within a few days of scaling and continued to increase; then the gingival index showed a plateau at about 12 months. Bleeding on probing and later spontaneous bleeding were common in buccal sites after 1 year. Loss of attachment rose rapidly up to 2 years, then increased more slowly and was more severe on upper teeth than on lower teeth. Plaque and calculus developed most severely in the premolar and molar teeth, starting at 1 month on the upper carnassial and first molar teeth and subgingivally by 6 months.

Cats

The general cause and effects of periodontal disease in cats are similar to those of dogs (see Figs. A-86 and A-87, p. 72). The teeth are smaller, and they are more difficult to scale and to keep plaque-free after scaling. A dry-food diet results in improved gingival health compared with a soft-food diet. Two specific abnormalities associated with periodontal disease in cats make the disease in this species more difficult and frustrating to treat. These abnormalities are described in Chapters 5 (oral inflammatory diseases) and

7 (external odontoclastic resorption). These conditions often result in a decision to treat by extraction rather than by scaling.

▶ SYSTEMIC DISEASE AND PERIODONTAL DISEASE

Anecdotal reports over many years have suggested that chronic periodontitis is a cause of chronic changes in the lungs, heart (myocarditis and valvular endocarditis), kidneys, and possibly liver, probably as a result of frequent bacteremia. Recently a statistically significant relationship has been demonstrated between the extent of periodontitis and the extent of microscopic changes in the kidneys, suggesting that periodontitis may be a common cause of chronic nephritis in dogs.

It generally is agreed that systemic conditions that depress metabolic activity will exacerbate periodontal disease by lessening the ability of the local tissues to defend themselves against the omnipresent bacterial population. In theory, this should be true of conditions and medications that suppress the immune system. However, drugs that specifically suppress the inflammatory response, such as nonsteroidal antiinflammatory agents, may have the opposite effect by blocking the prostaglandin cascade that results in release of tissue-destructive cytokines from bacteria and degenerating neutrophils. One form of immunopathy, neutrophil dysfunction, leads to rapidly destructive periodontal diseases. Other systemic diseases may have a deleterious effect for other reasons; for example, diabetes and autoimmune disease can lead to xerostomia.

The interrelationships of the immune system and the oral tissues are discussed further in Chapter 5.

Treatment

The overall purposes of treatment of periodontal disease are to restore physiologic anatomy and function and to obtain consistent plaque retardation on all unattached tooth surfaces, thus preventing further tissue inflammation, tissue loss, and eventual tooth loss. To achieve these objectives, a treatment plan appropriate for the individual animal must be developed. Teeth cleaning (scaling) is widely recognized as the principal means of treatment of periodontal disease, and the means to achieve this are available in most veterinary hospitals. It must be understood that teeth scaling is only a part—although a vital and universally required part—of treatment designed to permit retention of teeth.

▶ FACTORS IN PLANNING PERIODONTAL TREATMENT*

The Owner

It is helpful to know how responsive the owner will be to recommendations regarding long-term home care; complying for a week or two is of little value. Particularly for severe disease requiring involved procedures, long-term commitment is important. If the likelihood of compliance with home care instructions is not clear from an initial discussion, the owner should be advised to try brushing the animal's teeth for a week or two before proceeding with treatment, which facilitates a more realistic approach. If compliance with brushing or other plaque-control instructions is unlikely, extraction should be considered for severely compromised teeth.

The Animal

Even the most willing owner may be unable to comply with home-care instructions if the animal is vicious or uncontrollable. Other considerations include the anesthesia risk, medical condition, and expected life span of the animal. The clinician also should consider whether treatment of a disease that is rarely life-threatening is justified. Whether to admin-

---

*This section is adapted from Harvey CE: Treatment planning for periodontal disease in dogs, *JAAHA* 27:592, 1992.

ister an antibiotic during the treatment process is a further decision (see pp. 138-139).

The Veterinary Staff

Until the animal's mouth is examined thoroughly, the specific procedures required will not be known. Available equipment, expertise, and experience are factors. It is better to postpone or to refer the procedure than to leave it half done by scaling only coronally and skipping subgingival root planing and scaling. A second, related consideration is the time available; good quality periodontal work takes time!

The Mouth

Toy breed dogs have relatively little bone around and between teeth. They often have lips that are tight when their mouths are open, which makes it more difficult to obtain consistent and comfortable access to the premolar and molar teeth for brushing. This situation may shift the decision toward extraction of upper carnassial and molar teeth.

A second factor related to facial anatomy is the presence of the lip frenula. The clinically significant frenula in the dog attach to the maxilla or mandible just apical to the buccal surface of the MGJ over the upper second premolar teeth and lower first premolar teeth. As periodontal disease progresses and the attachment of gingiva to bone is lost, the effect of the pull of the weight of the lip by the frenulum is to cause a chronic distracting force, exacerbating loss of attachment of gingiva to bone (see Figs. A-68, p. 67; and A-80, p. 70). For these teeth, frenoplasty is indicated (see p. 135).

In addition to an examination of each tooth (see following discussion), the rest of the mouth should be inspected, particularly for asymmetric swellings or areas of abnormal coloration or texture. The cheeks and lateral margins of the tongue are examined for inflammation or ulceration. These ulcerations (see Figs. A-40 and A-41, p. 59) are painful, making home care less tolerable, and the ulcerations will recur unless plaque control is excellent (see Chapter 5).

The Teeth

There are 42 separate potential decisions to be made concerning a dog with a full set of teeth: each tooth must be considered as a separate entity. Infor-

mation to be gathered for each tooth includes mobility, structural normality, furcation involvement of multi-rooted teeth, and pocket depth. The area around each root should be examined, as well as the tooth's position in the arch—for example, rot owded, in functional alignment, or supernumary. ddition, the examiner evaluates whether opposing teeth are available for dietary abrasion, whether frenulum attachments affect a diseased tooth, and whether deep palatal pockets of maxillary teeth are present.

After induction of anesthesia

The clinician inspects the mouth to estimate the time required for a procedure. If extensive work is required, the teeth or segments of the mouth are separated into categories (such as most appropriate to treat, least necessary to treat) so that time and financial resources are used most effectively to treat the disease. Sometimes it is best to perform the necessary treatments as staged procedures (more than one anesthesia episode).

The extent of disease is recorded; several schemes have been described, and examples are given in Chapter 2. It is important to write down *something* so that there is information available for comparison later. Periodontal disease is a continuing problem; rarely will it be cured or completely prevented, only controlled to a greater or lesser extent.

Individual teeth are examined and treatment planned by use of a logical system for decision making (Fig. 4-9). Supragingival scaling may be needed to remove large calculus concretions, thus permitting accurate assessment of crown structure, pocket depth, furcation involvement and other factors. Radiographic studies of the teeth and jaws are obtained as necessary to supplement the clinical examination.

Fig. 4-9, *A* and *B* are algorithms designed to lead to a specific treatment decision, the object being retention of the tooth if practical. Included are realities of veterinary dental practice, such as the likelihood of the owner and animal complying with home care instructions. The algorithm might seem unnecessarily complicated at first glance; however, many of the decisions are made naturally and quickly.

The basic techniques for examination of the periodontium were described on p. 100. In Fig. 4-9, *B*, a pocket up to 4 mm is considered "shallow" whereas

A

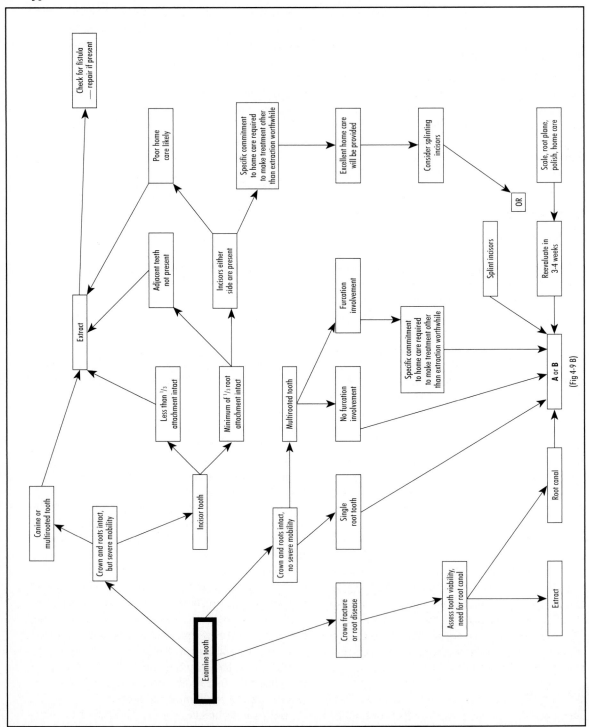

(Fig 4-9 B)

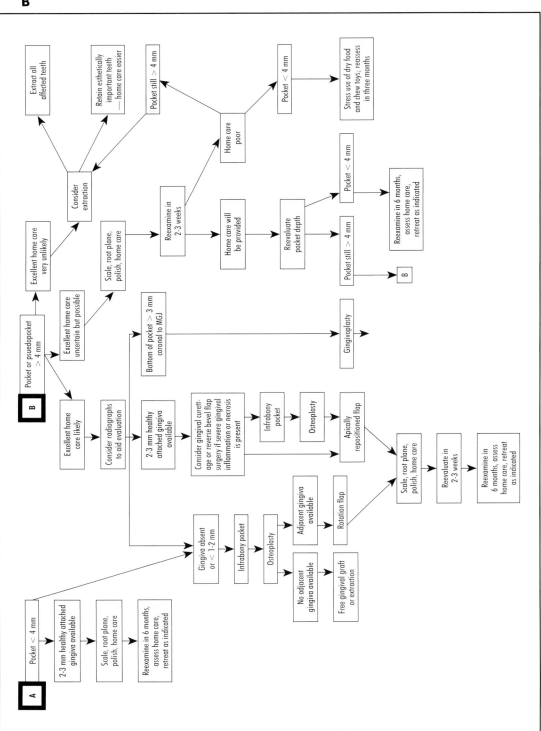

FIGURE 4-9

Algorithms for treatment planning for periodontal disease in dogs. **A,** Is the tooth treatable? **B,** Specific treatment for individual teeth. (**B** from Harvey CE: JAAHA 27:592, 1991.)

one greater than 4 mm is a "deep" pocket. This division is based on the inability of a toothbrush to effectively remove plaque in pockets more than about 4 mm in depth, as well as the increased likelihood of failure to remove calculus during scaling as pocket depth increases. However, a simple measurement of maximum pocket depth is insufficient; the conditions surrounding the pocket must be considered. In some instances, pocket depth will be expected to decrease after thorough scaling and root planing. Consider two pockets whose depth is 5 mm or greater. One has conditions that will prevent bony or soft tissue healing, for example, a one- or two-wall pocket in which the level of attachment is apical to the MGJ or a pseudo-pocket resulting from 4 mm of gingival hyperplasia, in which case pocket-reduction surgery is indicated. The second pocket has conditions that are likely to result in some reattachment during healing (for example, a three- to four-wall bony pocket that does not extend apical to the MGJ), in which case the pocket depth is likely to decrease to 2 to 3 mm over the next 2 weeks, making pocket-reduction surgery unnecessary. With experience, the likelihood of reattachment after scaling and root planing can be estimated at the time of initial inspection. The best way to obtain such experience is to "stage" several cases, treating with a thorough prophylaxis during the first anesthesia episode, with reexamination 2 to 3 weeks later to decide whether pocket-reduction surgery is necessary.

Specific circumstances may alter the treatment decision, for example, the presence of *buccal* or *lingual ulceration* (contact ulcers), or severe gingivostomatitis (in cats), conditions described in Chapter 5.

Major malocclusion is another factor. When occluding teeth have been extracted or are missing, or segments of the jaws have been resected, dietary abrasion as a means of controlling plaque accumulation is less effective. Either a greater commitment to home care must be made for involved periodontal procedures to be of long-term value or the affected teeth should be extracted if periodontal disease is severe.

▶ THE PRAGMATIC APPROACH TO PERIODONTAL THERAPY

Under most circumstances, human periodontal therapy starts with scaling, root planing, and polishing, followed by a 2- to 3-week interval to permit healing and reattachment to occur. This often significantly reduces pocket depth and the acute inflammatory response in tissues that may be surgically manipulated subsequently. Thus the necessity for involved procedures such as flap surgery or bone augmentation, for example, may be avoided. Because human patients are not given general anesthesia for periodontal procedures, there is little or no risk to staging periodontal procedures and considerable advantage. Under most circumstances, veterinarians will continue to perform most periodontal treatments as single procedures, much as they routinely perform root canal procedures in dogs in a single treatment session, compared with three to four visits for human endodontic treatment. In an old or systemically sick dog, compared with a healthy, younger dog, the specific treatment decision is shifted more readily to extraction, which reduces the need for subsequent anesthesia. In an animal that is medically severely compromised—one for whom anesthesia is a great risk—long-term or intermittent antibiotic therapy (see p. 139) may be the only practical treatment for severe periodontal disease.

▶ CONSERVATIVE TREATMENT— PROPHYLAXIS
Teeth Scaling
Supragingival scaling

To be performed adequately, teeth scaling requires general anesthesia because of the discomfort associated with subgingival manipulation. Prophylaxis begins with the removal of supragingival calculus with hand or mechanical instrumentation. This equipment, as well as basic principles for the use and care of this equipment, is described in Chapter 11.

Gross calculus deposits are easily removed with use of a pair of dental extraction forceps or old rongeurs. Being careful to avoid damaging the gingivae, the clinician closes the forceps across the calculus, which cracks off from the surface of the tooth (Fig. 4-10).

A sickle-shaped supragingival scaler or a periodontal hoe is used to pull the remaining visible calculus off the crowns of the teeth, always pulling away from the gingivae (Fig. 4-11).

A B

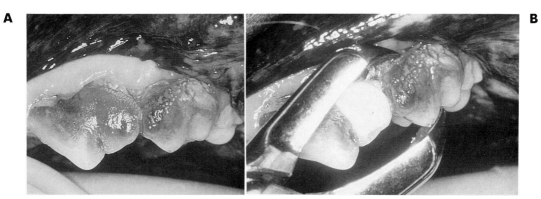

FIGURE 4-10
Teeth scaling. Cracking off gross chunks of calculus with dental extraction forceps. Before (**A**) and after (**B**) closing the forceps across the calculus mass.

The ultrasonic or sonic scaler is used to remove the residual plaque, calculus, and debris. A plentiful water flow is essential to cool the oscillating tip and to flush away the debris. When the frequency of oscillation and the water flow are correctly adjusted, an aerosol of water flows from around the oscillating tip (Fig. 4-12). Gentle stroking of the tooth with the side of the sickle-shaped scaling tip is best (Fig. 4-13). The tip must not be pressed firmly against the tooth surface or kept in contact with the same area for more than a few seconds, and the water spray must be functioning correctly. If these precautions are not taken, the tooth surface may be severely gouged and the pulp tissue may be injured by heat and subsequently undergo necrosis. Damage also results from using the point of the scaler instead of the side or holding it in one place; it should be moved gently and continuously over the tooth surface, always moving away from the gingivae. No more than 15 seconds of continuous scaling should be used for any one tooth. If the tooth is not clean in that time, the operator can return to it after scaling another tooth.

The units that generate ultrasonic frequencies cause contamination of the immediate environment with bacteria-laden water droplets (Fig. 4-13, *A*). Protective eyeglasses and face masks should be worn by all personnel in the immediate vicinity during use of this equipment, and sterile surgical procedures should not be scheduled in the same work area immediately afterward.

Ultrasonic teeth-cleaning devices and subsonic air-scaler handpieces that attach to an air-driven dental unit are designed to remove supragingival plaque and calculus. Once inserted into the gingival crevice or a pocket, the cooling water can no longer reach the oscillating tip, which results in thermal damage to both hard and soft tissues. Quick gentle dips into the pocket are permissible and may aid the removal of subgingival debris; however, hand instruments are required for most subgingival work. If the gingiva is gently held away from the tooth to allow the cooling water to reach the tip and to flush out debris, mechanical scalers may be used subgingivally.

Calculus and plaque also may be removed with a rotosonic bur (Roto-Pro) used in a high-speed dental handpiece (see Fig. 11-14). Roto-Pro burs are used supragingivally and, with care and gentleness, subgingivally. This is a controversial method of calculus and plaque removal because it entails the use of high-speed mechanical instrumentation that can easily damage crown and root surfaces unless care is taken. Veterinarians are urged to practice with this instrument before treating their first patients!

It is not possible to perform teeth scaling adequately by using only power equipment in animals with established periodontitis. Subgingival plaque and calculus (that is, below the free margin of the gingiva) is removed with hand instrumentation (subgingival curettage). The curet removes the soft and hard substrate as well as the diseased sulcal lining. Subgingival

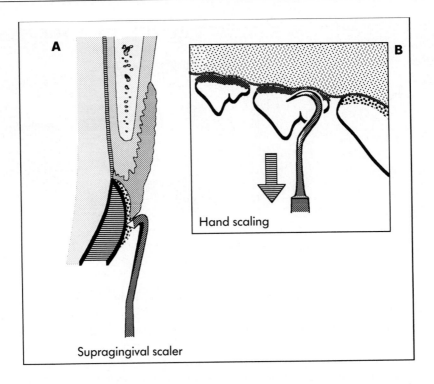

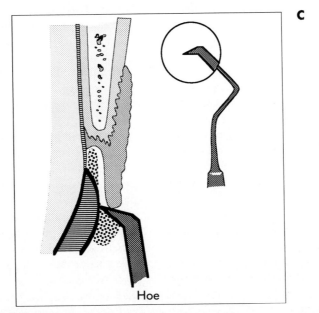

FIGURE 4-11
Supragingival calculus is removed with a scaler or hoe. **A,** Tooth in section showing the scaler at the start of the working stroke. **B,** The scaler is pulled coronally *(arrow).* **C,** The working edge of the hoe is engaged against the calculus at the gingival crest.

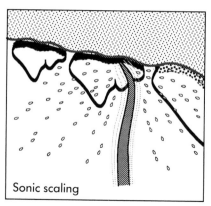

FIGURE 4-12
An ultrasonic tip oscillates and cavitates the calculus from the surface of the tooth, producing an aerosol of water droplets.

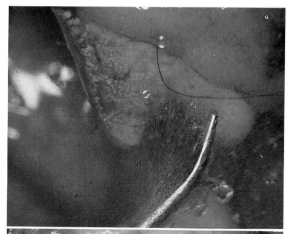

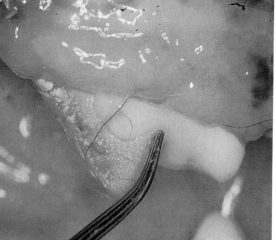

FIGURE 4-13
The tip of the ultrasonic scaler is moved gently over the surface of the tooth (**A**), causing plates of calculus to be loosened and flushed from the tooth (**B**).

scaling or curettage (closed curettage) is the primary form of periodontal surgery. Ultrasonic units produce clean white crowns rapidly and easily and, if used with considerable care, can start the subgingival cleaning process effectively, but hand scaling also is required in an animal with established periodontitis.

Thus some hand instruments are essential. The basic set consists of a periodontal scaler, curet, hoe, and chisel. Hand periodontal instruments are held in a modified pen grasp (see Fig. 11-21) for optimum control and support. The scaler, hoe, and chisel (see Fig. 4-25), which are used to remove supragingival calculus concretions, are not essential if ultrasonic equipment is available. The scaler and hoe are used with a pull stroke; they are inserted below the calculus mass then pulled forcefully toward the tip of the crown (coronally). The chisel is used with a push stroke toward the tip of the root (apically). Because an apical direction is required, the chisel can cause a great deal of soft tissue and bone damage if not used under close control.

Subgingival scaling

The most important hand instrument is the curet, which has a sharp working edge on the curved blade and a rounded tip (see Figs. 4-14 and 11-18). Many shapes and sizes are available; recommended instruments are listed in Chapter 11. The curet is inserted gently into the pocket with its curved side against the gingiva and its sharp edges faced toward the root, at an oblique angle, with the toe (tip) of the curet pointing apically. Resistance is felt when the rounded tip reaches the bottom of the pocket. The curet handle is then tilted away from the tooth, engaging one sharp edge against the debris and cementum on the root surface and the other sharp edge against the crevicular

A 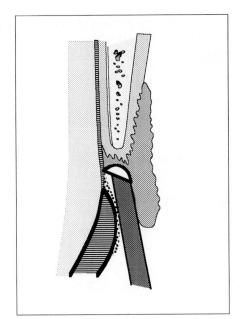 B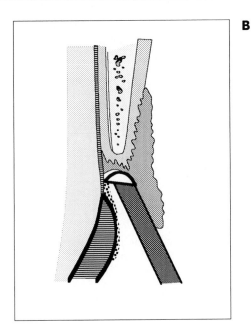

FIGURE 4-14
Subgingival curettage. **A,** The curet is inserted gently to the bottom of the pocket. **B,** The blade is rotated to engage the working edge against the surface of the tooth before starting the working withdrawal stroke.

epithelium as it is pulled out (Fig. 4-14). The face of the blade should be at an angle of 45 to 90 degrees to the cemental surface during the active coronal stroke. One such stroke with a curet will clean about 20% of the circumference of the root; thus several strokes are necessary to clean the entire circumference.

For teeth with deep (more than 4 mm) pockets, overlapping vertical strokes are used. For shallower pockets and for use in the furcation area of multirooted teeth, oblique or horizontal strokes are used. The key is to damage the tissue at the attachment as little as possible while ensuring that all subgingival calculus is removed. To determine if a root is thoroughly clean, the operator gently runs a curet or dental explorer over the surface. The instrument will skip over areas of remaining calculus, which must be removed by additional scaling with a curet. If the surfaces cannot be properly cleaned by means of closed curettage (for example, if pocket depth exceeds 4 to 6 mm), a flap is raised and open curettage performed (see p. 123).

Moderately deep pockets can be scaled with curets with longer than normal shanks (such as the "After Five" series; see Chapter 11). When a flap is raised, mechanical scalers may be used for root planing, inasmuch as the cooling water is able to reach the tip of the instrument and the tip can be kept in constant view.

For scaling the furcation area or other areas that are difficult to reach, a periodontal file or rasp (Sugarman file) is used (see Fig. 11-20).

Root planing

After subgingival scaling, the root is planed. The technique is the same as for scaling. The purpose of root planing is to remove irregularities and a thin layer of superficial cementum—loaded with bacterial toxins—that will inhibit healing if left in place. Root planing produces a smooth root surface that is less likely to accumulate additional debris. Numerous overlapping strokes are made, each time pulling the curet coronally out of the pocket, its cutting edge firmly engaged in the cementum of the root.

Gingival curettage

While one edge of a periodontal curet is engaged in a working stroke against the root surface, the other edge generally engages the soft tissues of the pocket lining (or bony surface of an infrabony pocket). Although often not thought of as a deliberate procedure, this gingival curettage has the beneficial effect of removing diseased soft tissue. Where there is extensive purulent debris and bleeding from a pocket before examination, firm gingival curettage is particularly useful. A finger tip is placed on the gingival tissue to permit the instrument to engage the soft tissue side of the pocket more fully. This procedure generally is performed closed, but open gingival curettage can be performed if the pocket lining is exposed by flap surgery.

Hand scaling and root planing take time; thorough scaling and planing in a dog with extensive pocketing and calculus accumulation often takes an hour or more. The temptation to consider the procedure completed once the externally obvious disease has been treated must be resisted if the result is to have more than cosmetic value only. Teeth may be more sensitive after scaling and root planing because the sensitive dentinal tubule nerve endings are now nearer the surface. Especially in cats, application of fluoride to enhance remineralization of exposed cementum is recommended; however, in dogs there is no objective evidence that this is beneficial.

Sharpening periodontal instruments

With use, periodontal hand instruments become dull and will burnish the surface of the calculus rather than remove it. Heat sterilization also dulls the sharp edge. Scalers and curets should be sharpened before use on each patient. The technique is described in Chapter 11.

Polishing

Tooth surface irregularities are created by hand and mechanical instrumentation during plaque and calculus removal. These irregularities serve to retain plaque and to permit additional accumulation of

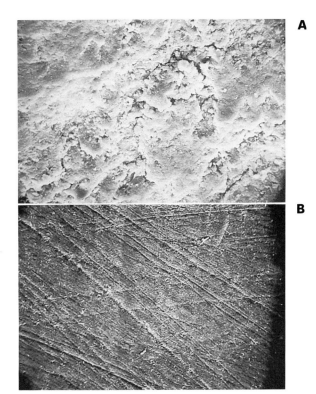

FIGURE 4-15
Scanning electron microscopic view of the surface of a tooth. **A,** After scaling but before polishing. **B,** After polishing.

plaque at a rapid rate. Polishing the teeth smoothes out these rough areas caused by the scaling procedure (Fig. 4-15). A mildly abrasive fluoride prophylaxis paste is applied to the surface of the teeth with a prophylaxis cup mounted in a prophylaxis angle in a slow speed (<5000 rpm) handpiece (Fig. 4-16; this equipment and materials are described in Chapter 11). The slow-speed handpiece can be driven by belt, air, or electricity. The cup, filled with a slurry of the paste, is moved over all unattached tooth surfaces, the operator pushing just firmly enough against the tooth to flare out the edges of the cup, which allows dipping below the gingival margin (Fig. 4-16). Excessive heat, produced by rubbing too hard or using insufficient paste, can produce pulpal necrosis. To avoid

A

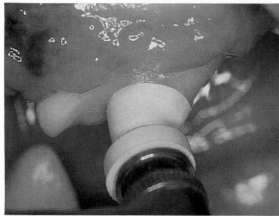

B

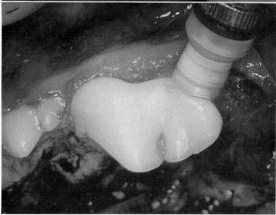

FIGURE 4-16
Polishing teeth. **A,** The prophylaxis cup is pushed against the tooth just firmly enough so that the edges start to flare. **B,** Unattached root surfaces, including subgingival areas, are polished.

this, the operator refills the prophylaxis cup when the slurry of prophylaxis paste is almost depleted, adjusts the speed control to less than 3000 rpm, uses soft prophylaxis cups that permit flaring to polish subgingivally without excessive pressure, and avoids more than 15 seconds of continuous polishing on one tooth. The prophylaxis cup is kept moving, with a return to large teeth several times if necessary to provide time for the tooth to cool.

Irrigation

After polishing, the gingival sulcus must be irrigated to flush polishing paste and debris loosened by curettage from the gingival sulcus. This can be accomplished with a blunt 18-gauge needle and syringe, a plastic bottle fitted with a perforated tapered cap, or a Water Pik device. The flushing solution can be saline or 0.5% chlorhexidine solution. It is not advisable to use pressurized water because particles become embedded in the inflamed tissues rather than flushed away.

Postoperative antibiotics rarely are necessary after a routine dental prophylaxis (see p. 139).

▶ HOME CARE

If there are no deep pockets, loose teeth, or other complicating factors, the complete prophylaxis is now finished. The next challenge is to extend by means of effective, long-term home care, the value of the professional attention the animal has received.

The most important aspect of home care is the compliance of owner and animal with a continuing program designed to retard plaque and calculus formation. Daily brushing is ideal. The veterinarian should demonstrate to the owner the importance of follow-up care at home by taking time in the office to demonstrate good application technique.

Clients can teach or train their animals to stay quiet for daily tooth brushing, especially on the buccal aspects of the upper premolar and molar teeth (the site of most rapid accumulation of plaque and calculus). Compliance will be improved if the animal is introduced gradually to brushing. A solution of water and a trace amount of garlic salt makes a palatable introductory brushing solution for dogs and cats. The following sequence works well for many owners:

With a finger and thumb of one hand placed gently around the muzzle to keep the animal's mouth closed, start by brushing only the external surface of the canine and incisor teeth (Fig. 4-17).

After a few days, extend the brush into the cheek pouch to reach the buccal surfaces of the premolar and molar teeth (Fig. 4-17, *B*).

When the animal is comfortable with the taste of

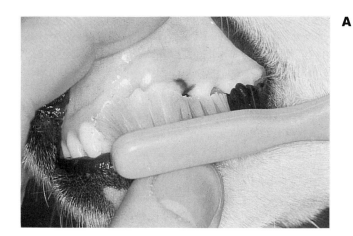

A

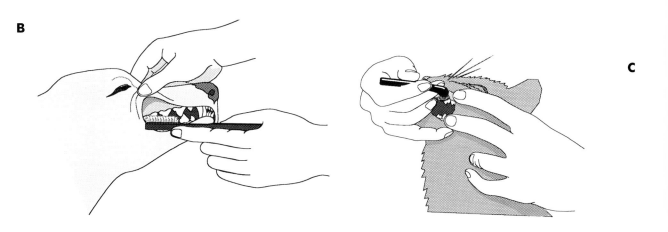

B

C

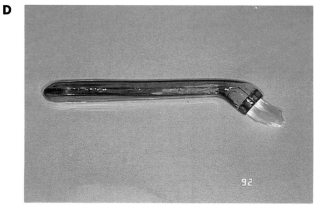

D

FIGURE 4-17
Toothbrushing. **A,** Initially the incisor and canine teeth are brushed with the jaws closed. **B,** The buccal surfaces of the premolar and molar teeth are reached by lifting the lip and inserting the brush into the buccal pouch. **C,** Using the short brush on the teeth of a cat. **D,** The short brush with forward-facing bristles designed for cats and small dogs.

the material and the sensation of brushing, open the mouth by holding the head back as far as possible with one hand, then brush the palatal and lingual surfaces of the teeth.

Even if the owner cannot become comfortable with brushing the lingual surfaces of the teeth, there is very good reason for continuing to brush the buccal surfaces only. The teeth are brushed in a circular motion that includes the gingiva, gingival sulcus, and the crowns of teeth, with the brush at a 45-degree angle to the long axis of the tooth at the gingival margin (Fig. 4-17, A). It is generally not appropriate for owners to remove the calculus deposits themselves with dental scalers or hand instruments, which can lead to injury not only to the periodontium and tooth surface but to adjacent sensitive structures if the instrument slips and can result in bite wounds to the owner.

Daily brushing is best. Powders or sprays that do not require brushing may suppress the halitosis odor but mask the continuing disease in the periodontal pocket. Several brushes, designed for veterinary use, are now available. Brushes intended to be "gentle" usually have bristles that are too soft to be of value in removing plaque and preventing accumulation of calculus. A soft human nylon bristle brush (pediatric size) is firm enough to be effective without causing discomfort. For very small dogs and for cats, a brush with forward-facing bristles is available (Fig. 4-17, C and D). Bristle brushes and rubber "gingival exerciser" tips also are available; they insert into short plastic or rubber sleeves that fit over a finger (Fig. 4-17, D). A flannel cloth folded over a finger may be more comfortable for the dog and owner, but it is less effective. Disposable plastic-backed paper "finger brushes" impregnated with a mild abrasive also are available. For some owners a reasonable option would be to bring in the dog once or twice weekly for a thorough brushing by a technician at the veterinary hospital.

Chlorhexidine has proved to be the most effective antiplaque agent to date. It is available in mint and other flavors in liquid and gel form for brushing, spraying, or smearing onto the teeth. Disadvantages of chlorhexidine are that it causes a gray-brown dark stain on teeth that are not mechanically cleansed regularly, and it is deactivated in the presence of organic material. The other chemical plaque retardant with demonstrated clinical effectiveness in dogs is an enzymatic glucose oxidase–lactoperoxidase system that is similar chemically to one of the natural antibacterial mechanisms in saliva. This retardant results in production of hypothiocyanate within oral bacteria, and it can be packaged in a paste or liquid-containing organic material. Other solutions marketed as chemical plaque retardants include zinc–organic acid combinations (ascorbic or citric acid); these products also promote tissue healing. Although not marketed specifically as plaque retardants, fluoride solutions or gels are moderately antibacterial, in addition to their desensitizing effect on cementum and enamel.

If the owner is unwilling or unable to mechanically or chemically clean the animal's teeth each day, the animal can be encouraged to "clean its own teeth" by chewing. Biscuits, rawhide strips or shapes, and rubber and nylon toys all help, but none of these are universally effective; the dog should be encouraged to use the product(s) daily. Rawhide strips have been shown to be the most effective material tested to date. Plaque retardation in dogs is a rapidly developing science; recent developments include the addition of chemical calculus-retardants (pyrophosphates) in biscuits or sprayed on the surface of rawhide chews.

▶ RESULTS OF CONSERVATIVE PERIODONTAL THERAPY

Several studies examine the effectiveness of scaling and plaque removal. When plaque removal is performed mechanically and thoroughly daily or every other day, the periodontal tissues remain clinically healthy for the duration of treatment, as shown by the difference between treated and untreated sides over prolonged periods (4 years in one study in dogs). Chemical plaque removal can produce similar results, although gradual accumulation of calculus is inevitable. The effect of diet in slowing accumulation of plaque and calculus was described on p. 97. The two factors that determine long-term results in dogs are the extent of disease existing before treatment (for example, presence or absence of furcation involvement that promotes plaque retention in areas that are difficult to clean) and the efficacy of long-term plaque retardation. Few owners are scrupulously conscientious, and thus the range of clinical effectiveness is broad.

Under some circumstances, periodontal disease will be exacerbated, and long-term brushing should be strongly recommended in the following instances:

1. After major jaw resections or repair of jaw trauma, in which the occlusion may no longer be normal, or for any condition that requires long-term feeding of a soft diet, inasmuch as dietary cleaning of teeth will be much less satisfactory than normal
2. Conditions resulting in ongoing oral or systemic immunosuppression, such as radiation therapy for oral tumors, or chemotherapy and immunotherapy for any reason

► MEDICAL MANAGEMENT OF PERIODONTAL DISEASE IN DOGS

Medical management consists either of control of (1) oral flora (see later discussion of antibiotic therapy in periodontal disease) or (2) the tissue-destructive chain of events initiated by the inflammatory response. In dogs, local or systemic flurbiprofen, a nonsteroidal antiinflammatory drug, has been shown to be a potent inhibitor of alveolar bone loss in experimental studies; long-term clinical use has yet to be evaluated.

► MANAGEMENT OF SEVERE PERIODONTAL DISEASE

Periodontal Surgery

Whether surgery is indicated and which technique to use depend on the extent of bone loss, pocket formation, pocket location, and the amount of remaining attached gingiva (Fig. 4-9).

Initial therapy

Initial therapy is the same as prophylaxis, described on pp. 114-115. It consists of those procedures designed to control the cause of the disease process: scaling, root planing, polishing, irrigation, and follow-up plaque control. Initial therapy is the most important phase of complete periodontal treatment. Periodontal surgery is designed to correct or eliminate the

consequences of the disease process. Several weeks may be required after initial therapy to allow for regeneration of tissue, although as noted previously, this is not always practical for veterinary clinical circumstances because of the risk and expense of anesthesia. Antibiotic therapy may be indicated as part of initial therapy (see p. 139).

After clinical and radiographic examination (if necessary) has been accomplished, a complete prophylaxis is performed before a treatment plan can be formulated. One cannot make a treatment plan with surgical intervention for a mouth in an acute inflammatory stage, full of debris and exudate, without risking overtreatment or potential failure of therapy because of wound breakdown resulting from treating acutely inflamed tissues. Theoretically, there is every reason to delay the decision to proceed with surgical periodontic therapy until the results of the initial therapy are clear, except for two major considerations in veterinary dental practice: cost and anesthesia risk.

When pocket formation or other anatomic abnormality exceeds the ability to eliminate the sulcular pathogens on a daily basis, surgical intervention is indicated. In planning a surgical procedure the attached gingiva must be considered (Fig. 4-9). After surgical elimination or correction of the pocket, a minimum of 2 to 3 mm of attached gingiva must remain to maintain the underlying alveolar bone and to separate the tooth surface from the thin, sensitive buccal or sublingual mucosa that is less able to resist dietary forces.

Periodontal surgical procedures include (1) gingivoplasty, (2) flap procedures (3) osteoplasty, and (4) mucogingival surgery.

Gingivoplasty

Gingivoplasty is the removal of gingival pockets by the excision of gingiva, or recontouring the gingival tissue to its proper anatomic form. Gingivoplasty can be used in combination with other surgical procedures such as flap operations. Gingivoplasty includes procedures in which some gingival tissue is resected, commonly known as *gingivectomy*. Because resection of the entire attached gingiva never is indicated and it is always important to ensure a correct recontouring of the gingival margin, *gingivoplasty* is

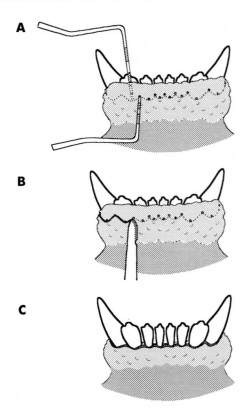

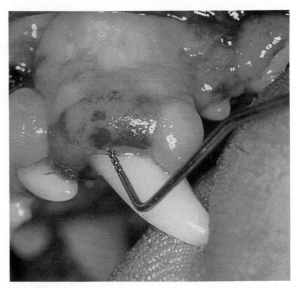

FIGURE 4-19
For legend see opposite page.

FIGURE 4-18
Diagram of steps in gingivoplasty. **A,** Measuring of pocket and indicating depth with a periodontal probe. **B,** Linking the bleeding points. **C,** Full exposure of unattached tooth substance.

the term used in this text for any procedure requiring resection of gingival tissue.

Indications for gingivoplasty are gingival hyperplasia and shallow suprabony gingival pockets that will permit retention of 2 to 3 mm of attached gingiva after the procedure.

Contraindications include absence of attached gingiva and horizontal or vertical bone loss below the MGJ. Gingivoplasty can be performed with an electrosurgical unit if an abundance of attached gingiva is present. The procedure should be performed with sharp dissection if there is any concern about retaining sufficient viable gingiva (minimum height, 2 mm).

Pocket depth is outlined with a periodontal probe on all surfaces of the tooth requiring gingivoplasty. The pocket depth is measured; then the probe is withdrawn from the pocket, held against the gingiva to show the depth of the pocket, and its tip is pressed into the gingiva perpendicular to the tooth (Fig. 4-18, *A*). This is repeated every few millimeters to create a series of bleeding points (Fig. 4-18, *A* and *B*). A pocket-depth marker makes this a quick and simple procedure. A line connecting the bleeding points is used to determine the incision line. The No. 15 blade is placed at an angle to the long axis of the tooth, producing a beveled incision that will result in an anatomically correct gingival margin (Fig. 4-19, *E*). To achieve the correct angle, the incision line externally is located 1 to 3 mm (depending on the thickness of the gingiva) apically compared with the line of bleeding points marking the attachment level (Fig. 4-19, *C*).

The operator should avoid making the angle of the incision too acute, which may place the blood supply of the gingiva at risk; 30 to 45 degrees generally is a safe angle. Because gingiva has little elastic tissue and there is no retracting force, it does not separate

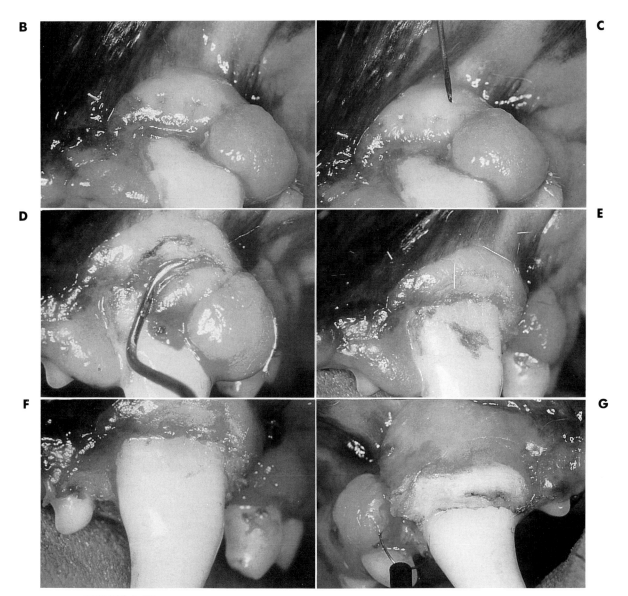

FIGURE 4-19

Gingivoplasty with an electroscalpel. **A,** Pocket depth measurement around a canine tooth with gingival hyperplasia. **B,** Bleeding points mark the pocket depth externally. **C,** The electroscalpel incision is commenced 1 to 2 mm apical to the line of bleeding points and angled toward the bottom of the pocket. **D,** Following a single pass of the instrument, a sharp dental scaler is used to complete the resection. **E,** The angled cut edge of the gingiva can be seen. **F,** The tooth is thoroughly scaled and polished. **G,** Gingivoplasty performed with the electroscalpel setting too high; further tissue loss occurs as a result of necrosis.

as it is cut. The separated tissue is removed by applying a sharp-edged dental scaler to the incision and levering coronally (Fig. 4-19, *D*).

For electrosurgical gingivoplasty, bleeding points are created as already described to mark the pocket depth. The electroscalpel is used to make the beveled incision (Fig. 4-19, *C*). In planning the incision, the operator should allow for tissue slough, 1 mm in thickness, when using an electroscapel. The electrode is activated at the minimal effective setting in *cut* mode and stroked across the gingiva at the required angle. If the setting was correct, the incised edge of the gingiva will be pink but not bleeding (Fig. 4-19, *E*); if the setting was too high, the tissue will stay blanched (Fig. 4-19, *G*).

Hemorrhage is controlled with gauze swabs and digital pressure. The newly exposed tooth surface is then scaled and polished (Fig. 4-19, *F*).

Gingival contouring. Ginival contouring is a gingivoplasty technique. Hyperplasia of the gingival tissues around and between the incisor teeth, which is common in large-breed dogs, is difficult to resect accurately with a cold scalpel blade. Large areas of excess tissue are resected as already described for gingivoplasty. Smaller areas, or where there is risk of overheating the tooth if the electrode is placed in the gingival pocket, can be resected by using the loop or diamond electrode like a clay sculpting loop or paintbrush (Fig. 4-20). The electrode is applied to the surface and activated as it is moved, causing

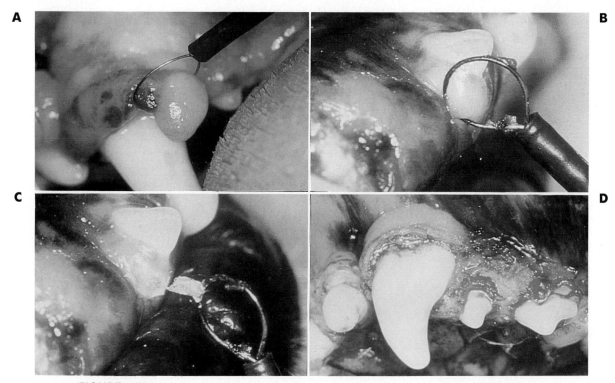

FIGURE 4-20
Gingivoplasty using a loop electrode. **A,** Resection of an isolated gingival margin mass. **B,** Uncovering incisor teeth: applying the electrode to stroke it across the hyperplastic tissue. **C,** A strip of gingiva is removed. This step is repeated as necessary, allowing approximately 15 seconds between each passage of the tip over any one tooth. **D,** Following extensive contouring of the gingiva of the incisors, canine, and first two premolar teeth.

a thin layer of gingiva to be incised and removed (Fig. 4-20, *B* and *C*). This process is repeated until the entire crown is exposed. To avoid overheating, the electrode should not be reapplied to the gingiva around the same tooth within 15 seconds. Usually several teeth require contouring; thus each tooth can be treated in turn with one stroke, with a return to the starting tooth after each round of single strokes is completed (Fig. 4-20, *D*).

The final and most important step in any periodontal procedure is to scale and polish the crown and exposed root surfaces.

Flap procedures

Flap procedures constitute the most common periodontal surgery. Gingival tissue is reflected to gain access to the deeper periodontal structures. A full-thickness flap (gingiva, mucosa, periosteum) ensures adequate vascular supply and regeneration. A partial-thickness flap may be indicated (discussed later), but its success is more dependent on technique; the simplest, most reliable procedure compatible with the desired end result is always preferable.

General indications for flap procedures include the following:
1. An active pocket deeper than about 4 mm after initial treatment
2. A pocket that extends apical to the mucogingival line
3. Bone loss covered by soft tissue that forms a deep pocket
4. Marginal deformity

Flap procedures are contraindicated when gingival hyperplasia is present; gingivoplasty is recommended instead.

Conservative (nonrepositioned) periodontal flaps. Flap procedures have the advantages of allowing direct vision and access to the pocket or defect for proper scaling and root planing. The pocket epithelium is severed with a reverse (internal) bevel incision. After scaling, the flap is replaced to its original position. Thus little gingival tissue actually is lost and there is no additional exposure of root structure.

An internal incision severing the sulcular epithelial attachment is made with a No. 11 or No. 15 blade, designed to preserve maximum attached gingiva (Fig.

4-21, *A*). The scalpel blade is used to make an incision at a slight angle (10 to 20 degrees) of the tooth (reverse bevel flap), separating the diseased pocket epithelium, which is excised as a separate layer (Fig. 4-21, *B*). If the incision is made only along the gingival margin, the procedure is known as an *envelope flap* (Fig. 4-21).

Greater access to the roots can be obtained by making vertical releasing incisions at one or both ends of the gingival section to be flapped (Fig. 4-22). If the flap is to be returned to its original position, the releasing incisions do not extend beyond the MGJ. The flap may be of one or more teeth in length. If it involves more than one tooth, the incision follows the gingival margin by "scalloping" to include the interdental papilla (Fig. 4-22, *A* and *B*). Generally, flaps are made on both the buccal and lingual sides of the tooth, although this technique often is impractical for maxillary teeth. The full-thickness releasing gingival flap is reflected from the coronal 1 to 2 mm of crestal alveolar bone by means of a small periosteal elevator (Fig. 4-22, *C*) following the scalloped line of the epithelial attachment incision. The released gingiva is then rolled back, exposing the roots and crestal alveolar bone (Figs. 4-21, *D* and 4-22, *C*). Fine curets are used to remove remnants of pocket epithelium and granulation tissue (Fig. 4-23, *C*). Thorough root planing is performed, with repeated irrigation (Fig. 4-21, *E*). Root planing is an important part of all periodontal surgical procedures. Corrections of osseous abnormalities (see Osteoplasty) are made at this time if needed.

Envelope flaps involving several teeth and releasing flaps are closed over the interdental areas without tension by use of interrupted absorbable sutures (Fig. 4-22, *D*). The flaps are adapted to the underlying bone and the necks of the teeth by the application of digital pressure for several seconds. New interdental papillae were created by the scalloped form of the initial incision if several teeth were flapped.

Apically repositioned flap. When the remaining gingiva must be saved because there is so little left, an apically based flap is used to permit repositioning of the gingival margin at the existing bone level. This eliminates the pocket. A reverse bevel incision at the gingival margin is made, as described for a nonre-

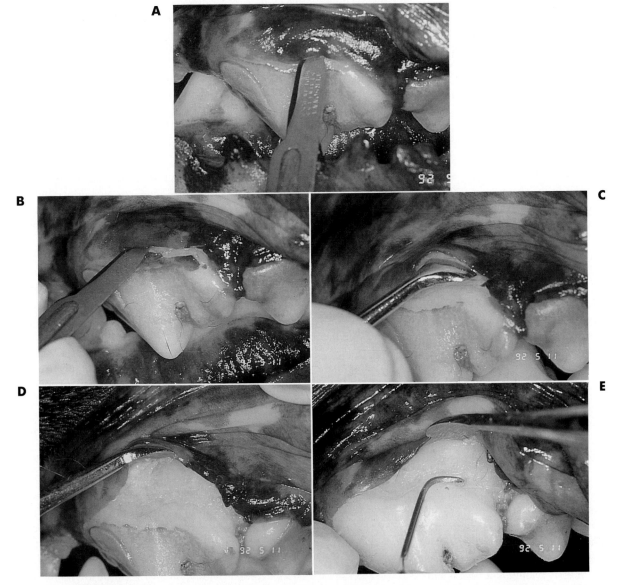

FIGURE 4-21
Conservative (envelope) flap surgery. **A,** The soft tissue attachment is incised. **B,** Incisions for reverse bevel flap surgery. **C,** The gingival tissue is dissected. **D,** The rolled-back gingiva exposes the crestal bone. **E,** The tooth can be scaled and root planed thoroughly.

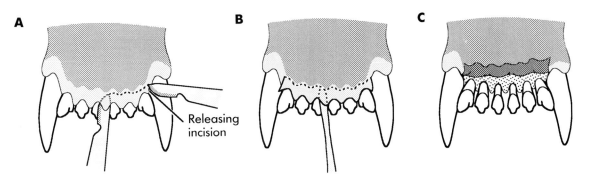

A Releasing incision

Incising to crestal alveolar bone

B Raising attached gingiva

C Exposing roots and alveolar bone

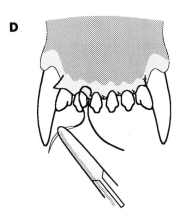

D

Suturing flap

FIGURE 4-22
Nonrepositioned flap surgery. **A,** The procedure commences with a releasing incision in the attached gingiva at the end of the proposed flap. **B,** The gingiva is dissected. **C,** This exposes the alveolar bone. **D,** Following thorough scaling, root planing, polishing and irrigation, and osteoplasty if indicated, the flap is sutured back in its original position.

positioned flap (Fig. 4-23, *A*). If the flap is designed to extend along several teeth, the gingival margin incision extends between the teeth to include the interdental papillae. Vertical releasing incisions are made at one or both ends of the flap, extending onto the alveolar mucosa apical to the MGJ. The gingival tissue and alveolar mucosa are elevated and reflected, dissecting deeply enough to sever the periosteal attachment of the mucosa (Fig. 4-23, *B*). The exposed roots are scaled, polished, and irrigated thoroughly (Fig. 4-23, *C*), and bony defects are treated as necessary by osteoplasty (Fig. 4-23, *D*,; see following section). If vertical releasing incisions are made, the flap is sutured at each end so that the gingival margin is now 1 to 2 mm coronal to and completely covering the

existing bony attachment (Fig. 4-23, *E* and *G*). The flapped gingiva is sutured between teeth to conform the new gingival margin to the attachment line around individual teeth. Absorbable suture material is used in a simple interrupted pattern. The gingival tissues are adapted to the bone and teeth with digital pressure for several seconds (Fig. 4-23, *F*).

A periodontal pack is a malleable, chemically cured or light-cured material formed around the teeth to maintain the position of the flap relative to tooth and bone structure and to protect the tissues during the first several days of healing. Periodontal packs rarely are used in veterinary periodontal practice because the shape of the crowns and the size of the interdental spaces do not permit the retention of the

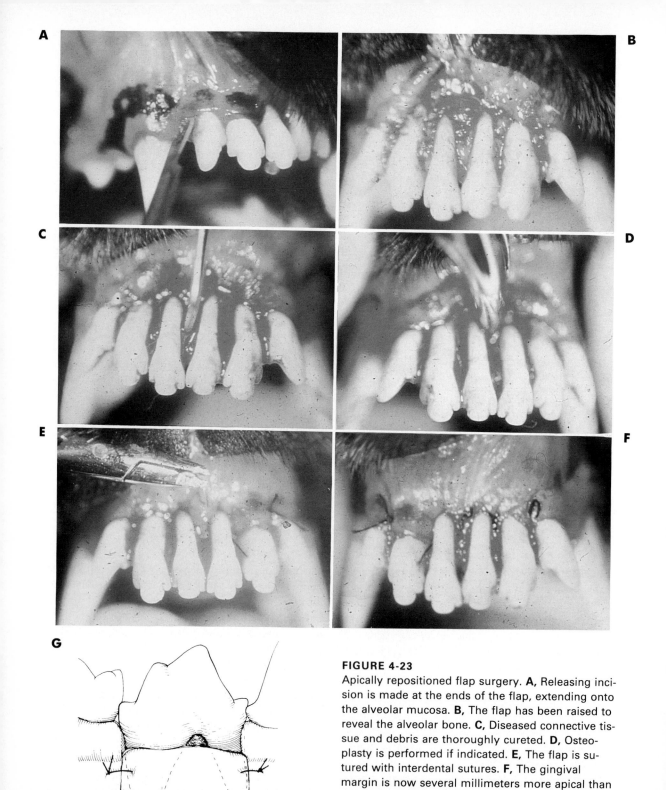

FIGURE 4-23

Apically repositioned flap surgery. **A,** Releasing incision is made at the ends of the flap, extending onto the alveolar mucosa. **B,** The flap has been raised to reveal the alveolar bone. **C,** Diseased connective tissue and debris are thoroughly cureted. **D,** Osteoplasty is performed if indicated. **E,** The flap is sutured with interdental sutures. **F,** The gingival margin is now several millimeters more apical than it was preoperatively. **G,** Diagram showing use of sutures at each end of the flap to maintain the apical repositioning of a single tooth flap.

pack for the several days necessary to achieve a beneficial effect. When used, they should be formed so that occlusal interference will not dislodge the pack.

Brushing is postponed for about a week after gingival surgery; instead irrigation with dilute chlorhexidine once or twice daily is recommended.

Coronally repositioned flaps occasionally are advocated in an attempt to re-create soft tissue attachment. Their use is not described here.

Osteoplasty

A reflected flap can provide access to areas in which osteoplasty (bone recontouring) is necessary. Indications for osteoplasty are lateral pockets extending beyond the attached gingiva or mucogingival line, reverse bony architecture (reverse of normal anatomic contours), and thickened bony margins in which the flap is to be repositioned. Osteoplasty is best performed with the use of slow-speed round burs. Sterile saline must be used for cooling during this procedure because heat is generated even at low speeds.

Bulbous bony margins are eliminated, especially between the teeth, by narrowing the buccal and lingual cortical plates. This permits repositioning of soft tissue flaps and physiologic regeneration of the gingival margin.

Ideally, the exposed crown and root surfaces are thoroughly polished 10 days after surgery; it is im-portant to remember that the wound-healing processes (regeneration, formation of the junctional epithelium) will not be complete at that time, and the prophylaxis paste and rubber cup should not be forced into the sulcular area.

Mucogingival surgery

Mucogingival surgery is performed when there is a need to widen the band of attached gingiva or to cover a denuded root surface ("gingival cleft"). A successful procedure requires development of a soft tissue attachment between the grafted gingiva and cementum of the tooth. Thus rotation or sliding grafts are more likely to be successful than are free grafts because the blood supply to the graft remains intact during the early healing stage.

Also included in this section is a description of frenoplasty, which prevents further attachment loss around teeth adjacent to a lip frenulum.

Sliding (rotation) graft. A rotation graft is used when sufficient adjacent gingiva permits the defect to be covered by gingival tissue that retains its blood supply. The most common location for use of a rotation graft is the upper canine tooth (buccal surface) (Figs. 4-24 and 4-25) and the mesial root of the upper fourth premolar tooth (Fig. 4-26). The tooth is thoroughly scaled and polished. The edge to which the flap will be sutured in the recipient area must be

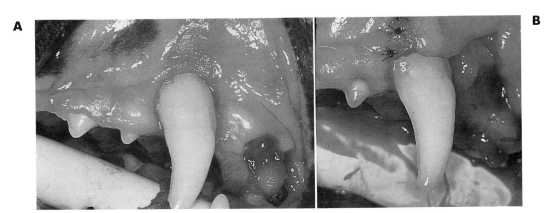

A   **B**

FIGURE 4-24
Rotating flap. **A,** Gingival cleft over an upper canine tooth following scaling, root planing, and polishing. **B,** Tissue has been rotated from the no longer needed third incisor area and sutured to provide some gingival coverage over the root of the canine tooth.

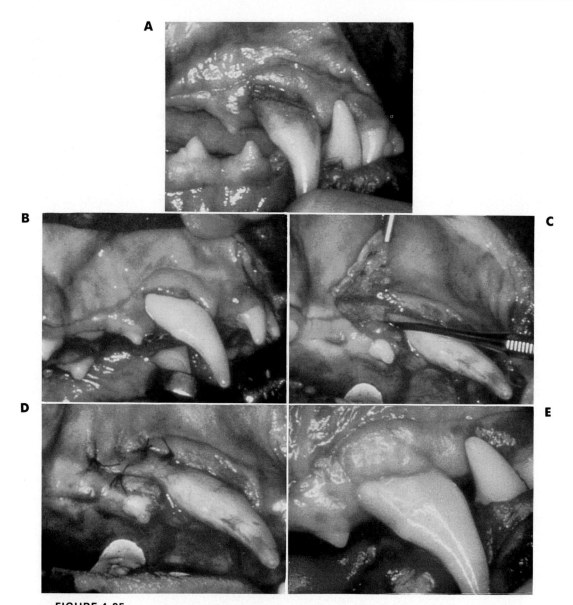

FIGURE 4-25
Rotating flap. **A,** The third incisor and first premolar teeth adjacent to this severely diseased upper canine tooth are present and healthy, so a split-thickness flap will be used. **B,** The canine tooth has been scaled and root planed. **C,** A partial-thickness flap is raised, leaving 2 to 3 mm of healthy attached gingiva over the first premolar tooth. **D,** The flap is sutured in place over the root of the canine tooth. **E,** At 6 months after the operation, the gingiva over the canine and first premolar teeth is healthy.

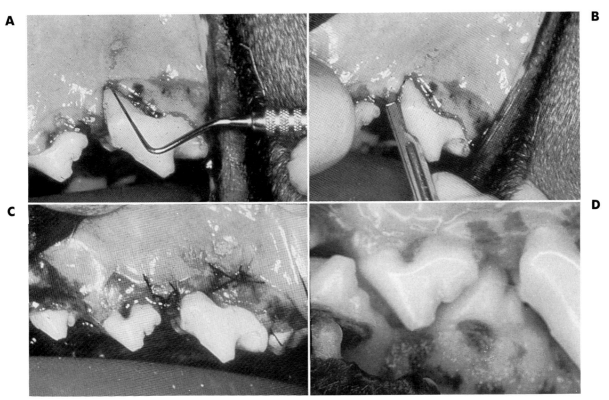

FIGURE 4-26
Rotating flap—upper carnassial tooth. **A,** The teeth on either side of the carnassial tooth with the gingival cleft (probe) are in place, so a partial-thickness flap will be used. **B,** An incision is made to create the flap apical to the third premolar tooth. **C,** The flap is sutured in place. **D,** Healthy gingiva over the recipient and donor sites is present 3 months later.

trimmed to provide a clean incised edge for optimal healing. This edge is continued apically as one side of the flap. A second incision is made at the other side of the flap (Fig. 4-25, *C*). Both incisions extend beyond the MGJ. The flap tissue is undermined, taking the full thickness of the soft tissue by dissecting with a periosteal elevator against bone. The flap is reflected, the unattached root surface is scaled thoroughly, and the flap tissue is rotated and maintained in position with synthetic absorbable sutures (Fig. 4-24, *B*). As already noted, a periodontal pack can be used, but there rarely are sufficient holding spaces between teeth to make it practical. A full-thickness flap is used if there is a large interdental space adjacent to the gin-

gival defect or if the adjacent tooth has been lost or is to be extracted. Tissue for a sliding or rotation graft can be created apical to an existing tooth if the gingival height will permit rotation of 2 to 3 mm of attached gingiva to the recipient site, or a partial-thickness flap can be made (Figs. 4-25 and 4-26).

Free gingival graft. The decision to proceed with a free gingival graft should be made very carefully because circumstances (the location, patient, owner) have to be optimal for success (Fig. 4-27, *F*). Typical locations for free grafts are the buccal surface of the upper canine tooth, lingual or buccal surface of the lower canine tooth, and buccal surface of the upper fourth premolar tooth. The recipient site is outlined

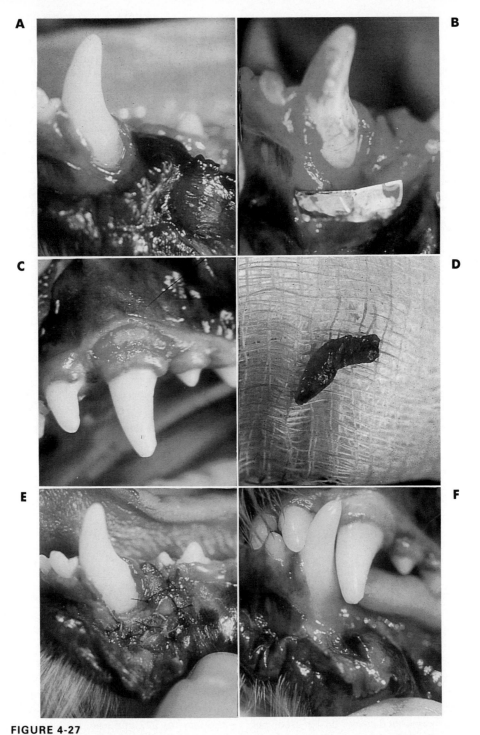

FIGURE 4-27

Free gingival graft. **A,** Lower canine tooth with a severe gingival cleft following scaling and root planing. **B,** Template of aluminum foil is cut to shape. **C,** The template is used to trace a graft site from the donor area (upper canine), and the graft is incised. **D,** The graft is sharply dissected free. **E,** The graft is sutured into position. **F,** A healthy gingival covering of the tooth and donor site is present 1 year postoperatively.

to make a template (Fig. 4-27, *A* and *B*), the template (for example, aluminum foil) is used to mark the graft in the donor site (typically the gingiva of the mandibular premolar teeth), and a partial-thickness graft is dissected (leaving the marginal gingiva and 2 to 3 mm of attached gingiva intact at the donor site; Fig. 4-27, *C*). The graft is transferred (Fig. 4-27, *D*) and sutured in place with synthetic absorbable sutures (Fig. 4-27, *E*). The epithelial surface must be sutured with the incised surface placed down in the recipient site.

For optimal development of new cemental attachment, the root surface must be thoroughly cleaned (scaled, root planed, polished, irrigated) and then chemically prepared by applying citric acid or tetracycline solution for 15 seconds, followed by further irrigation and flap closure.

Frenoplasty. To prevent further loss of attached gingiva in teeth close to a lip frenulum attachment, where the weight of the lip distracts the gingiva, frenoplasty (frenectomy) is indicated. This procedure is used most commonly to protect the lower canine teeth.

The mucosa of the frenulum is incised at its attachment to the mandible; then dissection is continued ventrally to free the fibrous frenular attachments. By means of blunt dissection, it sometimes is possible to identify and avoid transecting the mental artery. The mucosal incision gapes as the dissection continues. Dissection is adequate when there no longer is a more obvious attachment of lip in that location than in adjacent areas. To prevent reformation of the frenular attachment, the mucosa is sutured so that the labial mucosa is apposed as one suture line, leaving the alveolar mucosa of the mandible to heal by granulation and contraction.

Management of Deep Palatal Pockets

The buccal surface is a plate of cortical bone parallel to the long axis of the roots, whereas the palatal surface is cortical bone perpendicular to the long axis of the root. Thus a deep pocket palatally does not show any external gingival or bone recession, and it may fistulate into the nasal cavity. It is impossible to perform apically repositioned flap surgery on the palatal surfaces of the upper teeth. These deep palatal pockets may respond to thorough scaling and root planing, followed by packing the pocket with an osteoconductive agent (see next section) (Fig. 4-28). Etching the scaled and root-planed cemental surface

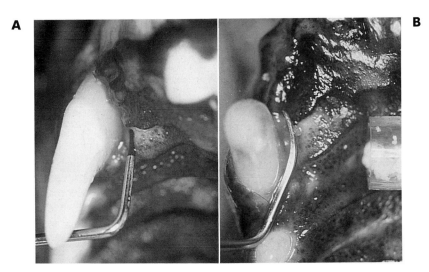

FIGURE 4-28
Management of deep palatal pocket. **A,** 12-mm pocket on the palatal surface of an upper canine tooth. **B,** Following thorough scaling and root planing, polylactic acid granules are gently placed to fill the pocket.

with citric acid or tetracycline may enhance connective tissue reattachment; long-term clinical results have yet to be reported for this technique in dogs. If simple flap surgery is used to obtain improved access for scaling, the palatal gingiva is sutured snugly around the tooth. If the palatal alveolar plate is resorbed, the root may be sitting exposed in the nasal cavity or maxillary sinus recess. Reformation of attachment in these circumstances is impossible. Nasal discharge may be evident clinically. Management of oronasal fistula is described in Chapter 10.

Periodontal bone grafting

Bone lost as a result of periodontal disease may be replaced to some extent in certain limited circumstances. Bone replacement procedures are most successful in four- or three-wall infrabony pockets (see p. 101), with a 50% to 75% likelihood of success. The next most successful bone grafting procedure is in two-wall infrabony pockets in which bone is present bucally and lingually; the root surfaces of the adjacent teeth are the third and fourth walls (less than 50% success rate). The least successful procedure is the one-wall infrabony pocket (up to 10% success rate). Generalized horizontal bone loss is rarely successfully aided by bone-grafting procedures.

Grafting materials are of natural bone and bone substitutes, such as hydroxyapatite, porous coral-derived material, and nonresorbable ceramic bone materials, all of which have osseous conductive properties.

Natural bony materials currently employed are usually allografts (interspecies), xenographs (species to species), or autografts (the host's own bone). Autografts are the most successful; bone can be harvested from the iliac crest, rib, ventral mandible, or dental extraction sites.

A full-thickness periodontal flap is raised, exposing the bony defect. The pocket is débrided, the root surfaces are thoroughly planed, and any lateral bony projections or irregularities are removed by osteoplasty. The bony pocket walls are fenestrated with a No. ½ round bur and dental handpiece with use of sterile saline irrigation to a bony depth of 1 to 2 mm. Sufficient fenestrations are made to ensure permeability of bone-forming elements from the underlying vascular tissue. Bone-grafting material of choice is placed

into the prepared defect, filling to the greatest height of remaining bony wall(s). Bone cannot be placed above the remaining natural alveolar crest. The gingival flap is replaced with simple interrupted sutures; the grafted bone or bone substitute should be covered completely with gingiva.

If the graft is located in an area of the mouth where adjacent teeth make it practical, a periodontal pack is placed over the grafted site for 1 week (see p. 129).

Guided tissue regeneration

An additional technique that may become useful in clinical veterinary dentistry is *guided tissue regeneration*. With standard periodontal treatment techniques, the current level of periodontal bone loss is accepted, and steps are taken to prevent further bone loss. Some epithelial reattachment does occur after root planing, but bone and periodontal ligament regeneration does not because the fibroblastic and osteoblastic activity is too slow to compete with the connective tissue and epithelial healing occurring from the gingiva. If a tissue barrier is placed to separate the gingival tissue from the root surface, the stem cells in the periodontal ligament and osteoblasts on the periodontal bone surface have the time available to form new bone and normal periodontal ligament. Tissue barriers used to date, such as Gore-Tex, are nonabsorbable and must be removed about 3 months after placement. Tissue barriers that are predictably absorbable, such as polylactic acid, are under development; these will be more practical for veterinary use inasmuch as only one anesthetic episode will be necessary.

Periodontal splinting

Upper and lower incisors, in groups or as a single tooth, may require stabilization because of bone loss from periodontal disease, particularly in toy-breed dogs. This stabilization is performed in conjunction with periodontal treatment. Mobile teeth interfere with postsurgical healing, often making it impossible to ensure remission of the periodontal disease.

Mobile teeth are stabilized by splinting or ligating the involved tooth or teeth to stable abutment teeth, provided there are no missing teeth in the incisor segment (Fig. 4-29). This can be accomplished in two ways: with the use of dental acrylics or composite filling material alone or with dental acrylic/composite and interdental ligation. After periodontal therapy the mobile teeth are placed in proper arch alignment.

Method 1. Dental acrylic is applied to the contact areas between teeth and over the labial and lingual surfaces, making sure to prevent subgingival seeping of the acrylic. The acrylic is best applied by dipping a camel's hair brush into the liquid, then dipping the brush into a small reservoir of powder. This small amount of mixed acrylic is then carried to the contact area. This is repeated until sufficient acrylic has been applied and allowed to cure.

Method 2. The crowns and roots are thoroughly scaled and polished with a nonfluoride dental polish. A groove is cut in the labial enamel of the teeth at the level of the lateral cusp tips (Fig. 4-29, *A*), the teeth are acid-etched (Fig. 4-29, *B*), and a length of transparent nylon or fiberglass material is glued

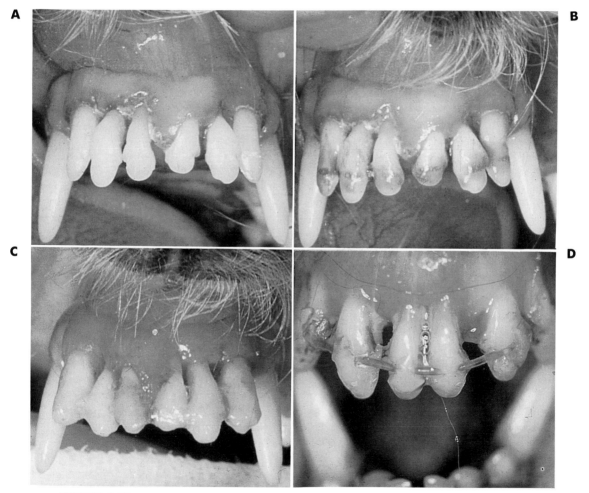

FIGURE 4-29
Splinting incisor teeth. **A,** Following thorough scaling and root planing, a groove is cut in the labial surface of the teeth. **B,** The teeth are acid-etched. **C,** A figure-eight nylon splint is held in place with composite restorative material. **D,** This nylon splint has been in place for 2½ years: the owner brushes the teeth twice daily. The composite has worn down, exposing more of the chlorhexidine-stained nylon.

into the groove and around the teeth in a figure-of-8 pattern with composite resin. Additional composite resin is placed to form a band 2 to 4 mm high and 2 to 3 mm thick along the coronal, labial, and lingual parts of the teeth and between the teeth. It is essential to leave sufficient space between the splint and the soft tissues to allow for proper oral hygiene. Finishing disks and burs are used to shape and smooth the surface of the teeth (Fig. 4-29, *C*). The bonding technique is described further in Chapter 7.

After stabilization, the mouth is closed to check for occlusal contact. If the splinted teeth or tooth is found to strike the opposing incisors, the incisal edge of each affected tooth or maloccluding bulge of the splint is reduced and the bite rechecked until the occlusion is normal. Composite resins are somewhat more rigid than are acrylic splints; this may be a problem for the lower jaw because the symphysis is fibrous. The result is that a rigid splint joining the right and left lower incisors may break.

Dental splints, depending on the severity of the disease or bone loss, may be retained for a short period or for several years (Fig. 4-29, *D*). Composite resins provide a more esthetic splint than does pink acrylic material; they will slowly wear down and require periodic reinforcement. When dental splints need repair, dental acrylic and composite resins bond to themselves, and thus repair is easily accomplished.

Odontoplasty

Odontoplasty is the removal of anatomically abnormal dental enamel, iatrogenically created restorative irregularities, or natural plaque-retentive areas on a tooth, with the use of dental burs, stones, or diamonds in a dental handpiece.

Natural tooth corrections are confined to those areas in which dental morphologic anomalies can create plaque-retentive areas. These morphologic anomalies are fused roots of multirooted teeth that exhibit an irregular profile, enamel pearls or projections located at the furcation entrance, and crowded teeth (especially incisors) that create hidden pockets of plaque.

Technique. With the use of coarse diamond burs, the overhanging buccal enamel projections or irregularities are removed. Fine diamonds are used for initial polishing. A fine rubber wheel is used for final polishing in a slow-speed handpiece with light pressure to eliminate overheating of the tooth and subsequent pulpal necrosis.

The use of odontoplasty should not be abused! In doubtful cases the procedure should be omitted.

Descriptions of odontoplasty in veterinary dentistry include two additional procedures. These are the flattening of the cervical bulge of enamel on upper fourth and third premolars and first molars (upper and lower) and removal of the contact area between the upper fourth premolar and first molar, creating an abnormally wide interdental space. Both procedures are contraindicated. Removal of the cervical bulge of enamel on molars and premolars removes the natural food-deflecting surface. Without this deflecting surface, food is forced into the lateral gingival sulcus, creating a periodontal defect (Fig. 4-30). One has only to observe the gingiva above a slab fracture of an upper fourth premolar tooth to see the long-term results of this loss of tooth surface. Effective frequent oral health care is a much better way of preventing plaque accumulation apical to the CEJ. Opening of the distal contact between the upper fourth premolar and first molar creates the same problem. The large cusp of the lower first molar drives food up into this open space, creating a severe gingival defect.

▶ ANTIBIOTIC AND ANTISEPTIC THERAPY IN PERIODONTAL DISEASE

The oral cavity is grossly contaminated; however, this does not justify the tendency to include antibiotic coverage as an automatic part of the management of oral disease in animals. The oral tissues are covered with an epithelium that is bathed in a fluid rich in potent antibacterial systems, and they have a well-developed blood supply.

Bacteremia is inevitable when oral procedures are performed in a mouth with gingival inflammation, gross plaque and calculus, and pocket formation. The most common organisms found in blood cultures during dental procedures are *Streptococcus, Staphylococcus, Pasteurella,* and *Bacteroides* spp. The bacteremia can be prevented or reduced in severity by

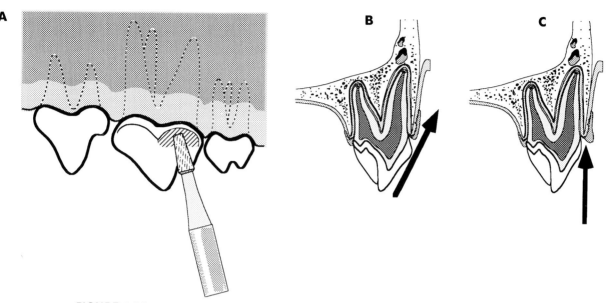

FIGURE 4-30
Odontoplasty. **A,** The procedure: the buccal enamel bulge of the carnassial tooth is removed. **B** and **C,** The effect. Normally, the enamel bulge deflects food particles from the gingiva (**B**). Following odontoplasty (**C**), food particles will continually hit against the gingival crest, opening the gingival sulcus.

gentle flushing of the oral cavity with chlorhexidine before the oral procedure is begun. This technique should be routinely employed whenever the procedure will uncover connective tissue—for example, periodontal therapy in animals with deep pockets—or when extractions, flap procedures, maxillectomy or mandibulectomy, or open fracture fixation will be performed.

During a typical scaling procedure, bacteremia occurs but lasts less than an hour because the bacteria are filtered out by the reticuloendothelial system. Thus when antibiotic administration is indicated, a single dose that produces a bactericidal serum concentration during the procedure is sufficient. This combination can be achieved by the concurrent administration of a drug such as ampicillin or amoxicillin and the preanesthetic medication.

Antibiotics should not be routinely used for management of oral diseases for numerous reasons. Generally they are not necessary; they are neither 100% safe nor 100% effective drugs (some organisms may not be susceptible to the antibiotic selected); and routine use of antibiotics results in development of resistant strains of bacteria that may cause disease at another body location, another time, or in another animal that will not be amenable to standard therapy. In addition, superinfections with fungal organisms can ocur. By temporarily lessening the severity of clinical signs, the antibiotic administration may mask the underlying problem and perhaps permit it to worsen or spread; antibiotic treatment may improve the mouth odor for a while but will delay definitive diagnosis and possibly worsen the prognosis.

When an antibiotic that is effective against periodontopathogens is given at the time of dental scaling, a measureable benefit is evident (lessened bone loss and gingival inflammation) several months later as compared with scaling without antibiotic therapy if no ongoing plaque-control measures are instituted. The beneficial effect of antibiotic therapy is not demonstrable, however, if ongoing plaque-control measures are not instituted.

Antibiotics should not be administered without a specific reason for their use.

Clinical Indications for Antibiotic Therapy

In the following situations, administration of antibiotics may be justified.

1. Oral ulceration is severe and causing sufficient pain so that the animal is not willing or able to drink but in which scaling is indicated as part of the therapeutic plan. Examples are cats with gingivostomatitis (see Chapter 5) or dogs with ulcerative stomatitis (see Chapter 5). A 5- to 7-day course of amoxicillin-clavulanate, clindamycin, or metronidazole will lessen the inflammation and encourage a rapid return to eating after the scaling procedure.

2. A dog has severe periodontitis, but its owner wishes to retain as much of the dentition as possible. A two-stage periodontal procedure is performed. The sequence is pretreatment for 5 days with amoxicillin-clavulanate, clindamycin, spiramycin-metronidazole, or metronidazole alone; scaling under anesthesia; continuation of the antibiotic administration and oral rinsing with chlorhexidine for 10 to 14 days; and then reanesthetizing the dog for the definitive periodontal procedure (for example, gingivoplasty, gingival flaps, splinting). Antibiotic administration generally is not necessary after the definitive procedures. A wait of several days after the initial scaling permits some healing, reattachment, and reduction of pocket depth, and the definitive procedures may not need to be as radical as would have been the case if the procedures were performed concomitantly.

3. Dental scaling is required in an animal with evidence of systemic disease that may be worsened by bacteremia. Examples are dogs with (a) chronic heart failure or cats with cardiomyopathy, in which the turbulent blood flow may increase the likelihood of development of endocarditis, and (b) chronic kidney or hepatic failure, in which metabolic instability may produce a secondary immunopathy or septic vascular aggregates may exacerbate the systemic disease. Animals with primary immunopathies are another example, as are animals that are on a regimen of immunosuppressive medication at the time of the procedure.

4. A scaling procedure is indicated for an animal in which a sterile clean or clean/contaminated surgical procedure will be performed during the same anesthetic episode as the dental procedure. An example is an older animal with a mammary neoplasm and extensive periodontal disease, for whom—because of anesthetic considerations relating to age and general condition—separate anesthesia episodes are not recommended. If no antibiotic drug is given, the surgical wound will be seeded with bacteria from the dental bacteremia, and infection, with potentially disastrous results, is likely. A regimen of antibiotics is commenced at the same time as preanesthetic medications and continued for 4 to 5 days until the surgical wound has completed the initial inflammatory phase of healing.

5. A pulp-capping procedure (see Chapter 6) suggests the need for antibiotics. Bacterial contamination of the pulp chamber at the time of pulp capping is the equivalent of seeding a closed cavity with bacteria, which may result in necrosis of the pulp contents and subsequent apical abscess or fistula because there is no room in the pulp chamber to accommodate the swelling that the inflammatory response causes as it attempts to deal with the bacteria. Contamination may occur despite efforts to perform pulp-capping with use of sterile technique. A single dose of a bactericidal antibiotic will prevent seeded bacteria from becoming a focus of infection.

Antibiotic Drugs and Dosages
Antibacteremic therapy

Antibacteremic therapy requires the use of any bactericidal broad-spectrum antibiotic with particularly good activity against gram-positive aerobic cocci and anaerobes, for example, ampicillin (10 mg/kg intravenously [sodium salt] at the time of preanesthetic medication or 20 mg/kg orally an hour or more before inducing anesthesia) or amoxicillin. For continuation of treatment to prevent development of infection in surgical wounds that may be contaminated by dentally induced bacteremia, an agent such as ampicillin, 10 mg/kg administered orally four times daily, can be used for 4 to 5 days.

Other drugs

Drugs used to treat periodontal bacterial infection or to suppress bacterial growth in inflamed oral tissues include clindamycin and tetracycline, selected principally for their broad-spectrum activity and activity against anaerobes, and metronidazole, chosen for its activity against anaerobes and its antiflagellate activity. Spiramycin is an excellent drug for oral use that is not currently licensed for use in the United States; it is available in other countries, in combination with metronidazole, as Stomorgyl.

Amoxicillin-clavulanate. Clavamox is a combination of amoxicillin and potassium clavulanate, a β-lactamase inhibitor. The broad spectrum of antibacterial activity of amoxicillin is extended by the addition of clavulanate to fight against β-lactamase−producing organisms. A recent study showed that amoxicillin-clavulanate is broadly effective against oral anaerobes. Dosage is 13 to 15 mg/kg orally twice daily. Maximum duration of treatment is 30 days.

Clindamycin. Clindamycin is given at a dose rate of 11 mg/kg orally twice daily. This drug is effective against a wide spectrum of organisms, particularly against obligate anaerobes. It is concentrated in neutrophils and found in bone at a concentration similar to that found in serum. It can be used for up to 28 days at a time, although shorter-duration administration is satisfactory in most situations.

Metronidazole. Metronidazole is administered in a recommended dose of 40 to 50 mg/kg orally as a loading dose on the first day, followed by 20 to 25 mg/kg three times daily. It is used for 7 days or less at this dosage. When used intermittently to control chronic gingival or buccal ulceration, it is given at 10 mg/kg twice daily, with a reduction to administration every second or third day on the basis of treatment response. The drug has antibacterial activity only against obligate anaerobes, with very few instances of development of resistance among susceptible microbes. It is absorbed most effectively when given with food. When metronidazole is used for high-dose initial therapy or prolonged intermittent low-dose therapy, the white cell count should be monitored periodically, and the animal should be observed for neurologic signs or signs that indicate exacerbation of known or previously undiagnosed liver disease. Other drugs in this group, such as tinidazole, also are effective in suppressing growth of oral anaerobes.

Tetracycline. Tetracycline has a broad spectrum of antibacterial activity, including anaerobic bacteria.

The oral dose is 20 mg/kg three times daily; it can be used for several weeks at a time at this dose. The drug chelates in bone and teeth, causing discoloration and slowed growth; tetracycline should not be used in skeletally immature animals. Other drugs in the tetracycline group (for example, doxycycline, minocycline) also are useful antibiotics in management of oral diseases.

Spiramycin. Spiramycin has a broad spectrum of activity against aerobic bacteria and an additive or synergistic effect with metronidazole against anaerobic bacteria; it is concentrated in secreted fluids such as saliva and in gingival tissue and bone.

Antiseptic Therapy

Chlorhexidine is a safe and effective oral antiseptic, active against all oral pathogens and particularly effective against plaque organisms. As a 0.5% solution, it can be used safely as an oral rinse during preparation for oral procedures. It is available as a palatable 0.1% solution and gel for daily home use for plaque retardation or cleansing after oral trauma. Its use also is beneficial when a metal or plastic device is required to be in the mouth for prolonged periods. As a 0.5% solution mixed with isopropyl alcohol, it is effective as a skin and oral mucosal disinfectant. Because it loses its effectiveness rapidly when mixed with organic debris, copious flushing is recommended. Long-term use causes dark staining of teeth surfaces, particularly of fissures, and junction lines between tooth structure and restorative materials.

Povidone-iodine surface disinfectants are effective antimicrobial agents in the mouth, but they stain oral tissues yellow-brown and thus are rarely used.

▶ SUGGESTED READINGS

Aller S: Basic prophylaxis and home care, *Compendium* 11:1447, 1989.

Arnbjerg J: *Pasteurella multocida* from canine and feline teeth, with a case report of glossitis calcinosa in a dog caused by *P. multocida, Nord Vet Med* 30:324, 1978.

Attstrom R, Beer MG, Schroeder HE: Clinical and histologic characteristics of normal gingiva in dogs, *J Periodont Res* 10:115, 1975.

Baxter CJ: A survey of dogs' mouths and the effects of hide chews, *Br Vet Dent Newsletter,* 1:2, 1991.

Bell AF: Dental disease in the dog, *J Small Anim Pract* 6:421, 1965.

Bieniek KW, Kupper H: Zur Atiologie und Therapie der Parodontopathien beim Kleintier—unter besonderer Berucksichtigung von parodontalen Implanteten, *Praktische Tierarzt* 11:11, 1988.

Black AP, Crichlow AM, Saunders JR: Bacteremia during ultrasonic teeth cleaning and extraction in the dog, *JAAHA* 16:611, 1980.

Bozzo L: Doenca periodontal em caes: aspectos clinicos e histopatologicos, *Rev Bras Odont* 165:228, 1970.

Boyce E: Microbiology of canine periodontitis, *Proc Vet Dent Forum* 6:59, 1992.

Brown MG, Park JF: Control of dental calculus in experimental beagles, *Lab Anim Care* 18:527, 1968.

Burstone MS, Bond E, Litt CR: Familial gingival hypertrophy in the dog (boxer breed), *Arch Pathol* 54:208, 1952.

Burwasser P, Hill TJ: The effect of hard and soft diets on the gingival tissues of dogs, *J Dent Res* 18:389, 1939.

Calvert DA: Valvular bacterial endocarditis in the dog, *JAVMA* 180:1080, 1982.

Carlsson J, Egelberg J: Local effect of diet on plaque formation and development of gingivitis in dogs, *Odontologisk Revy* 16:42, 1965.

Colyer F: Variations and diseases of the teeth of animal. In Miles AEW, Grigson C, editors: New York, 1990, Cambridge University Press.

Dean TS et al: Metronidazole in the treatment of gingivitis, *Vet Rec* 85:449, 1969.

DeBowes LJ: Systemic effects of oral disease, *Proc Vet Dent Forum* 6:65, 1992.

Duke A: The effects of a chewing device on calculus buildup in the dog, Nylabone Products, Neptune, NJ 1990.

Duke A: Nylon chew device reduces dental calculus, *Vet Forum*, March 1990.

Egelberg J: Local effect of diet on plaque formation and development of gingivitis in dogs, *Odontologisk Revy* 16:31, 1965.

Eisenmenger E, Zetner K: *Veterinary dentistry,* Philadelphia, 1985, Lea & Febiger.

Eisner ER: Treating moderate periodontitis in dogs and cats, *Vet Med* 84:768, 1989.

Emily P: Clinical periodontology, *Vet Focus* 2(1):23, 1990.

Ericsson I, Lindhe J, Rylander H, and Okamoto H: Experimental periodontal breakdown in the dog, *Scand J Dent Res* 83:189, 1975.

Esterre P: Flore buccale des carnivores domestiques et pathologie de la muqueuse associée, *Pointe Veterinaire* 12(56):73, 1981.

Fardal O, Turnbull RS: A review of the literature on use of chlorhexidine in dentistry, *JADA* 112:863, 1986.

Fitch R et al: A warning to clinicians: metronidazole neurotoxicity in a dog, *Prog Vet Neurol* 2:307, 1991.

Franceschini G: Traitement des pyorrhees alveolo-dentaires et parodontoses, *Point Veterinaire* 9(43):55, 1979.

Gad T: Periodontal disease in dogs, *J Periodont Res* 3:268, 1968.

Ghergariu S, Greblea A, Giuglea M, Pais C, Stroia S, Bundaru L: Periodontopathie carencielle chez les chiens, *Zbl Vet Med A* 22:696, 1975.

Golden, AL, Stoller N, Harvey CE: A survey of oral and dental diseases in dogs anesthetized at a veterinary hospital, *JAAHA* 18:891, 1982.

Gompf RE: Bacterial endocarditis, *Proc Kal Kan Symposium,* 4:73, 1983.

Goodson JM, Tanner ACR, Sornberger GC, Socransky SS: Patterns of progression and regression of advanced destructive periodontal disease, *J Clin Periodont* 9:472, 1982.

Grove TK: Periodontal therapy, *Compendium Contin Educ* 5:660, 1983.

Guelfi JF, Legeay Y, Pages JP, Pechereau D, Trouillet JL: Essai comparatif Stomorgyl, spiramycine, metronidazole, dans le traitement des affections oro-pharyngees du chien et du chat, *Rev Med Vet* 141:985, 1990.

Hamlin R: Presentation at Fifth Veterinary Dental Forum, New Orleans, September 1990.

Hamp SE, Lindhe J, Loe H: Long-term effect of chlorhexidine on developing gingivitis in the beagle dog, *J Periodontol Res* 8:63, 1973.

Hamp SE, Olsson SE, Farso-Maden K, Viklands P, Fornell J: A macroscopic and radiologic investigation of dental diseases of the dog, *Vet Radiol* 25:86, 1984.

Hamp SE et al: Prevalence of periodontal disease in the dog. I. Clinical and roentgenographical observations, *IADR Abstr* 53:L4, 119, 1975.

Harari J, Gustafson S, Meinkoth K: Dental bacteremia in cats, *Feline Practice* 19(4):27, 1991.

Harvey CE: The interrelationship of diet and dental health in cats, dogs, *DVM News Magazine* 19:21, 1988.

Harvey CE: Diet and periodontal disease in dogs, *Proc Vet Dent Forum* 1990.

Harvey CE: Treatment planning for peridontal disease in dogs. *JAHHA* 27:592, 1991.

Heigl L, Lindhe J: The effect of metronidazole on the development of plaque and gingivitis in the beagle dog, *J Clin Periodontol* 6:197, 1979.

Helderman WH: Is antibiotic therapy justified in the treatment of human chronic inflammatory periodontal disease? *J Clin Periodontol* 13:932, 1986.

Henke CL, Colmery BH: Treating canine dental infections with oral clindamycin hydrochloride, *Vet Med* 82:197, 1987.

Hennet P: Les inflammations du parodonte du chien et du chat, *Point Veterinaire* 21(125):763, 1989.

Hennet P, Harvey CE: Anaerobes in periodontal disease in the dog—a review, *J Vet Dent* 8(1):9, 1991.

Hennet P, Harvey CE: Anaerobes in periodontal disease in the dog—a review, *J Vet Dent* 8(2):18, 1991.

Hennet P, Harvey CE: Spirochetes in periodontal disease in the dog—a review, *J Vet Dent* 8(3):16, 1991.

Henrikson PA: Periodontal disease and calcium deficiency—an experimental study in the dog, *Acta Odontol Scand* 26:(suppl 50):1, 1968.

Hirst RC: Chlorhexidine: a review of the literature, *J West Soc Periodontol* 20:52, 1972.

Holmberg DL: Abscessation of the mandibular carnassial tooth in the dog, *JAAHA* 15:347, 1979.

Holmstrom SE: Periodontal disease, *Compendium,* 11:1485, 1989.

Hull PS, Davies RM: The effect of chlorhexidine gel on tooth deposits in beagle dogs, *J Small Anim Pract* 13:207, 1972.

Hull PS, Soames JV, Davies RM: Periodontal disease in a beagle dog colony, *J Comp Pathol* 84:143, 1974.

Jackson DA et al: Bacteremia following ultrasonic scaling in the dog, *Proc ACVS,* 1981.

Jeffcoat MK, Williams RC, Wechter WJ, Johnson HG, Kaplan ML, Grandrus JS, Goldhaber P: Flurbiprofen treatment of periodontal disease in beagles, *J Periodont Res* 21:624, 1986.

Johnson LA: A clinical study of the effects of clindamycin hydrochloride on canine dental infections, *J Br Vet Dent Assoc* 2:2, 1990.

Kamata H et al: Oral flora of the dog, *J Jpn Vet Med Assoc* 41:549, 1988.

Karlsson UL, Penney DA: Natural desensitization of exposed tooth roots in dogs, *J Dent Res* 54:982, 1975.

Kostlin VR: Zur Parodontopathia beim Hund, *Kleintierpraxis* 24:159, 1979.

Krasse B, Brill N: Effect of consistency of diet on bacteria in gingival pocket in dogs, *Odontologisk Revy* 11:152, 1960.

Krook L: Periodontal disease in dogs and man, *Adv Vet Sci* 20:171, 1976.

Lage A, Lausen N, Tracy R, Allred E: Effect of chewing rawhide and cereal biscuit on removal of dental calculus in dogs, *JAVMA* 197:213, 1990.

Lang N, Low H: A fluorescent plaque disclosing agent, *J Periodont Res* 7:59, 1972.

Legeros RZ, Shannon IL: The crystalline components of dental calculi: human vs. dog, *J Dent Res* 58:2371, 1979.

Lindhe J, Ericcson I: Effect of ligature placement and dental plaque on periodontal tissue breakdown in the dog, *J Periodont* 49:343, 1978.

Lindhe J, Hamp SV, Loe H: Plaque induced periodontal disease in beagle dogs, *J Periodont Res* 10:243, 1975.

Lindhe J, Rylander H: Experimental gingivitis in young dogs, *Scand J Dent Res* 83:314, 1975.

Lindhe J et al: Influence of topical application of chlorhexidine on chronic gingivitis and gingival wound healing in the dog, *Scand J Dent Res* 78:471, 1970.

Listgarten MA, Lindhe J, Parodi R: The effect of systemic antimicrobial therapy on plaque and gingivitis in dogs, *J Periodont Res* 14:65, 1979.

Loret J: Etude de l'efficacite in vivo in vitro de l'association spiramycine—metronidazole sur la flore parodontale apres induction experimentale d'une paradontite chez le chien, these, Toulouse, France, 1990. Universite Paul Sabatier de Toulouse.

Loux JJ, Alioto R, Yankell SL: Effects of glucose and urea on dental deposit pH in dogs, *J Dent Res* 15:1610, 1972.

Lyon KF: Feline caries, *Vet Focus* 2:27, 1990.

Mallonee DH, Harvey CE, Venner M, Hammond BF: Bacteriology of periodontal disease in the cat, *Arch Oral Biol* 33:677, 1988.

Meyer R, Suter G: Epidemiologische und morphologische Untersuchungen am Hundege-biss, *Schweiz Arch Tierheilkd* 118:307, 1976.

Morgan JP, Miyabayashi T, Anderson J, Klinge B: Periodontal bone loss in the aging beagle dog—a radiographic study, *J Clin Periodont* 17:630, 1990.

Morris RP, Person P, Cohen DW: Effects of soft dietary consistency and protein deprivation on the periodontium of the dog, *Oral Surg Oral Med Oral Pathol* 15:1061, 1962.

Nuki K, Cooper SH: The role of inflammation in the pathogenesis of gingival enlargement during the administration of diphenylhydantoin sodium in cats, *J Periodont Res* 7:102, 1972.

Nyman S et al: The effect of progressive tooth mobility on destructive periodontitis in the dog, *J Clin Periodontol* 5:213, 1978.

Page RC, Schroeder HE: Spontaneous chronic periodontitis in adult dogs: a clinical and histopathological survey, *J Periodontol* 52:60, 1979.

Page RC, Schroeder HE: Periodontitis in man and other animals—a comparative review, 1982, Basel, Switzerland, Karger Publishers.

Reed JH: A review of the experimental use of antimicrobial agents in the treatment of periodontitis and gingivitis in the dog, *Can Vet J* 29:705, 1988.

Richardson RL: Effect of administering antibiotics, removing the major salivary glands, and tooth brushing on dental calculi formation in the cat, *Arch Oral Biol* 10:245, 1965.

Rosenberg HM, Rehfeld CE, Emmering TE: A method for the epidemiologic assessment of periodontal health-disease state in a beagle hound colony, *J Periodontol* 37:208, 1966.

Rost DR, Baker R: Gingival hyperplasia induced by sodium diphenylhydantoin in the dog—a case report, *Vet Med / Small Anim Clinician* 73:585, 1978.

Rowland GN, Fetter AW: Nutritional secondary hyperparathyroidism. In Bojrab MJ, editor: *Pathophysiology in small animal surgery,* Philadelphia, 1981, Lea & Febiger.

Sangnes G: A pilot study on the effect of toothbrushing on the gingiva of a beagle dog, *Scand J Dent Res* 84:106, 1976.

Sarkiala E: Effect of scaling and tinidazole compared to scaling alone in dogs with periodontitis, *Proc Vet Dent Forum* 6:69, 1992.

Saxe SR, Greene JC, Bohannan HM, Vermillion JR: Oral debris, calculus, and periodontal disease in the beagle dog, *Periodontics* 5:217, 1967.

Schebitz H: Zur Parodontopathia beim Hund, *Kleinterpraxis* 24:159, 1979.

Schneider VE, Schimke E, Schneider HJ: Ergebnisse von Zahnsteinanalysen beim Kleinter, *Mh Vet-Med* 35:707, 1980.

Schroeder HE, Attstrom R: Effect of mechanical plaque control on development of subgingival plaque and initial gingivitis in neutropenic dogs, *Scand J Dent Res* 87:279, 1979.

Schroeder HE, Lindhe J: Conversion of stable established gingivitis in the dog into destructive periodontitis, *Arch Oral Biol* 20:775, 1975.

Schroeder HE, Lindhe J: Conditions and pathological features of rapidly destructive, experimental periodontitis in dogs, *J Periodontol* 51:6, 1980.

Silver JG, Martin L, McBride BC: Recovery and clearance of oral microorganisms following experimental bacteraemia in dogs, *Arch Oral Biol* 20:675, 1975.

Smith MM, Zontine WJ, Willits NH: A correlative study of the clinical and radiographic signs of periodontal disease in dogs, *JAVMA* 186:1286, 1985.

Soames JV, Davis RM: The structure of subgingival plaque in a beagle dog, *J Periodont Res* 9:333, 1974.

Studer E, Stapley RB: The role of dry foods in maintaining healthy teeth and gums in the cat, *Vet Med/Small Anim Clinician* 68:1124, 1973.

Survey on the health of pet animals, *Jpn Small Anim Vet Assoc* 1985.

Svanberg G, Lindhe J, Hugoson A, Grondahl H-G: Effect of nutritional hyper-parathyroidism on experimental periodontitis in the dog, *Scand J Dent Res* 81:155, 1973.

Svanberg G, Syed SA, Scott BW: Differences between gingivitis and periodontitis associated microbial flora in the beagle dog, *J Periodont Res* 17:1, 1982.

Syed SA et al: The predominant cultivable dental plaque flora of beagle dogs with gingivitis, *J Periodont Res* 15:123, 1980.

Whitney LF: Dog biscuits and clean teeth, *Vet Med* 55:56, 1960.

Withrow SJ: Dental extraction as a probable cause of septicemia in a dog, *JAAHA* 15:345, 1979.

Wright JG: Some observations on dental disease in the dog, *Vet Rec* 51:409, 1989.

Yankell SL, Moreno OM, Saffir AJ, Lowary RL, Gold W: Effects of chlorhexidine and four antimicrobial compounds on plaque, gingivitis and staining in beagle dogs, *J Dent Res* 61:1089, 1982.

Zetner K: Atiologie, Pathogenese und Therapie von Zahnbett-krankheiten beim Kleintier, *Wien Tierarztl Mschr* 68:130, 1981.

Zetner K: Etiology, pathogenesis and treatment of gingivitis and periodontitis in small animals, *Tierarztl Umschau* 36:414, 1981.

Zetner K: Der Einfluss von Kollagen-sticks ("Kauknochen") auf die Plaqueakkumulation beim Hund, *Kleinterpraxis* 28:315, 1983.

Zontine WJ, Sims S, Donovan ML: Bacterial environmental contamination associated with ultrasonic dental procedures in dog, *JAAHA* 5:150, 1969.

5

Oral Inflammatory and Immune-Mediated Diseases

Chapter 4 describes periodontal disease that results from inflammatory-mediated tissue responses to oral 2bacteria. The discussion in this chapter focuses on the other oral inflammatory diseases encountered in dogs and cats. This division might seem arbitrary. For instance, acute necrotizing ulcerative gingivitis in dogs and gingivostomatitis in cats are induced or exacerbated by oral microflora, yet they differ in important aspects from the typical sequential pattern of periodontal disease described in Chapter 4: gingivitis, periodontitis, exfoliation. These differences are of great clinical significance and deserve separate consideration for that reason.

The inflammatory response generally is considered to be a useful protective response. When, however, the response is exaggerated, or stimulated when no external threat exists, the inflammatory response can lead to deleterious effects. In addition, if an inadequate response is mounted, the initiating disease becomes more readily established and may overwhelm the local tissues. An additional factor at work in oral tissues is the constant but wide-ranging flora to which oral tissues are subject.

▶ CONDITIONS RESULTING FROM IMMUNE SYSTEM SUPPRESSION OR FUNCTIONAL DERANGEMENT

In otherwise normal animals, suppression of inflammation by use of nonsteriodal antiinflammatory drugs slows or stops tissue loss associated with plaque accumulation, and there is no clear clinical correlation between worsening periodontal disease and chronic use of steroidal antiinflammatory drugs for management of dermatologic conditions and other problems. Certain clinical syndromes, however, result from immunologic abnormalities and cause suppression of local or systemic immune responses.

Necrotizing Ulcerative Gingivostomatitis

Necrotizing ulcerative gingivostomatitis (ulceromembranous stomatitis, Vincent's stomatitis, trench mouth), which is a severe but uncommon form of gingivostomatitis in dogs, is associated with *Fusobacterium* spp. and spirochetes. Because many other bacteria also are usually present, no reliable evidence exists that *Fusobacterium* organisms and spirochetes are a prime cause of this condition. The feline equivalent may be gingivostomatitis (see p. 150), although this usually is a more chronic disease. Severe gingivitis, with painful bleeding gums, occurs initially. The first lesions, as seen in experimentally induced disease, develop as ulcers on acutely inflamed interdental papillae. The condition may progress to necrosis of soft tissues and exposure of bone, or it may remain largely confined to the gingival tissues (acute necrotizing ulcerative gingivitis [ANUG]). Sometimes it spreads to adjacent buccal tissues as a generalized stomatitis (ulceromembranous stomatitis). An underlying cause, often unidentified, decreases oral resistance to infection. Stress can lead to this condition in humans (for example, trench mouth in soldiers ordered into battle), and corticosteroid administration can precipitate episodes in beagle dogs known to be at genetic risk for this disease. Signs are halitosis, salivation, and severe hyperemia or necrosis of the oral mucosa (see Figs. A-39 and A-40, p. 59). Differential diagnoses include thallium toxicity, leptospirosis, and severe uremic periodontal disease. The lesions of the condition in dogs known as *ulcerative stomatitis* are more specific (see next section). Treatment consists of teeth scaling, other procedures indicated for management of such conditions as deep periodontal pockets (see Chapter 4), and antibiotic administration (amoxicillin-clavulanate, clindamycin, metronidazole, or tetracycline; see p. 140 for dosages), followed by a maintenance program of tooth brushing or irrigation with a plaque retardant if the dog is compliant. If the signs recur, long-term administration of metronidazole every other day or every third day (see p. 140) may control some cases. An attempt should be made to identify and correct possible causes of the decreased resistance, such as malnutrition, hypothyroidism, systemic infection, immunopathologic factors, and physical or emotional stress. Extraction of teeth is an appropriate salvage treatment for chronically recurrent cases with severe acute episodes, particularly if the response to antibiotic therapy is poor.

Ulcerative Stomatitis

Ulcerative stomatitis is a condition seen in dogs in which ulcers (contact ulcers, "kissing" lesions) form on the oral mucosal surfaces that are in contact with the plaque-laden surfaces of the teeth (see Figs. A-41 and A-42, p. 59). The most clinically obvious lesions are on the buccal mucosa of the upper lip, typically affecting the mucosa that lies against the upper canine and carnassial teeth. Lesions also can be found in some affected dogs on the lateral margins of the tongue (see Fig. A-20, p. 54), from contact with the lingual surface of lower teeth. The palatal mucosa immediately adjacent to the palatal surface of the upper premolar and molar teeth may be flattened and inflamed, depigmented, or ulcerated (see Fig. A-110, p. 78). The condition occurs in family clusters in Maltese dogs (recognized in this breed as a familial problem since at least the 1940s) and sporadically in other breeds. Typically, no detectable lesions are present elsewhere on the body. Affected dogs have significantly increased serum immunoglobulin concentration, and there is evidence of immune complex formation in the ulcerated tissues, which suggests a local (mucosal) immunopathy, with secondary bacterial invasion and antibody production by deeper immunoreactive cells. The flora cultured from the ulcers is a mixed aerobic-anaerobic bacterial population, with no predominant organism suggestive of an etiologic agent.

Affected dogs often have so much pain that drastic treatment is resorted to at an early age; many Maltese dogs from affected breeding lines have had all their teeth extracted by 4 years of age. Antibiotic therapy provides only temporary improvement. Antiinflammatory treatment (for example, prednisolone 1 mg/kg twice daily for 5 days, reducing to 0.5 mg daily or every other day for 2 weeks) gives more prolonged benefit, but recurrence is expected. Extraction of teeth is curative, but this is a demanding procedure because the periodontal fiber attachments rarely are affected by the disease. Particular care is necessary in young, small-breed dogs undergoing extensive extractions (see discussion of extraction in Chapter 10).

Immune-Mediated Mycotic Infection: Candidiasis

Candidal lesions are described in Chapter 3 (see Fig. A-7, p. 50). Treatment includes elimination of the underlying cause if identified; nonspecific stimulation of the immune system (for example, levamisole therapy) combined with local rinsing with an antifungal agent such as nystatin; or systemic antifungal therapy (ketoconazole 10 mg/kg daily by mouth for 4 to 6 weeks).

Neutrophil Dysfunction, or Neutropenia

Failure of function or lack of sufficient neutrophils results in development of overwhelming infections, particularly in tissues subjected to constant bacterial bombardment, such as the oral cavity. Causes are the gray collie syndrome (cyclic neutropenia), high-dose whole body radiation, drug therapy (for example, cyclophosphamide, doxorubricin, cephalosporin), exogenous estrogen toxicity, chloramphenicol toxicity in cats, phenylbutazone toxicity in dogs, and viral diseases such as parvovirus and feline leukemia virus (FeLV).

► AUTOIMMUNE ORAL DISEASES

Bullous Autoimmune Skin Diseases

Bullous conditions result from autoantibody production against specific squamous epithelial structures. Clinically, this leads to development of bullae within the skin and oral stratified squamous epithelium. Bleb formation, erosion, and ulceration of the skin and mucous membranes, especially the mouth (see Fig. A-111, p. 78), are seen, with frequent involvement of the mucocutaneous junctions. Several syndromes have been characterized microscopically by immunofluorescence techniques, although they are impossible to separate by clinical examination only. Oral lesions are significant aspects of the syndrome in dogs, with oral involvement in 90% of cases of *pemphigus vulgaris* and in 50% of cases of *bullous pemphigoid.*

Sometimes the oral lesions are the most prominent or the only lesions. The vesicles are characteristic but may no longer be present at the time of diagnosis, replaced by more nonspecific ulceration and inflammation. Diagnosis is by biopsy and immunofluorescence testing. Both conditions have been reported in cats, more commonly pemphigus vulgaris. These lesions are both confirmed and differentiated by standard microscopic and immunofluorescent examination. In pemphigus vulgaris the causative lesions are suprabasilar intercellular clefts, with formation of acanthocytes. In bullous pemphigoid the causative lesion is subepidermal, with no acanthotic formation. Both conditions result in local complement cascade activation, with secondary neutrophilic and/or eosinophilic infiltration and increased capillary permeability.

Lupus Erythematosus

Systemic lupus erythematosus is a multisystem disorder caused by autoantibody production against nuclear and tissue proteins. Oral lesions in dogs appear as gingivitis and shallow painful ulceration, with a surrounding erythematous margin; chronic ulcers may heal with fibrosis and scarring (see Fig. A-37, p. 58). No oral lesions have been described in the cat. Microscopic examination reveals immunoglobulin deposition at the dermoepidermal junction. Diagnosis is confirmed by antinuclear antibody test, lupus erythematosus preparation, biopsy, and immunofluorescence assay.

Discoid lupus erythematosus is a benign form of systemic lupus erythematosus, with lesions restricted to the skin and oral cavity of the dog. The lesions manifest as hypopigmentation of the nasal plane, lips, and gums, and oral ulceration, especially of the tongue, may occur in dogs (see Fig. A-3, *B*, p. 49). Diagnosis is by immunoserologic testing, biopsy, and immunofluorescence assay.

Other autoimmune skin conditions, such as pemphigus foliaceus and pemphigus erythematosus, rarely cause oral lesions, or the oral lesions are a minor part of the syndrome. Although autoimmune skin disorders occur rather commonly in oral tissues and sometimes are seen only as oral lesions, atopic disease (allergic skin disease) rarely causes oral mucosal lesions in dogs (except when the oral mucosa is traumatized by scratching or rubbing facial or ear lesions).

Management

Animals with autoimmune disease limited to or centered mainly in the oral cavity tend to respond well to immunosuppressive corticosteroid therapy (for example, prednisolone, 2 to 3 mg/kg twice daily, decreasing after 10 days, if the oral lesions are resolving, to a dose of 1 mg/kg every 48 hours over a 4-week period). If improvement does not occur in the first 10 days of prednisolone therapy, combination immunosuppressive therapy is substituted (such as azathioprine 2 mg/kg twice daily). In some cases, lifelong intermittent treatment (every second or third day) may be needed.

Miscellaneous Disorders

Sjögren's syndrome

Dogs with keratoconjunctivitis sicca (KCS) tend to have dry mouths and significant periodontal disease; this condition may represent a canine form of Sjögren's syndrome (a triad in humans consisting of KCS, xerostomia, and a generalized connective tissue disorder that is believed to be of autoimmune origin). If parotid duct transposition is considered, parotid function should be assessed before surgery. The mucosa around the duct papilla should be smooth and glistening, and reflex salivation should be obvious as increased wetness in the papillary area after stimulation with a drop of bitter-tasting ophthalmic atropine solution placed on the animal's tongue. Good oral hygiene (see Chapter 4), is necessary to eliminate discomfort in animals with xerostomia (see Fig. A-15, p. 52).

Thrombocytopenia

Whatever the cause of thrombocytopenia, petechiae on the oral mucosa or bleeding from the gingival margin can result. In addition, drug reactions can cause severe inflammation progressing to ulceration. The most common triggering drugs are antibiotics.

Gingivostomatitis in cats

Recently it has been suggested that one possible cause for this condition is autoimmunity to type I or III collagen that is induced by bacterial activity. This condition is discussed further on p. 150.

Masticatory Muscle Myositis

Masticatory muscle myositis includes the conditions known as eosinophilic myositis and atrophic myositis of masticatory muscles. The pathophysiology, clinical signs, and diagnosis are described in Chapter 3.

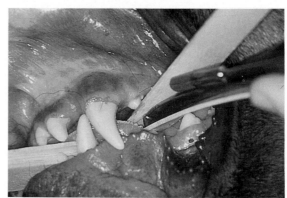
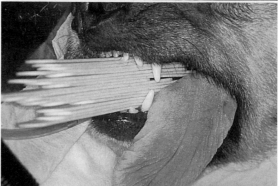
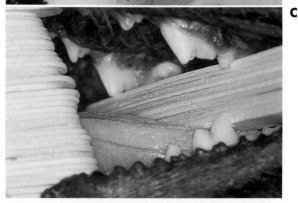

FIGURE 5-1

Masticatory myositis in a dog. Before starting the wedge-levering treatment, the mouth could be opened only 3 mm between the cusps of the upper and lower incisor teeth. **A** and **B,** Use of tongue depressors to lever the mouth open, starting at the incisor teeth. **C,** As the mouth is opened, the leverage point is moved caudally to the molar teeth to reduce the likelihood of jaw fracture.

Treatment consists of immunosuppressant medication (see p. 147) if there is still some ability to open the mouth; this therapy often needs to be continued for several months or used intermittently. If the mouth cannot be opened under general anesthesia, the only remaining option is forceful opening, followed by medical treatment as already described. Forceful opening of the mouth can be achieved by wedging, for example, tongue depressors (to prevent fracture of the enamel) between teeth (Fig. 5-1); the tongue depressors are tapped between the teeth with an orthopedic mallet or carpenter's hammer. As the mouth is forced open, the location for applying the wedging force is moved caudally to reduce the likelihood of fracturing the jaws (Fig. 5-1, *C*).

► HYPERSENSITIVITY CONDITIONS

Drug Eruptions

Acute hypersensitivity reactions can result from drug ingestion, especially sulfa drugs and antibiotics, including penicillins, chloramphenicol, cephalosporins, and tetracycline. Ulceration of oral mucosa occurs, sometimes with hemorrhage and edema, leading to massive soft tissue destruction; the nonulcerated adjacent mucosa may separate from the underlying connective tissue, resulting in necrosis. Diagnosis is made from a history of recent ingestion of a drug known to cause hypersensitivity response and resolution of the condition after cessation of drug therapy.

Toxic Epidermal Necrolysis

This eruption is the most extreme form of drug reaction; the animal is depressed, febrile, and inappetent, and the cutaneous lesions are painful. The oral epidermis sloughs, leaving an ulcer or ulcers (see Fig. A-13, p. 52); mucocutaneous junction and oral ulcerations are common. The only treatment necessary is to cease administration of the causative chemical and to provide nursing care (soft food by tube or parenteral nutrition; gentle oral irrigation with dilute chlorhexidine solution).

Insect Stings

Intraoral insect stings can cause hypersensitivity and significant inflammatory swelling, although this reaction is rare and short-lived. Antiinflammatory medication by injection hastens resolution of this condition. Snake bites can cause similar acute oral swellings, although these are more commonly extraoral (lip or muzzle) than intraoral.

Gingivostomatitis in Cats

Recent preliminary work suggests that some cats with this condition or set of conditions have elevated IgE concentrations, including antibodies to common household or seasonal antigens or both. This condition is described on p. 150.

► MISCELLANEOUS INFLAMMATION-ASSOCIATED CONDITIONS*

Eosinophilic Granuloma

Feline eosinophilic granuloma complex

In cats, this disorder may manifest as an eosinophilic ulcer starting on the midline of the upper lip (see Fig. A-36, p. 58) or as isolated raised firm ulcers on the tongue, palate, or pharynx. The surface often is speckled with small dense white areas (see Figs. A-5 and A-106). This is an idiopathic lesion, although clustering of cases in households suggests a possible infectious or allergic cause. It is three times more frequent in females than males. Diagnosis is by biopsy or cytologic examination of lesional tissue, which shows ulceration and proliferation of granulation tissue, with infiltration of eosinophils, histiocytes, and lymphocytes. Circulating eosinophilia is rare. Treatment is described later in this section.

Canine eosinophilic granuloma

A similar lesion is recognized as occurring primarily on the tongue of the dog, most often in huskies and malamutes. The lesions are raised, firm, brownish pink irregular masses that may be ulcerated and extend along the lateral margin and frenulum of the tongue (see Fig. A-19, p. 54). Microscopic examination reveals degenerated collagen surrounded by histiocytes and epithelioid cells, with infiltration of eosinophils as a constant feature. Peripheral eosinophilia is an inconsistent feature. The breed predilection for the

---

*This section is adapted from Harvey CE: Oral inflammatory diseases in cats, *JAAHA* 27:585, 1991.

canine syndrome suggests a possible hereditary factor. We have seen the same microscopic pattern in biopsies of scattered soft palate or pharyngeal lesion in two unrelated Cavalier King Charles spaniels and a beagle dog (see Fig. A-107, p. 77).

Treatment

Treatment of eosinophilic granuloma lesions initially consists of prednisolone (1 mg/kg daily in two doses, tapered after 1 week to 0.2 mg/kg every other day over a 4-week period). Injection of repository corticosteroid medication (for example, methylprednisolone or triamcinolone, 5 to 10 mg) can be used if oral prednisolone is not satisfactory or after recurrence. Radiation and cryosurgery will halt the disease process but are more destructive of surrounding tissue.

Feline Gingivostomatitis-Pharyngitis

The condition or collection of conditions known as feline gingivostomatitis, gingivopharyngitis, or plasmacytic-lymphocytic gingivopharyngitis is a major source of frustration for small animal veterinarians and cat owners. Plasmacytic-lymphocytic infiltration of local tissues and hypergammaglobulinemia occur; however, these features are expected responses to chronic infiltration of bacteria or other antigenic stimulants. This condition is separate from the sequential pattern of periodontal disease seen in dogs: plaque and calculus accumulation, tissue loss, and tooth loss. Some cats do show the more typical periodontal disease pattern (see Figs. A-86 and A-87, p. 71). The major differentiating clinical factor with gingivostomatitis in cats is the severity of the continuing acute inflammation: the affected tissues are fire-engine red.

Clinical Presentations

A wide range of clinical presentations may represent stages of the same disease process or may be separate diseases.

Acute "marginal" gingivitis

The only tissue affected is the gingiva itself (see Fig. A-88, p. 72). This condition is not specifically "marginal" gingivitis; it often affects the entire marginal and attached gingiva (the marginal gingiva is a narrow zone that covers the gingival sulcus; however, the total gingival height in cats is so small that the red line seen in this condition appears to be a margin when in many cases it affects the entire attached gingiva, which is less than 3 mm high around premolar teeth). This condition is common in young cats, possibly more so in pure breeds in which it may progress to more widespread disease. It is seen in severe form in the incisor area of some cats (see Fig. A-89, p. 72).

Severe gingivitis with stomatitis

The grossly obvious inflammation extends across the mucogingival junction onto the more sensitive buccal (and less often sublingual) mucosa, particularly in premolar and molar areas (see Fig. A-92, p. 73). Purebred cats are more likely to be affected.

Severe stomatitis with gingivitis-faucitis

The condition is most obvious clinically in the areas that are most visible on superficial inspection of a wide-open mouth: the glossopalatine fold (fauces) (see Fig. A-92, p. 73). Whether glossopalatine-fold stomatitis (faucitis) always is preceded by gingival inflammation is not known, although gingival inflammation is present as part of the established disease. Purebred cats appear to be more commonly affected.

Severe oropharyngitis

Severe oropharyngitis manifests grossly obvious inflammation of the caudal oral cavity and oropharynx (see Fig. A-93, p. 73). This caudally centered disease is most likely to be seen in chronically affected cats that have been treated by extraction of premolar and molar teeth, which may resolve or lessen disease centered on the gingival tissues.

External odontoclastic tooth resorption and eosinophilic granuloma also are inflammatory-associated feline oral diseases. Clinically, external resorption lesions are accompanied by gingival inflammation, which may be limited to the area of the tooth lesion. It is not known whether these lesions develop without inflammation and the subsequent inflammation is caused by the resultant rough, plaque-retentive surface or whether the inflammation is an essential step. External odontoclastic resorptive lesions are described further in Chapter 7. Eosinophilic granuloma is described earlier in this chapter.

In 1986 members of the American Veterinary Dental Society indicated that gingivostomatitis was a common occurrence; 72% of respondents reported seeing one or more cases each week, with a clinical impression that purebred cats, particularly Siamese and Abyssinians, are most commonly involved. Studies of 200 cats in Europe and of cats in California from a veterinary hospital, humane society, and commercial pure-breed cattery also showed an increased incidence of disease in purebred cats. As of January 1993, preliminary reports indicate that the prevalence of severe gingivitis-stomatitis may be decreasing in the United States and Europe.

Etiologic Factors

Possible causes of the plasmacytic-lymphocytic inflammatory oral conditions in cats include bacteria, viruses, and immunologic abnormalities.

Bacteria

The aerobic and anaerobic bacteria isolated from cats with gingivitis and periodontitis are similar in type and colony percentage to those found in humans and dogs with gingivitis and periodontitis (see Table 4-3). The predominant organisms in severely affected areas are black-pigmented *Bacteroides, Peptostreptococcus,* and *Fusobacterium* spp. Spirochetes are common in wet mount preparations. *Pasteurella multocida* isolates, which are common in the mouth and pharynx, are less prevalent in affected areas of the gingiva compared with unaffected areas. Antibodies to *Bacteroides gingivalis, B. intermedius,* and *Actinobacillus actinomycetemcomitans* were found in significantly elevated concentrations. However, *Pasteurella* sp. (very common in the mouth of cats) and *A. actinomycetemcomitans* antibodies cross-react. These studies suggest that if oral inflammatory diseases in cats are more severe than is generally the case in other species, infection by specific bacteria is unlikely to be the cause.

Viruses

FeLV infection is not associated with a higher prevalence of oral lesions, although FeLV-infected cats often have severe gingival inflammation.

Calicivirus is much more common in oral fluids of affected cats than in unaffected cats. However, virus isolation testing of washed gingival samples and im-

munoperoxidase staining for calicivirus antigen within affected gingival tissues have failed to reveal the presence of virus consistently in tissues overlain by virus-positive oral fluid. Strain-identification by means of serum-neutralization tests has shown no particular subgroup of calicivirus isolates from cats with chronic stomatitis. In a 10-month pilot study a calicivirus isolate from oral fluid of an affected cat caused acute oral ulceration in cats that were specific-pathogen free but did not lead to development of clinically obvious gingivostomatitis lesions. Calcivirus isolates from cats with faucitis do cause short-term faucitis and gingivitis in specific pathogen–free cats, although the lesions resolve after several weeks.

The evidence for feline immunodeficiency virus (FIV) as a causative agent or coagent also is unclear. Cats with chronic stomatitis often show FIV positivity and oral inflammation is the most common clinically obvious abnormality in FIV-positive cats. However, a high FIV-positive rate has been reported in one set of control cats matched for age, breed, and sex. Many cats with severe oral inflammatory disease are FIV-negative, including cats with a chronic history of oral lesions that do not develop any of the other lesions associated with FIV infection. It seems likely that FIV-induced immunosuppression may cause a predisposition to development of oral lesions, but no direct etiologic relationship exists between FIV and oral inflammatory disease in cats. One study found no correlation between feline calicivirus (FCV) and FIV infection in cats with gingivostomatitis. Another study, however, showed an increased severity of oral disease in FIV- and FCV-infected cats compared with FIV-positive but FCV-negative cats; challenge with FCV in FIV-infected cats caused increased severity of acute oronasal signs compared with FIV-negative cats challenged with FCV.

Immunologic abnormalities

There is a similarity between severe oral inflammatory diseases in cats and the oral syndrome seen in mink with Chédiak-Higashi syndrome, which affects function of neutrophils. No discernible differences, however, could be demonstrated in function of neutrophils from affected cats compared with control cats; both groups showed responses to stimulation within the expected range for human neutrophils. Serum IgA,

IgG, and IgM levels are all increased in affected cats. Circulating antibodies to *Bacteroides gingivalis, B. intermedius,* and *A. actinomycetemcomitans* were all increased in affected cats; however, because of biochemical similarity and antigenic cross-reactivity, the antibodies identified as *A. actinomycetemcomitans* may be *Pasteurella* spp. antibodies. There is no histologic evidence to suggest epithelial autoantigen autoimmunity as an etiologic factor. Hypersensitivity response to an unidentified antigen is possible but unproved; a recent pilot study showed increased circulating IgE in affected cats.

There are many similarities, clinical and pathologic, between severe feline oral inflammatory disease and idiopathic gingivostomatitis in humans who habitually chew gum; this condition is a hypersensitivity response to the essential oil flavorings. Cessation of gum chewing leads to resolution of the condition. However, hypoallergenic diets rarely are clinically useful as treatment of affected cats.

Clinical and Radiologic Studies

Mean gingival indexes are significantly higher in affected cats. Gingival inflammation progresses with increased amounts of plaque and calculus, but on the basis of the extent of the plaque and calculus present, gingival inflammation is relatively more severe than would be expected in other species.

In one study, radiographic evidence of loss of the tooth or severe periodontal bone loss was evident around 47% of incisor teeth; less than 10% of canine and upper second, third, and fourth premolar teeth and lower third and fourth premolar teeth; 39% of upper first molar teeth; and 53% of lower first molar teeth. The pattern of bone loss was generally horizontal. Irregular absence of tooth structure compatible with an external odontoclastic resorption (neck lesion) was seen commonly in both upper and lower incisor teeth (35%), upper second and lower third premolar teeth (26%), and upper and lower first molar teeth (35%). A radiographically visible root tip with no visible crown was present in 20% of upper incisor teeth, 22% of lower incisor teeth, and 7% of lower first molar teeth. Increasing severity of bone loss was correlated with increasing extent of loss of tooth structure as a result of external resorption.

Pathologic Studies

Biopsy samples were obtained from both most severely and least severely affected areas of the mouth of a group of affected cats. In the most severely affected areas, the predominant inflammatory cell type found in about half the samples was the neutrophil. Lymphocytes and plasma cells were each found to be the predominant inflammatory cell types in about a quarter of the samples. Although no significant correlation was found between the gingival index and the type of inflammatory cell predominating, a significant correlation could be demonstrated between the gingival index and the extent of plasma cell and neutrophil infiltrate. The biopsy specimens were categorized as "essentially normal," "mild-moderate acute disease," "mild-moderate chronic disease," and "severe chronic disease." Microscopic examination revealed a significant correlation between the gingival index and the microscopic extent of disease in the samples from the area that was most affected.

Much remains to be studied regarding the etiology and pathogenesis of chronic oral inflammatory diseases in cats.

Treatment of Gingivostomatitis

Many treatments have been used, which suggests that not one treatment has uniformly satisfactory results. Some subjective evidence exists that dry food prevents gingival inflammation and build-up of calculus compared with canned food. Also, a diet high in raw liver appears to increase gingival inflammation in young cats.

Antibiotic therapy

Antibiotic therapy almost always produces short-term benefit by restoring appetite and reducing discomfort, but rapid recurrence follows. For longer-term use, the antibiotic drugs of choice are amoxicillin-clavulanate, clindamycin, metronidazole, and tetracycline (see Chapter 4).

Periodontal prophylaxis

Treatment by teeth scaling (described in Chapter 4), followed by brushing several times weekly with 0.2% chlorhexidine, was assessed by periodic examination of periodontal indexes. All owners of pet cats reported that they were no longer willing or able to brush within 6 months of teeth cleaning. Brushing was continued in a closed colony of cats. The calculus index was significantly lower at 6 months compared with prescaling, as expected, but had increased close to prescaling values by 12 months; plaque index and gingival index were not significantly changed. This treatment regimen did not prevent redevelopment of the prescaling anaerobe-dominated gingival flora. Another study showed that brushing once or twice weekly significantly retards calculus formation on the brushed side compared with the unbrushed side. As has been shown in many human studies, the quality and duration of brushing is critical; many cats are not willing participants in oral home care.

Antiviral treatment

Preliminary results of antiviral (FIV) treatment with zidovudine (AZT) and 2-phosphorylmethoxy ethyl adenine (PMEA) suggest that further study may be valuable in FIV-positive cats.

Antiinflammatory drugs

Antiinflammatory drugs often have been used and usually produce improvement that lasts longer than does a course of antibiotics. Treatment with scaling and polishing, extraction of severely affected teeth, subgingival injection of triamcinolone (maximum 10 mg/cat), and oral spiramycin-metronidazole produced excellent long-term results in 90% of affected cats. This result, however, in part may be due to the extractions performed or to the prolonged effect of metronidazole on gingival pocket flora.

Local and systemic use of a nonsteroidal antiinflammatory drug (NSAID) in dogs has been shown to halt the destructive effect of plaque-induced gingival disease, prompting a recent pilot study of the use of NSAID in cats. Twelve cats with chronic gingivostomatitis had their teeth scaled and polished and then were treated with sodium salicylate (25 mg/kg) daily, either by smearing it on gingival margins or by capsule for 4 weeks, or they were given a placebo. The cats treated with salicylate were more comfortable than those treated with placebo. A dosage frequency as low as once every 3 days may maintain adequate tissue concentrations.

The concentration of lymphocytes in affected tissues suggests that antilymphocyte drugs such as cyclosporine may be useful; however, a preliminary trial in three cats did not produce significant or prolonged clinical improvement.

A recent study suggested that a beneficial response could be obtained in some cats with local application of PIND-ORF, a stimulant of paramunity; this material is not available in the United States.

Extraction of teeth

All teeth in arcades affected with severe gingivostomatitis should be extracted if extraction is selected as a salvage treatment. This generally requires extraction of all premolars and molars on both sides and both jaws (Fig. 5-2, A). This is not a simple, short procedure (see Chapter 10); however, significant improvement often occurs within a short period (Fig. 5-2, B and C). Good results after extraction of all teeth (or at least all premolars and molars) have been reported. In one series of nine cats, six did well, although one required intermittent prednisolone therapy to control continuing oral inflammation and three had recurrence of severe disease; continuous prednisolone therapy subsequently controlled the disease in one cat, and two were killed. In a series of 12 cats treated by extraction and cryosurgery, eight showed good long-term effects, one improved but was never completely normal, one improved but became diabetic and was killed, and recurrence of significant inflammation developed in two, requiring subsequent steroid or megestrol treatment. One possible reason for the approximately 25% poor or incomplete response in these two series is that root segments without crowns may have been left in place. If extraction is to be performed as a salvage treatment, the jaws should be radiographed after extraction to search for any remaining fragments. Aggressive removal of root fragments and radiographically confirmed diseased bone reduces the likelihood of recurrent disease to close to zero.

Miscellaneous treatments

Recently, use of a soft tissue laser has been proposed as a way of hastening resolution of severe lesions. In a preliminary series of eight cases, improve-

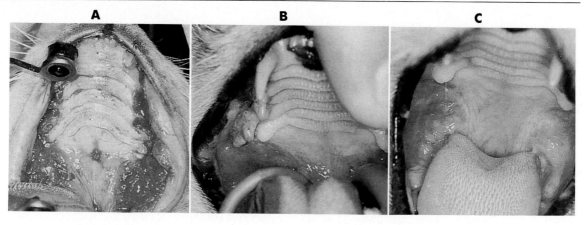

FIGURE 5-2
A, Immediate postsurgical appearance after extraction of all premolar and molar teeth in a cat with gingivostomatitis-faucitis. **B,** Cat with gingivofaucitis immediately before extraction. **C,** Same cat as shown in **B** 4 days after extraction; the fauces are significantly less inflamed.

ment was seen in some cats but not in others. Other proposed but undocumented treatments include vitamin therapy and acupuncture.

The current frustration with our attempts to treat and prevent oral inflammatory diseases in cats is not surprising given that there is much that we do not know about these conditions. Studies designed to investigate the responses of oral tissues to oral flora may be more successful than recent studies seeking a specific etiologic agent. Meanwhile, treatments based on attempts to control oral flora (antibiotic therapy, plaque control agents) and to suppress the inflammatory response provide the best conservative option. For nonresponsive cases, extraction of all premolar and molar teeth is recommended.

▶ SUGGESTED READINGS

Baldrias L, Frost AJ, O'Boyle D: The isolation of *Pasteurella*-like organisms from the tonsillar region of dogs and cats, *J Small Anim Pract* 29:63, 1988.

Barrett RE et al: Chronic relapsing stomatitis in a cat with feline leukemia virus infection, *Fel Pract* 5:34, 1975.

Bennet D: Autoimmune disease in the dog, *Practice*, 6:74, 1984.

Bennet D et al: Bullous autoimmune skin disease in the dog. I. Clinical and pathological assessment, *Vet Rec* 106:497, 1980.

Bennet D et al: Bullous autoimmune skin disease in the dog. II. Immunopathological assessment, *Vet Rec* 106:523, 1980.

Bennet M et al: Diagnosis of FIV infection, *Vet Rec* 124:520, 1989.

Borysenko M, Borysenko J: Stress, behavior and immunity: animal models and mediating mechanisms, *Gen Hosp Psychiatry* 4:59, 1982.

Bradley WA: Gingivitis in maltese terriers, *Vet Rec* 110:618, 1982.

Brogdon JD et al: Diagnosing and treating masticatory myositis, *Vet Med* 86:1164, 1991.

Brown N, Hurvitz AL: A mucocutaneous disease in a cat resembling human pemphigus, *JAAHA* 12:25, 1979.

Cheville NF: The gray collie syndrome, *JAVMA* 152:6, 1968.

Coles S: Prevalence of buccocervical erosions in cats of Australia, *J Vet Dent* 7:14, 1990.

Cotter SM et al: Association of feline leukemia virus with lymphosarcoma and other disorders in the cat, *JAVMA* 166:449, 1975.

Durr von UM, Reichart P: Gingivitis der Katze—medikamentose und chirurgische Therapie, *Kleinterpraxis* 23:231, 1978.

Eriksen T, Harvey CE, Venner M: Palliativ behandling of felin parodontal syndrom, *Dansk Vet Tidsskr* 75:429, 1992.

Frost P, Williams CA: Feline dental disease, *Vet Clin North Am* 16:851, 1986.

Gaskell RM, Gruffydd-Jones TJ: Intractable feline stomatitis, *Vet Ann* 17:195, 1977.

Gelberg HB et al: Antiepithelial autoantibodies associated with the feline eosinophilic granuloma complex, *Am J Vet Res* 46:263, 1985.

Harvey CE: Effect of extraction of cheek teeth in cats with gingivitis-stomatitis, *Proc Am Vet Dent Soc*, 1986.

Harvey CE: Oral inflammatory diseases in cats, *JAAHA* 27:585, 1991.

Harvey CE, Campbell DE: Neutrophil function in cats with chronic gingivitis-stomatitis, *Proc Vet Dent Forum*, 3:12, 1989.

Harvey CE, Hennet P: Feline dental resorptive lesions: prevalence patterns, *Vet Clin North Am, Small Anim Pract* 22:1405, 1992.

Huritz AL, Feldman E: A disease of dogs resembling human pemphigus vulgaris, *JAVMA* 166:585, 1975 (Case reports).

Jeffcoat MK et al: Flurbiprofen treatment of periodontal disease in beagles, *J Periodont Res* 21:624, 1986.

Johnessee J, Huritz A: Feline plasma cell gingivitis-pharyngitis, *J Am Anim Hosp Assoc* 19:179, 1983.

Kaplan ML, Jeffcoat MK: Acute necrotizing ulcerative gingivitis, *Canine Pract* 5:35, 1978.

Kaswan RL et al: Keratoconjunctivitis sicca: immunological evaluation of 62 canine cases, *Am J Vet Res* 46:376, 1985.

Kerr DA, McClatchey KD, Regezi JA: Idiopathic gingivostomatitis, *Oral Surg* 32:402, 1971.

Knowles JO, McArdle F, Dawson S et al: Studies on the role of feline calcivirus in chronic stomatitis in cats, *Vet Microbiol* 27:205, 1991.

Knowles JO, Gaskell RM, Gaskell CJ, Harvey CE, Lutz H: The prevalence of feline calicivirus, feline leukemia virus and antibodies to FIV in cats with chronic stomatitis, *Vet Rec* 124:336, 1989.

Madewell BR et al: Oral eosinophilic granuloma in Siberian husky dogs, *JAVMA* 177:701, 1980.

Mallonnee DH, Harvey CE, Venner M, Hammond BF: Bacteriology of periodontal disease in the cat, *Arch Oral Biol* 33:677, 1988.

Mayr B, Beininger S, Buttner M: Treatment of chronic stomatitis of cats by local paramunization with PIND-ORF, *J Vet Med* 38:78, 1991.

McClelland RB: X-ray therapy in labial and cutaneous granulomas in cats, *JAVMA* 125:469, 1954.

McKeever PJ, Klausner JS: Plant awn, candidal, nocardial, and necrotizing ulcerative stomatitis in the dog, *JAAHA* 22:17, 1986.

Mikx FHM, Hug HU, Maltha JC: Necrotizing ulcerative gingivitis in beagle dogs, *J Periodont Res* 19:76, 1984.

Ochs DL et al: Eosinophilic granuloma in the cat: two cases involving the tongue, *Vet Med/Small Anim Clinician* 73:1275, 1978.

Pederson NC: Immunosuppressive drugs and their role in the treatment of immunologic diseases of the dog, *Gaines Vet Symp* 28:13, 1978.

Pederson NC: Inflammatory oral cavity diseases of the cat, *Vet Clin North Am, Small Anim Pract* 22:1323, 1992.

Pfeifer EG et al: Die Behandlung der chronischen Gingivitis der Katze, *Prakt Tierarzt* 22:29, 1988.

Potter KA et al: Oral eosinophilic granuloma of Siberian huskies, *JAAHA* 16:595, 1980.

Quimby FW et al: A disorder of dogs resembling Sjögren's syndrome, *Clin Immunol Immunopathol* 12:471, 1979.

Reichart PA et al: Periodontal disease in the domestic cat, *J Periodont Res* 19:67, 1984.

Rerebel GH, Hoffman DE, Pederson NC: Acute and chronic faucitis of domestic cats: a feline calicivirus-induced disease, *Vet Clin North Am, Small Anim Pract* 22:1347, 1992.

Richardson RL: Effect of administering antibiotics, removing the major salivary glands, and toothbrushing on dental calculi formation in the cat, *Arch Oral Biol* 10:245, 1965.

Roenigk WJ: Radiation therapy. In Kirk RW, editor: *Current veterinary therapy,* ed 4, Philadelphia, 1971, WB Saunders.

Schlup von D: Epidemiologische untersuchungen an Katzengebib, *Kleinterpraxis* 27:87, 1982.

Schlup von D, Stich H: Morphologische untersuchungen der "neck lesions," *Kleinterpraxis* 27:179, 1982.

Schneck von G: Eosinophiles Granulom bei einer Katze, *Deutsche Tierarztl Wochenschr* 82:162, 1975.

Scott DW: Observations on the eosinophilic granuloma complex in cats, *JAAHA* 11:261, 1975.

Seawright AA, Hrdlicka J: Severe retardation of growth with retention and displacement of incisors in young cats fed a diet of raw sheep liver high in vitamin A, *Aust Vet J* 50:306, 1974.

Shelton GD et al: Canine masticatory muscle disorders: a study of 29 cases, *Muscle Nerve* 10:753, 1987.

Sims TJ, Moncla BJ, Page RC: Serum antibody response to antigens of oral gram-negative bacteria in cats with plasma cell gingivitis-stomatitis, *J Dent Res* 69:877, 1990.

Stannard AA et al: A mucotaneous disease in the dog resembling pemphigus vulgaris in man, *JAVMA* 166:575, 1975.

Stebbins K, Goldschmidt MH, Harvey CE: Unpublished data, 1988.

Studer E, Stapley RB: The role of dry foods in maintaining healthy teeth and gums in the cat, *Vet Med/Small Anim Clin* 68:1124, 1973.

Tannock GW, Webster JR, Dobbinson SS: Feline gingivitis, *NZ Vet J* 36:93, 1988.

Tenorio AP, Franti CE, Madewell BR, Pedersen NC: Chronic oral infections of cats and their relationship to persistent oral carriage of feline calici-, immunodeficiency, or leukemia viruses, *Vet Immunol Immunopathol* 29:1, 1991

Thompson RR, Wilcox GE, Clark WT, Jansen KL: Association of calicivirus infection with chronic gingivitis and pharyngitis in cats, *J Small Anim Pract* 25:207, 1984.

Van Campen GJ: The occurrence of acute necrotizing ulcerative gingivitis in a beagle dog colony, *IADR* 55:12, A45, 1977.

Walsh KM: Oral eosinophilic granuloma in two dogs, *JAVMA* 183:323, 1983.

Wessum van R, Harvey CE, Hennet P: Feline dental resorptive lesions: prevalence patterns, *Vet Clin North Am, Small Anim Pract* 22:1405, 1992.

Willemse A, Lubberink AAME: Eosinophilic ulcers in cats, *Tijdschr Diergeneeskd* 103:1052, 1978.

Williams C, Aller S: Gingivitis/stomatitis in cats, *Vet Clin North Am, Small Anim Pract* 22:1361, 1992.

Wouters SLS: Experimentally induced acute necrotizing ulcerative gingivitis in beagle dogs, *IADR* 13, 1977 (abstract).

Yamamoto JK et al: Epidemiologic and clinical aspects of feline immunodeficiency virus infection in cats from the continental United States and Canada and possible mode of transmission, *J Am Vet Med Assoc* 194:213, 1989.

Zetner K: Diagnostik und Therapie des Pemphiguskomplexes in der Mundhohle, *Praktische Tierarzt* 5:66, 1987.

Zetner K, Kampfer P, Lutz H, Harvey CE: Vergleichende immunologische und virologishe untersuchungen von Katzen mit chronischen oralen Erkrankungen, *Wein Tierartztl Mschr* 76:303, 1989.

Endodontics

Endodontics (root canal) therapy is the treatment of the internal components of the tooth, the dental pulp. Whenever possible, to maintain appearance and function of the tooth, it is the preferred alternative to dental extraction.

▶ DENTAL PULP

Anatomy

Dental pulp occupies the interior cavity of the tooth. It consists of loose connective tissue, intercellular substance, vessels, nerves, and fibers. The pulp (the endodontic system) is divided into a coronal pulp and root pulp, corresponding to the anatomic crown and the root (Fig. 6-1). In older animals the distribution and density of cells and fibers of the root canal are different from that of a young animal. As an animal ages, the pulp chamber and root canal narrow as a result of continual deposition of dentin (Fig. 6-2). This occurs more rapidly if the pulp is stimulated, such as in areas of dental attrition.

The pulp connects with the periapical tissue through the apex. In young animals, in which the apex is not yet fully developed, the pulp connects with the surrounding periapical tissue through a wide opening (Figs. 6-2 and 6-3). After the root lengthens, the opening at the apex (tip of the root) narrows (Figs. 6-2 and 6-3). During this period the walls surrounding

the apex still consist entirely of dentin. Root lengthening occurs as a result of activity of a ring of tissue (Hertwig's root sheath) surrounding the root apex. With increasing age and exposure to physiologic functioning, a layer of cementum gradually covers the dentin and the pulp chamber and root canal narrow. Root apex development continues and results in a series of small openings referred to as an *apical delta* in dogs and cats (Fig. 6-4 and Table 6-1).

Lateral or accessory canals are uncommon in dogs and cats. They connect the pulp tissue with the periodontal ligament at any level of the root but most frequently are found in the apical third of the root. Endodontic therapy success depends on obturation of the apical delta and lateral canals. In teeth with significant periodontal attachment loss, if the bacterial plaque reaches and involves the soft tissue of lateral canals, pulp involvement will result.

Histology

Pulp tissue consists of four layers: (1) the odontoblastic layer covering the periphery of the pulp chamber, with processes extending into the dentinal tubules; (2) Weil's basal layer (cell-poor layer), which lies next to the odontoblastic layer in mature teeth; (3) a cell-rich layer, located between the cell-poor layer and the central pulp; and (4) the central pulp, which has fewer cells per unit area than the cell-rich layer. The dental pulp is a blood-rich organ. Vessels

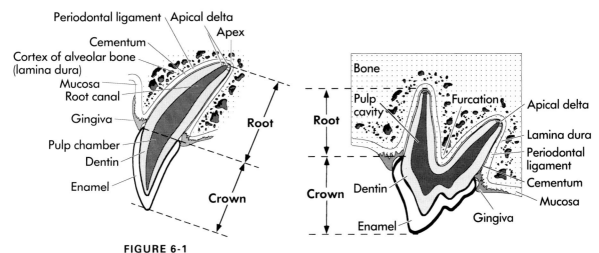

FIGURE 6-1
Drawings of mature teeth showing the pulpal tissue and apical delta.

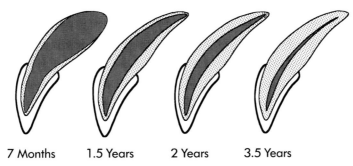

7 Months   1.5 Years   2 Years   3.5 Years

FIGURE 6-2
Diagram of the changes in pulpal tissue and dentin with age in the canine tooth of a dog.

that pass through the apical foramina are distributed throughout the pulp. Most vessels are thin walled with large lumens. Pulp contains lymph vessels, permitting rapid uptake of calcium hydroxide into the pulp during pulp capping and pulpotomy procedures.

Function

Pulpal functions are formative, nutritive, sensory, and defensive.

Formation

Pulpal tissues produce dentin. When a lesion involves the dentin, the odontoblastic processes and the pulp are involved. As maturation occurs, additional layers of dentin are added, with each odontoblast enclosed and remaining vital in its dentinal tubule that extends to the dentinoenamel/dentinocemental junction. The dentinal tubules and the odontoblastic process narrow toward the periphery of the tooth, tapering

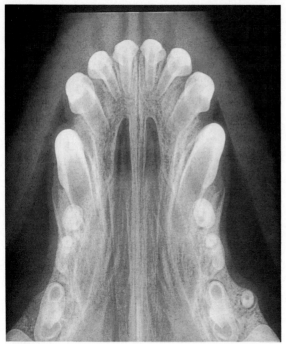

FIGURE 6-3
Radiograph of the canine and incisor teeth of a 6-month-old dog. Short roots and open apexes are evident.

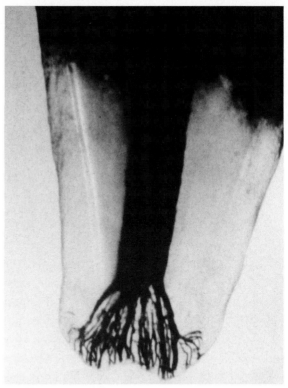

FIGURE 6-4
Photomicrograph of the apex of a mature tooth of a dog. Indian ink stain was used to demonstrate the vascular channels that form the apical delta. *(Courtesy of Dr. Philippe Hennet.)*

TABLE 6-1	Apical delta configurations in mature teeth of dogs and cats			
Species/teeth	Number of teeth	Mean number of apical ramifications	Mean length of apical ramifications	Lateral canals observed?
Dogs				
Canines*	23	16 (11-22)	2 mm (1-3.5)	No
Incisors, canines, premolars, molars†	240	ND (5-20)	ND	ND
Upper lateral incisors‡	22	16.4 (9-30)	1.8 mm (1-2.5)	No
Cats				
Canines§	61	12.5 (7-22)	1.75 mm (1-3)	No
Premolars, molars‖	54	10.4 (4-18)	ND	Yes

ND, Not done.
*Hennet P, Harvey CE: Extracted teeth from dogs age 1 to 17 years, Unpublished data, 1992.
†Masson E, Hennet P, Calas P: Apical root canal anatomy in the dog, *Endod Dent Traumat* 8:109, 1992.
‡Hennet P, Golden A, Harvey CE: Unpublished data, 1992.
§Hennet P, Harvey CE: Apical root canal anatomy in the cat, in preparation, 1992.
‖Hennet P, Harvey CE: Unpublished data, 1991.

to an almost closed structure at the enamel junction or cemental wall. The cellular content of the dentinal tubules is significant in endodontic treatment inasmuch as open dentinal tubules can lead to pulpal disease.

Normal healthy pulpal tissues continue dentinal deposition at a slow rate throughout life. Pulpal disease decreases dentinal deposition, which ceases entirely after pulpal death.

Nutrition

The pulp provides nutrients to the surrounding tissues during development. After development, dentin metabolism continues via the odontoblastic processes. The narrow pulp canals of older animals continue to remain vital, with pulpal circulation intact.

Sensation

The sensory function of the pulp is a response to pain via nerves that enter the apical foramen and divide into finer bundles that penetrate the odontoblastic layer and dentinal tubules as unmyelinated fibers. Pulpal nerves remain unchanged in older animals, although there is increased thickness of nonsensory mineralized tissue between the external environment and the sensory nerve endings. After necrosis of the coronal pulp with apical inflammation, nerves may still persist in the apical area. The sensory nerves are branches of the trigeminal nerve (V).

Defense

Pulpal response to injury is inflammation. Continued severe irritation results in pulpal death because hypervascularity and swelling in a closed space effect necrosis once arterial inflow ceases, a consequence of excessive pressure within the pulp space. Reparative dentin results from stimulation of the pulp by extrinsic factors, such as attrition, abrasion, and trauma. It is a response to any low-grade chronic irritant—protecting the remaining pulp from that irritant—and can narrow the pulp chamber and root canal in the area of the irritation.

Pathology

A basic understanding of pulpal disease is needed to establish the indications for specific endodontic procedures and to predict the results of treatment. When circulation is cut off, as occurs with inflammatory swelling that restricts blood flow, traumatic severance of vascular supply to the pulp or periodontal involvement of the apical area, pulpal necrosis results from lack of gas exchange and nutrients to the pulp.

As the animal ages and new dentin is laid down by odontoblasts, pulp tissue is reduced in volume, cellular components, nervous tissue, odontoblasts, and vascular supply. With this closing down of pulpal dimensions, the ability of the pulp to respond to injury is impaired (Figs. 6-2 and 6-3).

Pulpal insult can result from extension of the inflammatory process through the dentinal tubules, by direct dentinal insult from topical irritants, through localization of blood-borne bacteria in hyperemic pulp, or as a result of periodontal disease in combination periodontic-endodontic lesions (see Fig. 6-48).

Pulpal damage is the result of trauma (pulpal exposure resulting from coronal fracture or intradental hemorrhage without pulp exposure), penetration by bacteria from such factors as caries or external resorption, or iatrogenic factors, or it can be idiopathic in origin (for example, internal resorption from unknown factors, hematogenous seeding of bacteria).

Pulpal disease passes from reversible hyperemia to an irreversible pulpitis and ends in suppurative pulpitis and necrosis. Periapical inflammation and abscess formation (apical periodontitis—inflammation of the part of the periodontal ligament around the apex of the root) are extensions of the pulpal inflammatory response. Acute periapical abscess occurs when bacteria invade the pulp and overwhelm the local inflammatory response, with suppuration extending through the apex following the path of least resistance. Bacterial contamination also can result in a chronic apical periodontitis or granuloma (Fig. 6-5) and possible cyst formation or drainage via a fistula or through the coronal exposure of the root canal (Figs. 6-7 to 6-9).

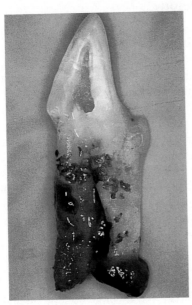

FIGURE 6-5
Periapical granuloma surrounding the root of a carnassial tooth in a dog. The crown was hemisected during extraction. There is extensive root calculus that extends to the level of the granuloma. This could be a primary endodontic lesion with secondary periodontitis or a combined periodontal-endodontic lesion.

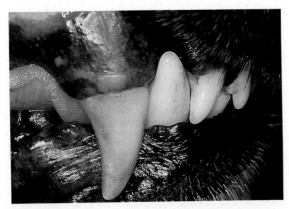

FIGURE 6-6
Intact but discolored coronal third of the crown of the upper canine tooth in a dog, indicating pulpal disease at the area of discoloration. Some enamel staining can be seen at the gingival third of the tooth.

► CLINICAL FACTORS

The diagnosis of endodontic lesions in veterinary dentistry is complicated by the lack of diagnostic procedures based on subjective symptoms of pain, sensitivity to hot, cold, or percussion, and foul taste or odor. Veterinary dentists must rely on input from the owner of the animal and their own clinical and radiographic evaluation. Many endodontic lesions go undetected.

Signs

The clinical signs of pulpal disease include (1) broken teeth with pulpal exposure (see Fig. 7-12), (2) abnormal coloration of the crown (usually reddish-purple to gray-black [Fig. 6-6]), (3) refusal to chew or eat, (4) chewing on one side only, (5) constant or frequent licking and tooth chattering, (6) drooling, (7) sensitivity to hot and/or cold food or fluids, (8) sensitivity to percussion of the tooth or palpation of that part of the face, (9) bleeding from an exposed canal, (10) general malaise, (11) clinical appearance of an infection or fistula around the tooth root (Fig. 6-7; see also discussion of Carnassial Abscess that follows), and (12) cystic swelling around the root tip (Fig. 6-8). Many endodontically involved teeth are not clinically apparent. Signs such as mucogingival fistula will be obvious only to a careful observer.

An actively bleeding tooth resulting from a fresh coronal fracture can be treated with vital pulpotomy therapy. Prognosis after pulpotomy is inversely proportional to the time of exposure to the oral environment and directly proportional to the size of the pulp chamber. Exposure beyond 1 hour diminishes the chances of a successful pulpotomy. An open canal exposed for a prolonged period usually requires complete root canal therapy, although the reparable period is longer in a young dog with a wide pulp because more space is available for absorbing the effects of the swelling associated with the inflammation and the apical blood supply is abundant (see later discussions, Vital Pulpotomy and Complications of Endodontic Therapy).

A dark hole in the center of the fractured or worn tooth that can be entered with a dental explorer indicates a long-standing pulp exposure that requires root canal therapy no matter what the age of the animal.

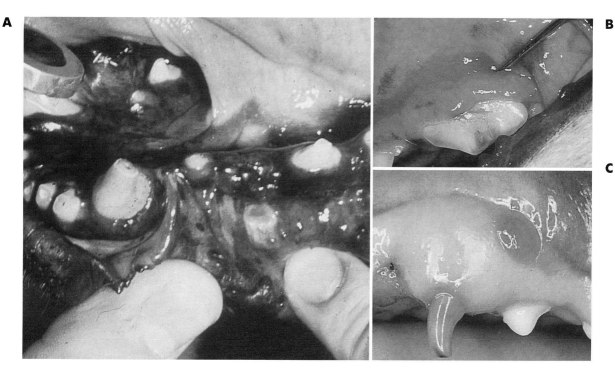

FIGURE 6-7
Endodontic fistulae at or apical to the MGJ. **A,** Lower canine tooth. **B,** Upper carnassial
tooth (with probe in the mucogingival junction fistula). **C,** Deciduous upper canine
tooth. *(Courtesy of Dr. S. Holmstrom.)*

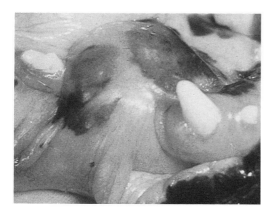

FIGURE 6-8
Endodontic cyst affecting the apical area of the
lower canine tooth of a dog.

Carnassial abscess

The inflammatory process may have spread beyond the confines of the pulp and root canal system into the periapical tissues in both immature and mature pulps. This inflammatory spread can occur long before it is observed clinically. Once it becomes clinically evident that severe apical inflammation is present, emergency treatment should be provided to eliminate the diseased contents of the root canal system. Inflammatory and necrotic tissue can be encouraged to drain through the root canal and coronal pulp exposure by enlarging the pulp exposure with a dental bur. These animals should be given antibiotic therapy until the acute symptoms have resolved, followed by root canal therapy.

Suborbital (facial) swelling (often known as carnassial or malar abscess or facial sinus) generally indicates a periapical abscess of the upper fourth premolar tooth, which results from a coronal slab fracture with pulpal exposure, apical extension of a deep periodontal pocket, or concussive disease of the root apex.

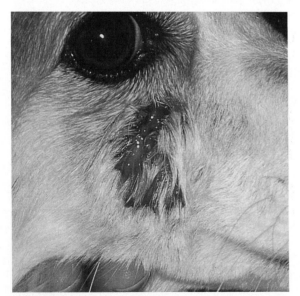

FIGURE 6-9
Carnassial abscess (facial fistula or sinus) in a dog, located immediately ventral to the medial canthus of the eye.

This condition is seen as a swelling or draining tract below the medial canthus of the eye, typically in middle-aged or older dogs, most often mongrels (Fig. 6-9). Soft tissue lesions always should be radiographed. A similar condition occasionally occurs that affects the upper first molar tooth or lower carnassial tooth. Fistulae resulting from endodontic disease almost always occur apical to the mucogingival junction; the fistulation may occur through the oral mucosa into the mouth (Fig. 6-7) or through the skin of the jaws (Fig. 6-9). Carnassial abscess may recur if extraction is used as treatment and a root tip is left in place (Fig. 6-10).

Clinical and Radiographic Examination

Clinical evaluation should include examination for swelling, fistula formation, tooth crown color or coronal appearance that reflects tooth vitality, palpation over the apex to determine swelling, and percussion along the long axis of the root to check for abnormal response that indicates the infection has extended beyond the pulp into the periodontal ligament space, creating an apical periodontitis. The pressure caused by an increase of fluid in this small space produces pain on percussion. Tooth mobility may increase when an endodontic lesion is present.

Radiographs are essential to good diagnosis; however, many oral structures, such as foramina and bony trabeculae, appear similar to endodontic lesions (Fig. 6-11). Accurate radiographic diagnosis is not always possible. A valuable landmark to endodontic radiographic diagnosis is the lamina dura, the compact layer of bone lining the tooth socket that appears as a thin white line next to the periodontal ligament (see Fig. 2-12). As the contents of an infected pulp exude through the apex, they cause changes in the shape and continuity of the lamina dura and width and shape of the periodontal ligament. These are common radiographic indications of pulpal and periodontal necrosis (Fig. 6-12). As the disease process extends, it causes an enlarging apical osteolytic lesion (Fig. 6-13). The extent of radiographic change does not correlate well with the duration of endodontic disease; if purulent debris is able to drain through a large pulp exposure, endodontic pressure will not build up sufficiently to force fluid through the apical foramina.

Radiographic positioning can fail to show a radio-

FIGURE 6-10
Recurrent carnassial abscess caused by a retained root tip following an attempted extraction of the carnassial tooth. **A,** Facial drainage. **B,** Radiograph showing root tip surrounded by a wide radiolucent space. **C,** Healed gingiva covering the root fragment. **D,** Gingival incision and exploration reveals the root fragment. **E,** The tip following extraction.

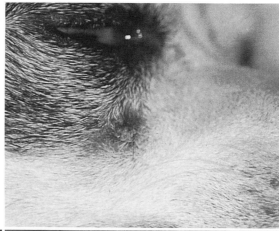

A

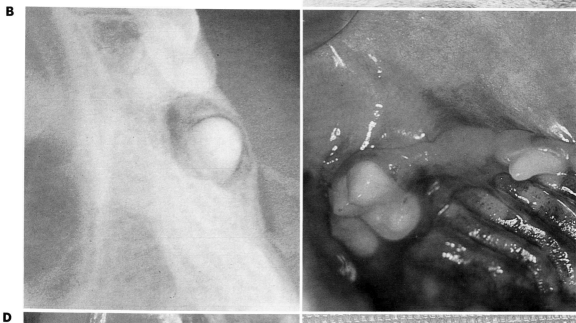

B

C

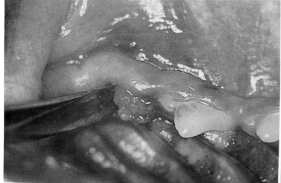

D

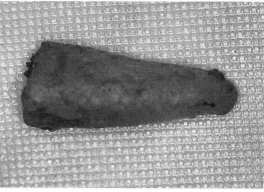

E

A

B

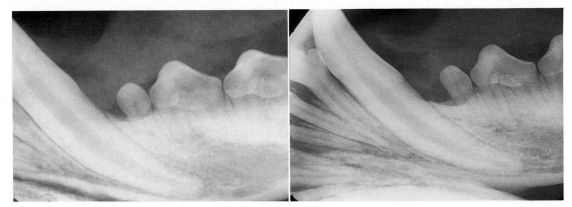

FIGURE 6-11
Radiographs of the apex of the lower canine tooth. **A,** Oblique view with the mental foramen located over the apex appearing as a periapical lucency. **B,** Slightly changed oblique view separates the mental foramen from the canine tooth apex.

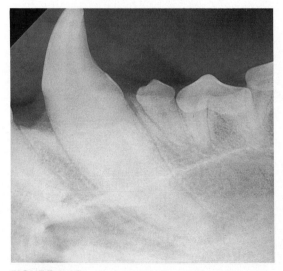

FIGURE 6-12
Radiograph showing an early periapical loss of lamina dura and increased radiolucency in a canine tooth.

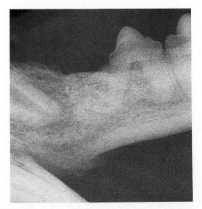

FIGURE 6-13
Radiograph of a severe osteolytic periapical lesion of a canine tooth in a cat.

lucency because of foreshortening of the image from incorrect placement of the tooth, radiograph, and tube head relative to each other (see Radiographic Examination, Chapter 2). Although the periapical lesion is in contact with the apex and cannot be displaced, often it can be hidden by poor radiographic technique. If there is doubt as to whether an apical lucency is a lesion or an anatomic feature, an additional view of the same tooth should be obtained and the contralateral tooth examined from the same radiographic position.

Indications for Root Canal Therapy

Indications for root canal therapy in *hard tissue* include (1) pulpal exposure through fracture, attrition, and caries and (2) discolored teeth, with the crown intact, as the result of trauma (heat or a direct blow) or hematogenous seeding of bacteria into the pulp (Fig. 6-6).

Indications for root canal therapy in *soft tissue* are (1) facial swelling, (2) intraoral or extraoral fistula, and (3) gingival inflammation with pocket formation (periodontal lesion) in a combined periodontal/endodontic lesion.

Contraindications to endodontic therapy are limited to the risk of anesthesia (for example, age and systemic health of the patient), lack of client compliance with postoperative care (for endodontic-periodontal lesions, for example), poor endodontic prognosis (restricted canals, root resorption, long axis fracture), and limitations of the operator or equipment and available supplies. There is rarely sufficient duration of benefit for endodontic treatment of deciduous teeth to be beneficial in dogs and cats.

Endodontic therapy deals with the contents of the tooth; however, the surrounding structures and their response to therapy determine the success or failure of endodontic treatment.

▶ ENDODONTIC TECHNIQUES

Conventional Root Canal Therapy

Conventional root canal therapy is the most common root canal procedure. It is indicated when there is an intact root apex and no root fracture is present. When the tooth is immature or the root is fractured, alternative procedures are indicated (see pp. 189-190).

Minimal equipment consists of a dental handpiece and burs, root canal files, flushing solutions, drying materials, canal-filling materials, and materials to restore the access site (see Chapter 11).

Many methods and materials are employed in the preparation and filling of tooth canals, but the objectives of conventional root canal therapy remain the same:
1. Antiseptic preparation of the oral cavity and root canal site
2. Access to the root canal
3. Removal of all diseased pulpal contents and necrotic dentin
4. Irrigation with an antiseptic agent
5. Drying the canal
6. Filling the canal
7. Restoration of the access site

In veterinary endodontics, it generally is unnecessary to isolate a tooth with a rubber dam before treatment. The tooth is disinfected with chlorhexidine solution. The new "paint on" rubber dam material may prove to be useful for animals.

Access cavity preparation

An adequate access cavity is the essential first step. A poorly planned or an improperly performed access preparation increases the difficulty of the entire procedure.

The objective is to gain access to the root apex so that complete débridement of the pulp cavity contents can be accomplished. A working knowledge of the internal anatomy of the tooth is essential to locate the pulp chamber and the orifice of the root canal(s). The internal or pulpal anatomy (pulp chamber and root canals) has approximately the same shape as the outside of the tooth. Preoperative radiographs are essential to show the shape and location of the chamber and root canals in the tooth to be treated, as well as the internal pulpal diameter.

The access preparation is made as small as possible to minimize any further weakening of an already weakened tooth; however, it must be large enough to accommodate the file shafts. Otherwise a false sensation of reaching the apical stop may be encountered as a result of a file shaft becoming jammed in the access preparation.

Access cavity preparation weakens the crown of

the tooth structurally. This is particularly true if any of the cusps have been weakened by trauma undermining the remaining dentin that supports enamel. A slight reduction of the crown height at the time of access preparation can lessen the occlusal stress that these teeth must withstand, thereby reducing the chance of subsequent fracture. Tooth structure, however, is not to be sacrificed unnecessarily.

A sterile bur in an air turbine handpiece is preferred; however, slow-speed electrical dental units can be used to penetrate the enamel and roughly shape the outline of the access opening to provide free accessibility to the root canal. A round (No. 1 or 2) or pear-shaped (No. 330 or 331) bur is used to make the access. In drilling into enamel, the initial 0.5 mm depth is cut perpendicular to the surface (Fig. 6-14, *A*); the drill is then angled toward the apex (Fig. 6-14, *B*). This reduces the risks of slipping while starting the cut. The hole is drilled directly over the pulp chamber as described later. The pear burs combine the penetrating advantage of the round burs, yet keep to a minimum the tendency to gouge the walls, as

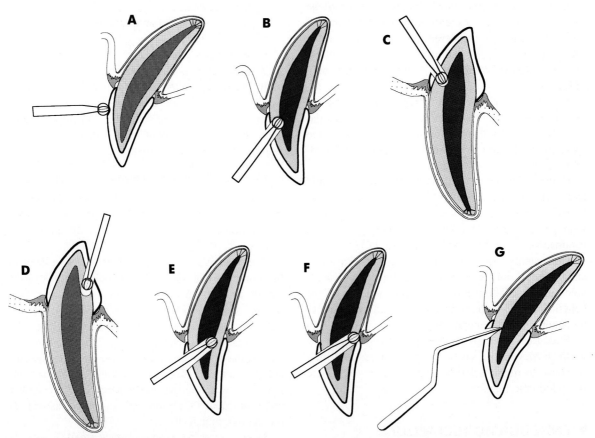

FIGURE 6-14
Access preparation for canine and incisor teeth. **A** and **B,** Initial entry for canine tooth; the bur is initially perpendicular to the tooth surface, then is angled to the direction of the root apex. **C,** Labial surface entry for incisor tooth. **D,** Palatal/lingual entry for incisor tooth. **E,** Excessive deep penetration causes gouging. **F,** Continued excess penetration causes exit through distal surface of canine tooth. **G,** Use of endodontic explorer to locate the pulp chamber.

often happens with the use of round burs and flat-end fissure burs. In young teeth the access opening is larger because the pulp chamber is larger. Older calcified pulp chambers require careful access to avoid unnecessary tooth structure removal, thereby weakening the crown in the search for small root canal orifice(s).

Locating the pulp chamber. Generally, most access preparations are begun by cutting the approximate shape of the access cavity into the occlusal or facial surface or into an exposed pulp canal. This initial cut is made for about 1 to 2 mm into the dentin, and then the preparation is narrowed until the pulp is reached.

The operator aims for the easiest place to locate the chamber; with teeth that have larger chambers, this is the center of the chamber. In those teeth with small or calcified chambers (as indicated by radiographs), a deeper penetration may be necessary to locate the pulp chamber. Even though the pulp has receded, the approximate shape of the final access cavity opening should be cut 1 to 2 mm into the dentin, with the opening narrowed toward the pulp. The size of the opening should not be kept deliberately small in an attempt to conserve tooth structure. Familiarity with the normal-sized opening will be an aid in locating the pulp. Also, a smaller opening limits the ability to see the floor of the preparation, and the opening must be large enough to accommodate the shaft of the final root canal file without binding (Fig. 6-15).

The operator, in attempting to locate a small-diameter pulp chamber or root canal, should take additional radiographs to check the size and direction of the canal. It is easy to head in the wrong direction (Fig. 6-14, *E* and *F*). Radiographs indicate bur or file direction and may prevent lateral root canal perforation. A sharp endodontic explorer can be used to penetrate into the roof of the chamber to locate the root canals (Fig. 6-14, *G*). Dull, bent, or restorative explorers (shepherd's hook explorers) are not suitable for this purpose.

Once the canal is located, a No. 10 or No. 15 root canal file is inserted into the pulp chamber and root canal through the access hole. It is worked in and out against the sides of the access hole to smooth the passage between the access, pulp chamber, and root

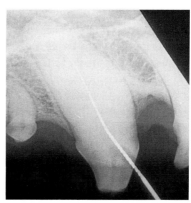

FIGURE 6-15
Radiograph showing effect of too narrow or poor direction of access preparation. The endodontic file binds at the access site.

canal. With larger pulp chambers, larger files may be used. The operator always should start with a small size and gradually work up to the larger size.

Fiberoptics. A fiberoptic light can be used to help locate the canal entrance of a calcified small-diameter pulp canal. The tip of the light source is held at a right angle to the proposed access site of the tooth. The room lights should be turned off to concentrate light that will emanate from the pulp chamber. If the fiberoptic tip is properly placed, the pulp chamber will glow with a reddish-orange hue. The tip of an endodontic explorer is directed into the newly located canal. Then a No. 10 or No. 15 root canal file is directed into the canal and worked in and out in a gentle probing motion to establish the pathway to the apex.

Many teeth that appear inoperable from the two-dimensional view of an intraoral radiograph frequently are manageable when manipulation is performed. An access preparation and attempt to locate the canal should be made before giving up and resorting to extraction.

Accessing root canals of specific teeth

Canines and incisors. Access cavity preparation for the maxillary and mandibular canines is similar. The pulp is oval, wider mesiodistally than buccolingually, extending incisally to provide direct line access to the root canal apex. On the mesial surface, 2 mm coronal to the gingival margin, the operator drills into the pulp chamber, starting at 90 degrees to the enamel surface, then turning to point the bur in the direction of the apex (Fig. 6-14, *A* and *B*). The apex of a dog's canine tooth lies apical to the mesial root of the second premolar. Allowance is required for the divergence of the canine teeth, particularly the lower canine teeth, and for the curve of the root relative to the crown (Fig. 6-14). For the incisor teeth the access is similar to the canine teeth but at a slightly reduced scale proportionate to the size of the incisor. On the buccal surface, halfway down the crown, the operator drills into the pulp chamber, starting at 90 degrees to the enamel surface, then turning to point the bur in the direction of the apex (Fig. 6-14, *C*). Because these are small teeth, with small pulp chambers, it may be necessary to use a smaller bur (round, No. ½).

It may be possible to make the access into the pulp chamber of the central incisors on the caudal (lingual) aspect, drilling almost vertically at the level of the cingulum (Fig. 6-14, *D*).

Premolars and molars. Premolar and molar endodontic involvement occurs most commonly in the upper fourth premolar and less often, the lower first molar. This is due primarily to the powerful occlusal contact of these teeth during mastication.

Upper carnassial. Endodontic involvement of the upper fourth premolar usually results from trauma exposing the dental pulp (slab fracture) or occlusal concussion of the root tips against bone. Access to the upper fourth premolar endodontic system varies, contingent on the amount of coronal destruction and operator preference. If a large amount of tooth structure has been lost, entrance to all three root canals can be gained through the fracture site directly into the exposed pulp chamber (Fig. 6-16).

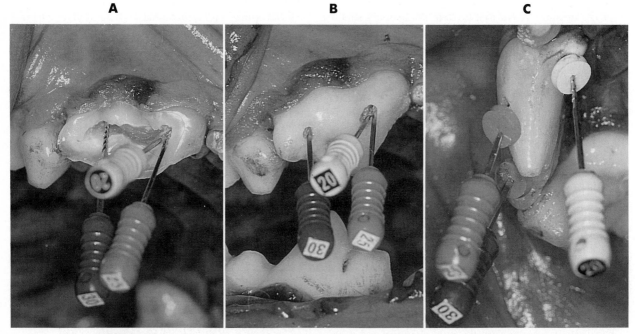

FIGURE 6-16
Access sites for carnassial tooth. **A,** Single opening if a substantial amount of crown is lost as a result of the fracture. **B,** Single transcoronal site for mesial and palatal root and separate site for distal root. **C,** Separate sites for all three roots.

If the crown is largely intact, the distal root canal usually is accessed from a site 1 to 2 mm coronal to the gingival margin and 1 mm distal to the buccal groove. The buccomesial (laterorostral) root and the palatal root can be accessed from a common entrance site on the buccal aspect of the crown (transcoronal approach) (Fig. 6-16, *B*). Access is gained directly over the mesial root halfway from the gingival margin to the cusp tip. The bony juga over this root can easily be palpated to give the operator location and direction for the access opening. After the initial penetration of the enamel perpendicular to the tooth surface, the bur is directed to the pulp chamber and then angled toward the palatal root entrance across the rostral pulpal section. The operator should be careful not to penetrate to the furcation of the mesial roots (laterorostral and palatal) when making the approach to the palatal root; a fine root canal file or root canal explorer is used to locate the canals and to indicate angulation for enlargement of the access.

The palatal root may be accessed separately from the occlusal surface (Fig. 6-16, *C*). The access opening is made into the buccal plane of the palatal cusp directed parallel to the buccomesial root. The palatal root and the buccomesial root usually show a slight apical divergence. The palatal root of the upper fourth premolar is small and tends to flare out medially. It is easy to drill the access for this root into the furcation (Fig. 6-17). The operator directs the bur toward the apex (medially in this case) and stops drilling as soon as the pulp chamber is reached. Gentle exploration with a No. 10 root canal file or a root canal explorer will lead to the canal. If the furcation has been entered or the canal cannot be found, the palatal root may be amputated and extracted, as described later.

Palatal root section. The palatal root is separated from the crown in a midcaudal to laterorostral direction through the furcation with a straight fissure bur. Usually, attempted elevation of the root will fracture the palatal root cusp tip, leaving the root fragment in place, and continued elevation of the root fragment likely will result in driving the root fragment into the nasal tissues. The root fragment is best extirpated with a No. 331L bur. The bur is directed along the long axis of the root fragment in a circular motion to remove all the root tissue to the apex (see also discussion

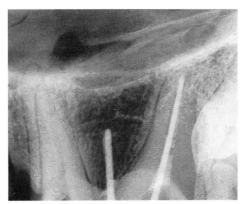

FIGURE 6-17
The furcation was penetrated during access preparation or canal instrumentation, and a gutta-percha point has penetrated the furcation.

of extraction technique). The entrance to the pulp chamber from the palatal root can be restored with a composite or amalgam filling, although the entrance to the pulp chamber is often obscure (Fig. 6-18). An injectable restorative material (such as glass ionomer using the capsule and applicator system) can be squeezed into the main pulp chamber and extruded through the palatal root pulp chamber connection; excess is wiped from the cut tooth surface at the extraction site.

Other premolars. All other premolars are accessed by a buccal entrance directly over each root.

Molar teeth. The lower first, second, and third molar access is made into the distal and mesio-occlusal pits to the root canals that are directly under the access sites (Fig. 6-19). The root canals diverge apically slightly.

Root canal therapy for the upper molar teeth rarely is required. These teeth do not receive the same occlusal forces as the upper fourth premolars, and their coronal anatomy makes them less susceptible to fracture. Access to the three roots of the upper first and second molars is gained from one common site in the central occlusal pit. The accessing bur is directed to each root canal to create a pathway to establish direction to the root canals after gaining entrance into the pulp chamber (Fig. 6-20).

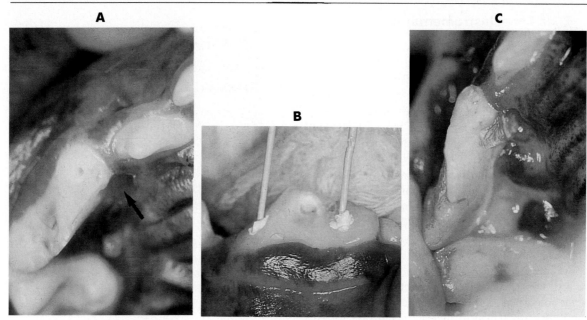

FIGURE 6-18
Section of the palatal root of an upper carnassial tooth. **A,** The palatal root has been extracted (*arrow*). **B,** The mesial and distal root canals are prepared and obturated. **C,** The access site has been restored with amalgam.

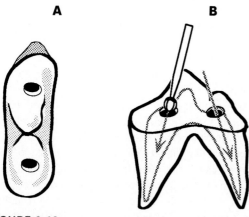

FIGURE 6-19
A and **B,** Access sites for lower premolar and molar teeth.

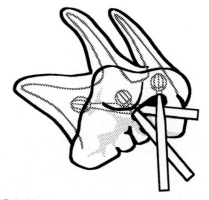

FIGURE 6-20
Access sites for upper first molar tooth.

Root Canal Instrumentation

Pulp extirpation

Débridement of vital pulp tissue, except in narrow canals, is best performed with barbed broaches (Fig. 6-21). Successful extirpation of the entire pulp in one piece depends on proper selection of the broach and on the adequacy of the access opening. Very young animals possess large pulpal canals. Two or three broaches used at the same time may be needed to extirpate a vital canal. Diseased pulp cannot be extracted as a single mass through an access opening that is narrower than the pulp.

Short-handled disposable barbed broaches are available in many styles and sizes. Broaches should be wide enough to engage the pulp effectively; broaches that are too narrow penetrate the pulp without securing enough tissue to remove the complete pulp in one piece. The broach should not be so wide as to make contact with the walls of the canal. Barbed broaches are not designed to cut dentinal walls and may fracture if wedged into a canal. Barbed broaches should be used sparingly in strongly curved canals and should never be inserted more than two thirds of the way into the canal. Proper engagement of the incisal two thirds of the pulp usually is sufficient to extirpate the apical third of the pulp without entailing risk of inserting the broach to the apex. The appropriately selected broach is placed two thirds of the way into the canal and rotated 180 to 360 degrees before attempting to extract the broach from the canal. An intact pulp will become entangled in the barbs without shredding and will be detached from the canal walls in one piece. When the vital pulp is successfully removed in total as one piece (Fig. 6-22), continued débridement of the canal is not necessary. The operator irrigates with sodium hypochlorite, dries the canal with sterile root canal paper points, and completes the conventional root canal procedure described next.

Débridement of necrotic material

Necrotic material is more difficult to remove from the canal. Barbed broaches are not recommended for use in cases of pulp degeneration because the necrotic tissue remnants are not amenable to removal in one piece. Broaches in such instances may be useful only

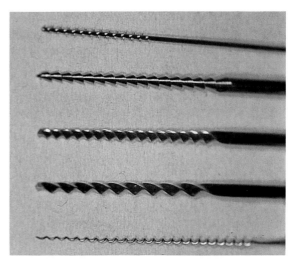

FIGURE 6-21
Working end of barbed broach *(top)*, Hedstrom endodontic file, K-file, reamer, lentulo spiral filler.

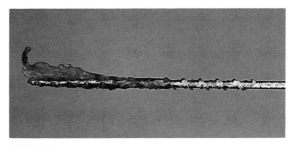

FIGURE 6-22
Pulpal soft tissue is entwined in a barbed broach.

to remove the occasional larger pieces of intact tissue or bits of food that have invaded root canal systems open to the oral environment. Débridement of necrotic and infected tissue depends on the effectiveness of the overall cleaning and shaping-filing procedure and on the thoroughness of irrigation during treatment.

Determining length to apex

Root canal length is best determined radiographically. A small-diameter root canal file (Nos. 8 to 15) of sufficient length to reach the apex (based on knowledge of tooth anatomy and palpation of the root juga) is inserted into the access opening until the estimated apical length is reached or the file cannot be advanced further. A premeasurement of apical length of an upper or lower canine tooth can be obtained by placing a curved file on the lateral aspect of the canine (over the canine juga) to a point directly over or under the mesial root of the second premolar. The length is measured and recorded. The same procedure can be employed for premolar and molar dentition. A small file is inserted to this length, left in place, and radiographed to confirm that the tip of the file has reached but not penetrated the apex (Fig. 6-23). The radiolucent root canal space ends 0.5 to 1.5 mm from the external root apex; the radiodense space between is the dentin surrounding the vascular channels in the apical delta. Because of the deltoid apical anatomy of mature canine dentition, it is difficult to penetrate the intact apex of mature teeth with an endodontic file. Apical root resorption can allow apical penetration of an overlong file in a mature tooth (Fig. 6-24). The apexes of immature teeth can be penetrated readily;

immature teeth must be verified radiographically for apical length.

Once apical length has been determined, all files are worked to that length (unless the step-back technique is used; see p. 175). The length is marked by a rubber endodontic file stop, a small circle of rubber or plastic with a hole in the center, which is available color-coded to match file size. An alternative is to use a small piece of rubber band or discarded surgical glove. The stop is pushed onto the shaft of the primary endodontic file before it is inserted into the tooth. It is pushed down the shaft of the file to the access opening when the file can be advanced no further. A radiograph is taken. If the file is at full length (Fig. 6-23), it is withdrawn and the distance from the stop to the tip of the file is recorded (Fig. 6-25). All subsequent larger files are measured or compared against the primary file distance during canal preparation.

Root canals are prepared by feel; the file can be manipulated with a greater sense of security if a stop is placed to prevent the instrument extending beyond the precise apical destination. When using movable

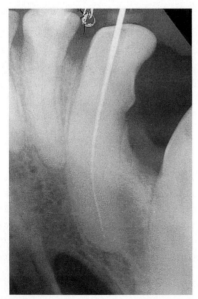

FIGURE 6-23
Radiograph is taken to determine that the initial file has reached the apex.

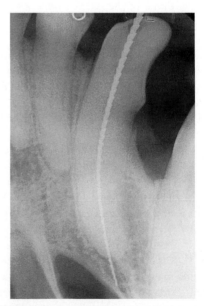

FIGURE 6-24
Radiograph showing penetration of an endodontic file through the apex of an incisor tooth.

stops, the operator must watch the stopping point of the instrument. This requires close visual observation and tactile sense.

Use of Lubricants, Chelates, and Irrigants

Lubricants and chelates

A few drops of surgical soap (such as chlorhexidine or povidone-iodine) can be placed in the access opening with an irrigating syringe. The soap is carried to the depth of the canal with the initial fine root canal file. After root canal length has been established and recorded, additional lubricant can be inserted into the access opening and an expanded diameter file is inserted into the root canal, carrying the lubricant to the apex. The surgical soap solution not only lubricates the instrument, making subsequent filing of the canal wall easier, but also dissolves necrotic pulp canal tissue. The canal is scrubbed with the file as is done with a surface wound. Wider-diameter instruments are introduced into the root canal as the instruments meet decreasing resistance against the dentinal wall.

Chelates such as R-C Prep (Premier Dental, Norristown, Pennsylvania) often are used as canal lubricants. They tend to soften the dentinal walls of the canal, however, making it more difficult to condense the filling material. Chelates should not be left in a root canal for an extended period and should never be used to try to advance a small instrument into a tight canal with the intention of moving beyond a blockage. Because the chelate softens dentine, the instrument may create a new canal rather than follow a blocked canal, thus resulting in root perforation.

Irrigants

Irrigants should be used freely during preparation of the root canal (Fig. 6-26). They also lubricate the root canal instruments to facilitate removal of vital and necrotic tissue. Root canals with necrotic tissue should be irrigated with sodium hypochlorite. Commercial full-strength chlorine bleach can be used for this purpose; diluted sodium hypochlorite is not as effective an antiseptic agent.

Hydrogen peroxide alternated with sodium hypochlorite has been recommended; however, sodium hypochlorite is most satisfactory used alone. Chlorhex-

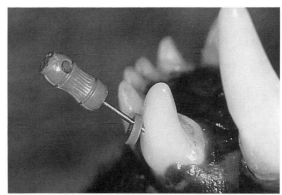

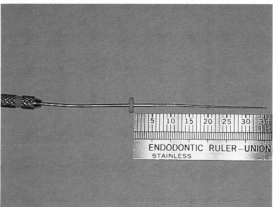

FIGURE 6-25
The distance (working length) of an endodontic file from the tip to the endodontic stop is measured in millimeters and recorded. **A,** The endodontic stop is pushed flush against the tooth. **B,** The file is withdrawn and measured.

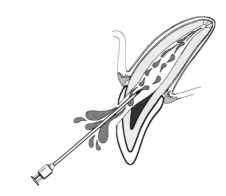

FIGURE 6-26
The instrumented root canal is irrigated.

idine (0.5%) solution is another excellent canal irrigant. The irrigant can be injected into the canal with a 3-ml syringe and 25-gauge needle, preferably long enough to reach close to the apex and curved to follow the shape of the canal. The canal is thoroughly flushed with sodium hypochlorite solution, which is left in the canal for 15 to 20 seconds. One purpose of canal irrigation is to remove dentinal shavings that are freed during canal preparation. Some of these chips inevitably are packed at the junction of the dentinal and cemental canals. These chips are matted together by the irrigating solution into an impervious dentinal plug, or "mud." It is almost impossible to prevent the filling of the narrow apical delta channels with this material. This dentin chip barrier adds to the impervious layer of the root canal–filling material and aids in perfecting an apical seal in a mature root apex.

During treatment of a tooth by pulpotomy, irrigation with sterile normal saline helps to reduce the inflammatory effect of instrumentation on the severed vital pulp stump left in the root canal.

Canal Exploration and Filing

The technique of canal exploration is important, particularly in small canals of molars and premolars, as well as canals of teeth in old animals with a narrow or radiographically absent root canal. Extremely fine No. 8 and No. 10 files are available, which are useful in exploring very fine canals, but they tend to bend easily at the tip (Fig. 6-27). Few root canals are straight, even when the radiograph makes it appear so. Canals that appear to be straight should not be instrumented with straight, stiff files. To prevent possible root ledging, gouging, or perforation (Fig. 6-28), it is important to preshape all files to follow the root canal anatomy before it is entered. The bend is a gradual curvature estimated to resemble the curvature of the root in the radiograph. A fine file usually will assume and retain the shape of the root canal. The easiest way to penetrate a diffusely calcified small root canal is to use small files placed to the apex, coated with lubricating solution, and used with gentle pressure.

Depending on their design, endodontic files are constructed for use in a specific manner. Most endodontic instruments are made by twisting an instrument blank in a clockwise direction. If the instrument binds in a tight canal, counterclockwise movement of the instrument handle beyond two complete turns frequently will cause fracture. A Hedstrom file (Fig. 6-21) is manipulated with an up-and-down circumferential motion; it never is rotated on entering a fine curved root canal. A rotary action will result in fracture of a Hedstrom file; there also is the risk of screwing the file against the tight walls of the root canal. A file that is forcibly turned or twisted counterclockwise after binding and partially unwinding is more likely to fracture. The cutting effect is mostly on the upstroke; however, some excess packing of dentin filings can occur if the instrument is not returned to the predetermined apical depth each time it is introduced.

Kerr files, generally known as K-files (Fig. 6-21), can be used in a rotary motion as well as an up-and-down action. In general they may be better suited to

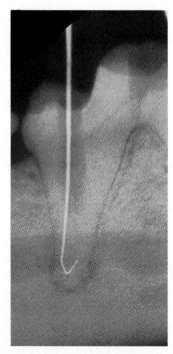

FIGURE 6-27
Radiograph showing a fine endodontic file that is bent at its tip.

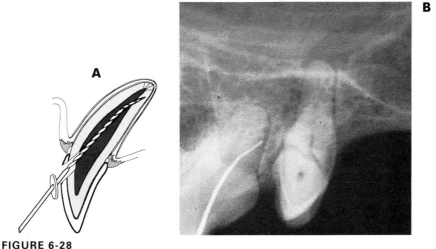

FIGURE 6-28
A and **B,** An incorrectly directed file is gouging the dentinal wall of the root canal.

veterinary dentistry than the more easily fractured Hedstrom files. In tight canals, K-files tend to unwind when a twisting force is applied. This fault can be detected by observing a shiny area on the file (usually 1 to 4 mm from the tip) where the flutes have started to unwind. K-files should be examined frequently and replaced as soon as a defect is seen because these defects are potential fracture sites of the file. The K-type files can be used in a twisting, up-and-down motion.

With both Hedstrom and K-files, the angle of insertion is changed slightly with each insertion, following a gradual circular pattern. The purpose of this change in direction as the file is pumped in and out is to ensure that the entire circumference of the canal is cleaned (Fig. 6-29). Failure to change the angle during insertions will result in the file carving out one pathway, leading to ledging or gouging and possible perforation (Fig. 6-28). Hedstrom or K-files are better for this purpose than reamers because reamers (Fig. 6-21) have a planing action and are most effective when twisted. If the canal is straight, it is safe to use the reamer; however, reamers should not be used in curved canals.

Once the initial file can be manipulated easily within the canal to full working length, the next-size

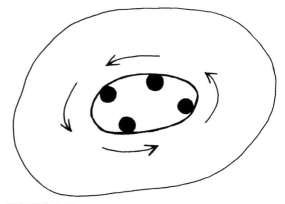

FIGURE 6-29
The entire surface of the root canal wall is filed by angling the file circumferentially as it is worked in and out.

file is used, and so on until the desired prepared canal diameter is achieved (see discussion later in this section). Each time a new, larger file is to be used, the original (smallest size) file is inserted to full working length and a few filing motions are made to free any compacted dentinal debris from the apical area. The

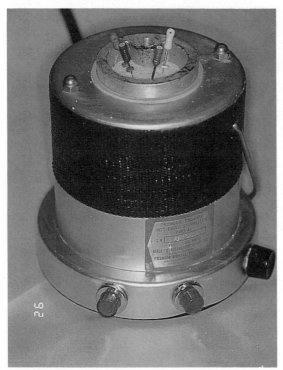

FIGURE 6-30
Bead sterilizer with endodontic files.

debris is flushed out with copious irrigation. This process is referred to as *recapitulation*. K-type files rather than Hedstrom files are recommended for recapitulation, although they may not be available in sufficient length to reach the apex of some long canine teeth.

To prevent carriage of contaminated material deeper into the canal, root canal instruments should be sterilized between insertions. This is best accomplished with a bead or salt sterilizer (see Chapter 11), a small electrically heated metal container into which the filing end of the instrument is inserted for several seconds (Fig. 6-30). An endodontic file organizer helps to keep the in-use files in orderly fashion during a procedure (Fig. 6-31).

Step-Back Preparation

In this technique the desired objective is a tapered apical preparation. With each change to a larger file size, the working length is reduced by 1 mm. It is important that the preparation is recapitulated between file changes with use of the original file size at the original file length. This technique is useful for roots that are sharply tapered in the apical one third; however, this rarely is the case in canine and feline dentistry.

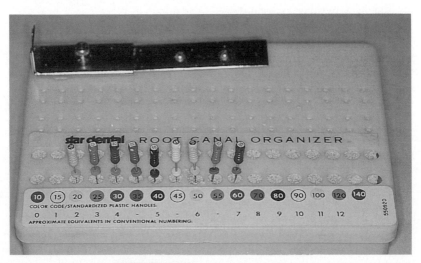

FIGURE 6-31
Endodontic file organizer with files.

Proper Diameter of the Prepared Root Canal

Proper diameter is determined by factors that control effectiveness of filling the root canal space. First, all soft or necrotic tissue in the canal must be removed. Usually, this is determined by observing clean white dentinal shavings as the file is withdrawn (Fig. 6-32). An absence of further necrotic debris after prolonged instrumentation and multiple flushes, or lack of black stain on a paper point inserted to the apex, is another indication. Following the curvature of the original canal, the canal is widened to a diameter in which a sufficient bulk of gutta-percha can easily be placed and condensed to the apical extent of the preparation. A properly prepared canal must maintain sufficient thickness of dentin along the length of the root canal to give strength to the remaining tooth structure while producing smooth tapering walls. Final file size and working length in a large series of canine and feline root canal procedures are shown in Table 6-2.

Management of Straight Canals

Straight canals need little special consideration. A reaming action can be used (the file is rotated on its long axis). This cuts the dentin in a fine planing action. The K-file can be rotated on its long axis one-quarter turn on insertion, withdrawn, and cleansed; the canal is irrigated and lubricated, and the file is reinserted to the desired prepared depth. Files of progressively larger diameter are used carefully, with recapitulation. This reaming motion should be used only for full-length straight canals. Because of the whipping action at the file tip, this type of rotation in a curved canal can cause the apical aspect of the root canal to be prepared to a greater diameter than the middle portion of the root canal.

Management of Curved Canals

Most root canals are curved. A thorough knowledge of the management of curved canals is necessary for endodontic success. In the treatment of curved canals, the files used in preparing the curved canal must all terminate at the same place in the root canal preparation. A reaming action must never be employed in preparing curved canals. Curved canals are cleaned with curved files. As a curved canal is pre-

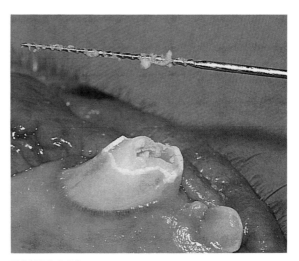

FIGURE 6-32
Clean dentinal shavings withdrawn from a root canal indicate that the canal has been cleaned of organic debris.

pared, dentin is removed selectively so that some of the curvature is reduced. It often is necessary to shorten the working length to prevent penetration of the apex by an instrument that is now longer than the new, straighter preparation.

Use of Mechanical Instruments

Mechanical instruments, such as the Gyromatic contra-angle, and long-shank burs, such as Gates-Glidden burs and Peeso reamers, have been used to facilitate canal preparation. The advantage of mechanical root canal preparation is reduced operative time, which is an important factor, but this approach lacks accuracy. Most mechanical devices have a tendency to overfile the root canal, particularly in curved canals, creating a canal outline that did not previously exist. A portion of the original root canal usually has not been cleaned by the mechanical device, and residual tissue remains to contaminate the root canal. At this time mechanically operated files of sufficient length to reach the apexes of canine teeth of dogs are not available. Mechanical instrumentation should be followed by hand instrumentation. Hand instrumentation can be followed by mechanical instrumentation.

TABLE 6-2	Final file size and working length in canine and feline root canal procedures

Tooth	Number of root canals	Type of animal*	Master apical file size and length (mm)			
			Mean		Range	
			File size	Length	File size	Length
Upper canine	8	Small dog	25	23	20-70	12-30
	23	Medium dog	55	33	25-100	22-42
	66	Large dog	50	36	30-140	30-47
	18	Cats	35	18	25-55	13-30
Lower canine	3	Small dog	60	19	25-90	15-23
	10	Medium dog	70	29	45-100	20-39
	40	Large dog	55	39	20-120	30-47
	7	Cats	45	16	30-90	12-19
Upper fourth premolar			*Distal:*			
	12	Small dog	35	18	15-50	10-21
	26	Medium dog	35	18	20-55	15-24
	19	Large dog	40	22	25-90	17-30
			Mesiobuccal:			
	12	Small dog	30	14	15-50	10-21
	26	Medium dog	30	17	20-55	15-23
	19	Large dog	35	21	20-60	15-23
			Palatal:			
	12	Small dog	25	13	15-35	10-17
	26	Medium dog	30	14	15-55	5-21
	19	Large dog	25	14	15-35	15-21
Lower first molar			*Distal:*			
	5	Medium dog	40	25	35-45	24-27
	4	Large dog	55	19	45-60	11-22
			Mesial:			
	5	Medium dog	40	25	30-45	23-29
	4	Large dog	50	20	45-60	11-29
Upper first molar			*Distal:*			
			45	11		
	1	Large dog	*Mesiobuccal:*			
			45	11		
			Palatal:			
			45	13		
Upper third premolar			*Distal:*			
	1	Large dog	70	10		
	1	Large dog	*Mesial:*			
			70	9		
Lower fourth premolar			*Distal:*			
	1	Medium dog	25	16		

Data courtesy of E. Eisner, Denver Veterinary Dental Service, Denver, Colo.
*Size of dog: small, <9 kg; medium, 10-27 kg; large, >27 kg.

TABLE 6-2	**Final file size and working length in canine and feline root canal procedures—cont'd**					
			Master apical file size and length (mm)			
Tooth	**Number of root canals**	**Type of animal***	**Mean**		**Range**	
			File size	**Length**	**File size**	**Length**
			Mesial:			
			25	17		
Upper first incisor	1	Small dog	50	14		
	3	Medium dog	45	14		
	5	Large dog	45	16		
Upper second incisor	11	Large dog	35	18		
	1	Cats	10	5		
Upper third incisor	1	Small dog	25	18		
	4	Medium dog	40	17		
	8	Large dog	50	19		
Lower first incisor	2	Large dog	60	12		
Lower third incisor	1	Medium dog	45	15		
	2	Large dog	55	21		
TOTAL	283					

Regardless of the type of instrument used in preparing the root canal, if a proper access opening has not been established and principles of canal preparation followed, the canal will be poorly prepared and eventual clinical failure is likely.

Instrument Fracture

In spite of all precautions, instrument fracture can result from file failure, canal stricture, or several other causes (Fig. 6-33). Such fracture is caused by the restricted lumen in aged animals binding the file tips, improper use of endodontic files, stress fractures at the file flutes and shaft union, or manufacturing flaws in file construction. Generally files that are fractured and that lodge in restricted canals are the result of overtwisting or rotation of files that are not designed to be twisted (such as Hedstrom files). File fragments in a small diameter are rarely removable. If the fracture occurs in a mature root canal that has been prepared to a size No. 30 or larger, there is an excellent chance that the apical aspect of the root canal preparation was filled with a plug of dentinal shavings, and fracture of the file will not alter the seal of the root canal. If the file segment has lodged at the apical

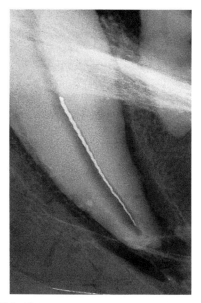

FIGURE 6-33
Radiograph reveals a broken tip of an endodontic file trapped in the root canal.

end of the canal, root canal therapy is completed to the base of the file segment. A thin mixture of endodontic filling cement is inserted, followed by gutta-percha that is condensed to the base of the retained segment. The cement forced past the file fragment can seal the file segment and apex. The prognosis is based on how clean the canal was before file fracture and how well the file segment has sealed the apex. The file fragment in effect becomes an endodontic filling cone, similar to a silver point.

If the fractured instrument was small (No. 20 or smaller) during the initial stage of cleansing pulp tissue, the chances of leakage are great and successful endodontic therapy is less likely; failure eventually may require an apicoectomy with retrofill to seal the apex and salvage the tooth (see p. 203). First an attempt is made to bypass the file fragment with a smaller file, establishing a new, lateral channel to the apex. Care must be taken in bypassing a retained file fragment. It is quite easy to perforate the root lateral to the file fragment, creating an illusion that the fragment has been bypassed, when in fact the file tip has penetrated into the periradicular tissues. A radiograph is taken with the smaller file in place after the file segment has been bypassed to ensure that the smaller file has reached the apex, properly bypassing the broken file segment. The bypassing file should be bent to follow the curvature of the canal. This will help to prevent lateral canal wall perforation. The retention of a bypassed file fragment does not affect the prognosis for the root canal procedure. Retained file segments in contaminated canals that cannot be bypassed are treated by conventional and surgical endodontic techniques. The remaining root segment coronal to the retained file fragment is cleaned and obturated in a conventional manner; a surgical endodontic technique seals the apical portion of the affected root.

Drying the Canal

Most pulpal canals can be dried with the use of sterile paper points of proper length and size. Paper points are available in lengths of 30 and 40 mm. Size is described as xx-fine (used in instrumentation with files smaller than No. 25), x-fine (for Nos. 25 to 30), fine (for Nos. 30 to 35), medium (for Nos. 40 to 45), coarse (for Nos. 50 to 55), and extra coarse (for those

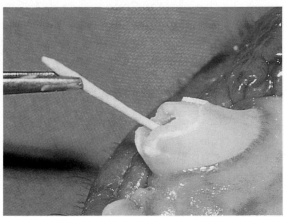

FIGURE 6-34
A paper point is inserted to dry the root canal.

larger than No. 60) or in diameters that correspond to the file diameter (No. 20 paper point for a No. 20 canal preparation).

The appropriate size of paper point is inserted into the irrigated canal to the apex and then withdrawn (Fig. 6-34). The procedure is repeated until the paper points are dry on removal. A moist paper point is gray rather than white and bends rather than folds when pushed gently against a flat surface. To ensure that the canal is thoroughly dry, the canal can be irrigated with either 95% ethyl alcohol or 99% isopropyl alcohol to remove additional moisture. Alcohol is flushed into the root canal with a needle and syringe. The alcohol is allowed to remain for approximately 2 or 3 minutes and then removed with sterile paper points.

▶ ROOT CANAL OBTURATION

The objective of obturation in endodontics is to seal permanently the cleaned and shaped root canal. Most commonly, an inert solid or semisolid material (such as gutta-percha) is used in combination with a root canal cement. Ideally the cement should constitute only a small fraction of the obturating material to reduce the possibility of dissolution and dimensional instability associated with most pastes and polymer fillings.

Fitting the Master Cone

A *master cone* is a piece of malleable, nonabsorbable material that is custom-sized and shaped to fit the apical area of the canal. Gutta-percha points are composed of 19% to 30% gutta-percha, with fillers of zinc oxide, barium salts, resins, waxes, and dyes. Under magnification, these materials combine into a solid mass with macroscopic and microscopic voids throughout the mass. Viewed under high magnification, numerous air spaces are seen throughout the content of a gutta-percha master cone. In the process of filling a root canal, gutta-percha is compacted as it is compressed.

There are two ways to fit a master gutta-percha cone. In small-diameter root canals, it often is difficult to get enough compression on the master cone to feel "tug-back" (resistance to nonforceful removal of a properly sized cone before cementation). Good lateral condensation with vertical pressure will obliterate the apical root canal space nonetheless. When it is possible to prepare the root canal to a larger diameter, a gutta-percha cone can be fitted with tug-back. This requires having a master cone one size larger than the last root canal file used to prepare the apical segment of the canal.

For a large-diameter root canal (greater than a No. 80 file) and particularly one that may have an immature apical foramen, it is possible to customize the apical fit of the master cone. One method requires the use of chemical solvents such as chloroform or eucalyptol to alter the shape of the master gutta-percha point. Two or more large gutta-percha points are sealed together with a few drops of the solvent in the bottom of a sterile dappen dish. The master cone should be slightly oversized compared with the diameter of the last root canal instrument. A slightly oversized cone will bind against the canal walls about 2 to 4 mm short of the apical preparation. The apical 2 to 3 mm of the cone is placed in the solvent for a few seconds, then introduced into the root canal as deep as it will go. The master gutta-percha point is reintroduced into the solvent and then back into the root canal in the same line of insertion until the altered gutta-percha cone reaches the depth of the last file used to prepare the root canal. The customized cone should have good tug-back and be an impression of

the apical termination of the canal preparation. The canal walls should be coated with hypochlorite irrigant when customizing techniques are used, so that chemically softened gutta-percha does not stick to the walls of the root canal preparation.

The disadvantages of this technique are that (1) most solvents such as chloroform are cytotoxic to some degree, (2) there is some shrinkage to the chemically treated gutta-percha after the solvent has dried; (3) the flow of material is hard to control, and (4) the chemically treated gutta-percha is more porous and more subject to fragmentation during trial fitting.

The gutta-percha point can be altered by heating instead of by use of chemical solvents. The master gutta-percha point is formed by heating the end of the gutta-percha to a temperature that makes it soft and pliable. This type of customization of the master point can be done by taking a gutta-percha point that is slightly smaller in diameter than the root canal preparation so that it will reach easily the apex of the root canal preparation. Because gutta-percha softens when heated, the apical 2 to 3 mm of a master gutta-percha cone can be dipped in sterile water that has been heated and introduced into the canal preparation. The bulk of the master cone remains cold and acts as a plunger against the softer 2- to 3-mm apical segment. A locking forceps is used to hold the gutta-percha cone, which is now inserted into the prepared root canal. This process is repeated as often as necessary to get the prepared cone to assume the shape and diameter of the apical preparation of the root canal. A Bunsen burner or butane cigarette lighter can be used to soften the apical 2- to 3-mm segment, which is then inserted into the root canal. The soft gutta-percha flows under the thrust of the colder bulk of gutta-percha cone, forming an impression of the root canal preparation in the same manner as with the chemically treated gutta-percha. The gutta-percha point is thus customized individually for that root canal preparation. Finally, the selected gutta-percha cone is fitted into a cement-filled canal and then condensed (see next section).

Root Canal Cements
Zinc oxide–eugenol

Zinc oxide–eugenol paste flows and does not stain the tooth structure it contacts. If root canal cement

A
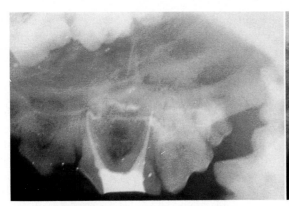
B
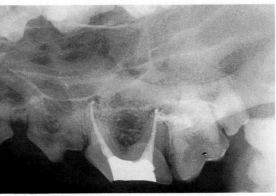

FIGURE 6-35
A, Radiograph showing extrusion of root canal cement through the apexes in the peri-apical area; the palatal root has been resected. **B,** After 18 months some of the extruded root canal cement has been absorbed, and there is no radiolucency indicating active inflammation. *(Courtesy of Philippe Hennet.)*

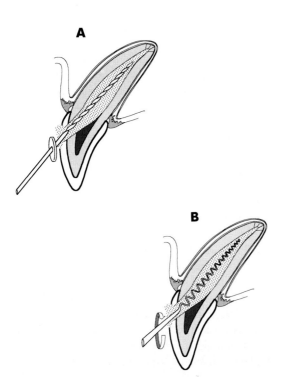

FIGURE 6-36
Loading cement to the tip of the root canal. **A,** Rotated hand file. **B,** Lentulo driven by a dental handpiece.

escapes beyond the apex of the root canal, it can cause an initial painful response but usually resorbs and causes little if any postoperative discomfort. Apical extrusion is rare in dogs with mature teeth because of the structure of the apex (Fig. 6-35). If the root canal has been properly prepared, none of the cement should escape through the apex but may flow into the apical delta and lateral canals. The zinc oxide paste and eugenol liquid are spatulated for 15 to 20 seconds to produce a homogeneous, light cream–colored paste. The setting time of zinc oxide–eugenol cement is long (several hours), giving excellent working time. The cement is introduced into the root canal in one of four ways:

1. A sterile file smaller than the last file used in preparing the root canal introduces the cement by spinning the loaded file counterclockwise (Fig. 6-36, *A*).
2. Rotary instruments such as lentulo paste fillers (Figs. 6-21 and 6-36, *B*) may be used, although there is always the risk of fragmentation of this type of instrument, particularly in small-diameter canals; they should not be used in canals of less than No. 35 file size because they will not pass to the end of the prepared canal.

3. The cement is injected into the canal by a pressure syringe through a long narrow needle that can reach the apex.
4. The paste can be introduced into the root canal with the fitted master point.

Sufficient cement should be introduced into the root canal to ensure that all the walls of the root canal preparation are covered with cement. As the file, lentulo paste filler, needle, or master point is withdrawn, some of the cement also is removed from the surface of the wall. Reintroducing cement two or three times may be necessary. As the gutta-percha and cement are introduced into the canal, the excess will exude from the coronal access opening (Fig. 6-36).

Root canal cement can be used as the only sealing material, but this is not recommended. It cannot be condensed firmly to fill irregularities in the canal and may be absorbed (although this takes many months or years).

Other root canal cements

Many other cements have been used, including Sargenti's paraformaldehyde paste and Wycoff's iodoform paste. Pastes with exotic chemical ingredients continue to be introduced. The appeal of these materials is that they can be extruded into canals that have been inadequately cleaned and shaped or that have not been cleaned and shaped at all. Although a certain degree of success can be achieved with paste fillings, no amount of chemical disinfection will neutralize a grossly contaminated root canal system. A thoroughly débrided canal requires little in the way of pharmacologic assistance. Pharmacologic pastes are a poor choice for root canal obturation.

Gutta-Percha Techniques for Filling Root Canals
Lateral condensation with gutta-percha cement

The term *lateral condensation* of gutta-percha means compression of gutta-percha against the tapering side walls of the prepared root canal. However, in compressing gutta-percha, it is impossible to compress against the side walls of the root canal without compressing vertically (apically) also. Thus lateral condensation refers to a compression of gutta-percha toward the apex of the tooth, as well as toward the lateral tapering walls of the root canal (compression in all directions).

After the cement has been thoroughly applied to the walls of the root canal preparation, the master point is seated (Fig. 6-37, *A*) and locked in place with a finger plugger (see Chapter 11). Currently, gutta-percha cones of proper length and size to reach the apex in dog canine teeth are not available. The length of commercial gutta-percha is 30 mm, and most canine

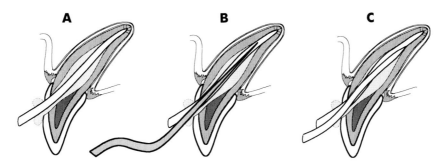

FIGURE 6-37
Condensation technique for obturation of a root canal with gutta-percha. **A,** The master point is placed to the apex. **B,** An endodontic spreader condenses the master point vertically and laterally. **C,** An auxiliary gutta-percha point is placed in the space created by the endodontic spreader.

teeth in dogs are 40 to 50 mm in length. Therefore the 30-mm gutta-percha point must be "boosted" into the apex with a plugger of proper size. Once the master gutta-percha point has been properly seated, a small-diameter (No. 1) finger spreader is placed between the wall of the root canal preparation and the master point and pressed apically, in an attempt to force the master point against the lateral wall and apical termination of the root canal (Fig. 6-37, *B*). When the small spreader has been removed, a medium (No. 2) and then large (No. 3) spreader is inserted and rotated, thus creating space for an auxiliary point. Each size enlarges the space for the auxiliary point to a greater diameter. A medium-fine auxiliary point lightly coated with sealer is introduced into this space (Fig. 6-37, *C*). Auxiliary cones come in various sizes (medium fine, fine fine) and are used to "stack" the root canal by continuing the sequence of insertion of the spreader and placement of another auxiliary point.

The gutta-percha is thermoplastic. This technique requires heating the finger spreaders by placing them in a bead sterilizer or under a flame. The spreader is introduced into the root canal immediately after removal from the sterilizer or flame. When the spreader reaches the previously placed auxiliary points and master point, it will soften the cones of gutta-percha. The spreader is then rotated. If the spreader is smooth and clean, the gutta-percha in the canal should not cling to it and become dislodged. Initially, the heated small spreader is placed; then the medium and next the large spreader are used. Another tapered auxiliary gutta-percha point is then coated with cement and introduced into the space left by the No. 3 finger spreader. This process is continued until the tip of the spreaders will not reach more than 1 or 2 mm beyond the junction of the pulp chamber and the opening of the canal orifice. At this time the root canal should be filled thoroughly—as verified radiographically (Fig. 6-38).

In the process of filling the root canal and using the thermoplastic quality of the filling material, the master and auxiliary points have been warmed and

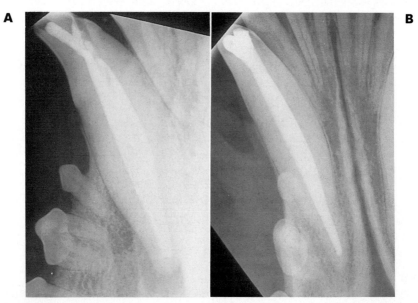

FIGURE 6-38
Radiographic verification of fill of the root canal. **A,** The root canal to the apex is completely and smoothly filled. **B,** Remineralization of lamina dura is evident 8 months later, and the periapical radiolucency is narrower.

are compressed on each other, with an intermediary layer of cement between each gutta percha-cone placed into the root canal. This produces a partially homogenized mass of gutta-percha and cement. In the process the auxiliary points have been forced apically as well as laterally.

During the process of lateral condensation, attention should be given to the size of the root canal spreader used for laterally condensing the gutta-percha. If the root canal spreader is as large or larger than the root canal diameter, it will bind against the walls of the dentin near the entrance to the pulp canal, rather than create a space between the gutta-percha and the dentin for an auxiliary cone. If binding occurs, it is not uncommon to produce a root fracture. Usually the root will fracture vertically, and this necessitates the removal of the tooth (or root, if the fracture involves one root of a multirooted tooth). If the instruments used for lateral condensation are smaller than the prepared canal, fracture will not occur.

After condensation of the gutta-percha, the excess root canal filling material and cement must be removed from the coronal aspect of the tooth (Fig. 6-39) by use of a curet that has been heated in the bead sterilizer or bur rotating at slow speed. Care must be taken, however, not to remove additional tooth structure—only gutta-percha and cement. If the tooth is to receive an endodontic post for crown construction, the post hole is prepared after removal of the excess gutta-percha from the pulp chamber (see Chapter 7). All root canals that require post space should first be thoroughly filled.

Miscellaneous endodontic filling techniques, which can be expected to produce a certain degree of clinical success, are available. Chloropercha techniques use the solubility of gutta-percha in chloroform and in certain essential oils to produce a plastic mixture that, with lateral condensation, can be expected to replicate reasonably well the internal anatomy of the root canal system. Although these techniques, properly applied, are effective, they are more demanding technically because of the difficulty of curtailing the apical movement of the chemically softened material, the potential irritant effects of the chloroform of the periapical tissues, and the measurable shrinkage that occurs when chloroform or essential oil volatilizes posttreatment.

Silver points and heavy sealer cements have been used in the past as root canal filling materials. Silver points have the advantage of being able to negotiate narrow and severely curved canals. They are radiopaque (a small advantage) and in some cases are able to seal the apexes of very narrow root canals because of the rigidity of the material. Silver points are preformed and thus cannot adapt to the intricacies of most root canal systems. It is impossible to seal canals without relying heavily on cement because a round silver cone may bind on two points only, without completely obturating an oval-shaped root canal system. Failures can occur when cement has washed out, resulting in seepage not only apically but also along the entire body of the silver cone.

Lateral condensation of gutta-percha in conjunction with nonsolvent cement has long been used. The objective is to press gutta-percha cones laterally against each other and against the dentinal walls of the canal to produce a dense and well-adapted filling. Usually the gutta-percha cones do not merge into a homogeneous mass after this technique (as occurs with gutta-percha solvent techniques). The cones glide and slip over each other until they are bound in cement as the cement sets in the later stages of the condensation procedure. This leads to a large amount of cement in the final filling. Also, little improvement over the initial fit of the master gutta-percha cone apically is

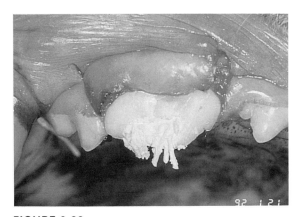

FIGURE 6-39
Excess length of gutta-percha points emerging from a filled root canal.

possible if condensation is lateral and primarily in the middle and cervical thirds of the canal. Apical seal with lateral condensation is enhanced when the spreader is used very close to the apex. In these instances the spreader is acting as a vertical condenser.

Vertical condensation with warm gutta-percha

Vertical condensation of warm gutta-percha combines ease with maximal effectiveness in consistently sealing simple and complex root canal systems. Gutta-percha can be softened by chemical action and by heat. This fact, combined with improved methods of cleaning and shaping, permits root canal systems to be filled more completely than was previously possible.

The use of vertical condensation of warm gutta-percha depends on the ability to place vertical compactors directly into root canals for proper gutta-percha positioning. The technique involves prefitting appropriate gutta-percha pluggers into the prepared root canal, selecting and preparing a master gutta-percha cone, placement of the master cone into the canal with a small amount of sealer, controlled softening of the gutta-percha with a heat-transfer instrument, and the gradual vertical compaction of the softened gutta-percha into the cleaned and shaped root canal system. A film of cement should surround the final gutta-percha filling. Vertical condensation produces dense homogeneous gutta-percha fillings with minimal cement content. All apical delta foramina are generally permanently sealed.

The technique produces the maximum cushion of softened gutta-percha, with appropriate pluggers moving the gutta-percha toward the apex. The pluggers must not contact the dentin walls of the canal preparation because a plugger wedged into the canal preparation cannot compact the gutta-percha apical to it. Vertical pressure also is essential to compact the mass, thus compensating for potential contraction as the material returns to body temperature. Any thermoplastic technique that does not include vertical compaction will result in gradual reduction in volume of the original root canal filling.

The technique is simple but should be carried out exactly for optimum results. The armamentarium consists of a series of pluggers or compactors. The pluggers are marked with 5-mm serrations so that the depth can be known at all times (see Fig. 11-24). Pluggers of sufficient length and diameter for canine teeth in dogs can be made of file shafts, Kirschner wires, or orthodontic wire, although these homemade pluggers do not have the length markings of a true endodontic plugger. Most premolar and molar teeth can be compacted with the shorter series of pluggers, the longer ones being reserved for unusually long canines or incisors.

A minimal amount of cement is desirable to ensure maximum sealing of the canal system. This technique produces a canal obturated in three dimensions. The gutta-percha is at no time chemically bound to the dentin surface. Any nonirritating cement may be used with this technique inasmuch as the cement constitutes only a microfilm around the completed gutta-percha filling.

The small amount of cement that is used in this technique is placed into the prepared canal with a lentulo paste filler. Although these instruments have been designed to fit into contra-angles, they should be used only by hand in this technique.

Heat transfer can be provided by a Bunsen burner flame or cigarette lighter. The master gutta-percha cone should be selected carefully. Preparation of the cone is the starting point for a good root canal system obturation. Most gutta-percha cones that appear to bind on initial placement into the root canal system do not bind apically; rather, they bind laterally somewhere short of the root apex. Either the length of the point should be measured against the known canal length, or the apical position should be verified radiographically. About 5 mm of the tip of the original cone should be cut off and placed into the canal to maximize apical gutta-percha bulk. Apical gutta-percha should be compacted effectively to fully seal the canal. This is more easily achieved with vertical compaction than with lateral condensation.

The gutta-percha master cones can be cones of standard size. Fine gutta-percha cones rarely are required, and fine-fine cones never are used. The apical portion of the gutta-percha cone should be cut back so that the narrow-pointed end is removed. This portion of any gutta-percha cone is of little value in effectively sealing the canal. By selective removal of varying amounts of the apical tip of a gutta-percha cone, the size of the cone can be easily adjusted to provide a great variety of master cone sizes. During adjustment, the tips of the gutta-percha cones are cut off with sterile dental scissors. The fit should be verified radiographically.

The objective is to compact gutta-percha apically. A narrow plugger in the wide portion of a canal preparation is ineffective because such a plugger will penetrate the gutta-percha without compacting it effectively. A wide plugger in the narrow portion of a canal preparation, which will bind against the dentinal walls, cannot compact the softened material.

Obturation can be effected by a sequence of condensing softened gutta-percha with pluggers, reheating the instruments, additional condensation with pluggers, reheating, and condensation deeper into the canal. With this process an exact impression can be taken of the apical half or apical one third of the root canal system. The shaped master cone is then removed, and a small amount of cement is introduced into the prepared canal by hand with a lentulo spiral filler. Care should be taken to apply the cement evenly along the length of the canal without using too much of the material. The objective is to attain a true gutta-percha filling—not one that consists primarily of cement. The apical third of the prepared master cone is coated with cement and is reinserted gently into the root canal until maximum depth has been achieved.

The plugger is compressed centrally into the mass, moved 2 or 3 mm apically, withdrawn slightly, and reinserted so as to capture any material that has been bypassed by the previous stroke. This process is repeated once or twice before additional heat is added to the gutta-percha.

The plugger is heated to cherry red, inserted directly into the central portion of the gutta-percha to a depth of 3 or 4 mm, and quickly withdrawn. Each time the plugger is used, it is hot enough to transfer heat to the gutta-percha mass and to be withdrawn easily from the gutta-percha before it "freezes" on the plugger, resulting in inadvertent removal of the gutta-percha cone at an early stage of the compaction process. Once compaction has proceeded more deeply into the canal, the gutta-percha is not likely to be removed accidentally.

The plugger repeats the vertical compaction process; first it is compressed centrally into the softened mass and then brought out slightly to recapture the softened material, with compaction repeated once or twice. The plugger is removed and reheated, reapplied to the approximate depth of 3 or 4 mm, and withdrawn. The apical portion of the preparation is sealed when compaction is appoximately 5 to 7 mm from the apex. It is not normally expected that apical movement of the gutta-percha will occur when compaction is taking place in the cervical (coronal) third of the canal, nor should it be necessary to work closer than 5 mm from the apex.

A commercially available system (Thermofill) consisting of a plastic or metal rod embedded in a gutta-percha point can be used. The gutta-percha is heated and then placed and condensed by pressing on the rod. This system gives a quick and radiographically adequate fill in incisor teeth of dogs; however, apical voids were found on microscopic examination more commonly than in canals obturated with nonheated but vertically and laterally condensed gutta-percha. The system is not yet available in sizes appropriate for canine teeth in dogs.

Back-packing. This technique consists of inserting 3- to 4-mm segments of softened gutta-percha and compacting them in a manner similar to that already described. The gutta-percha segments are obtained by cutting ordinary gutta-percha cones. Only two to four segments may actually be used for the compaction in any given case. The sequence of heat application and compaction has been rhythmically carried apically into the canal preparation and now is repeated coronally until the preparation is entirely filled.

It is more effective to use relatively narrow segments in the deeper portion of the preparation and wider ones in the wider portion of the preparation. Use of wide gutta-percha cones in the deeper portion of the preparation may lead to voids in the final filling, although they usually are of little significance. Voids also may occur if cement or gutta-percha was left on the walls of the preparation during vertical condensation. The gutta-percha segments may adhere to this lateral residual material.

Use of warm gutta-percha injectors

Injection into the root canal of small amounts of semimolten gutta-percha containing a small amount of cement can be an effective obturation technique.

A modification using a warm gutta-percha gun

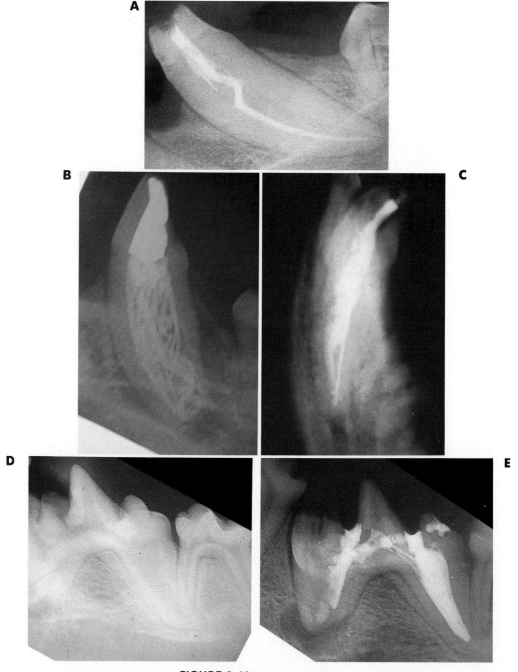

FIGURE 6-40
For legend see opposite page.

(similar to the heated glue guns) is carried out as described for the thermoplastic technique that condenses small amounts of warm gutta-percha to the apex with a heat transfer instrument. The warm gutta-percha technique, however, is designed to inject a semifluid gutta-percha mass to the apex, which is condensed while still soft, or to fill the entire canal by injecting gutta-percha through a fine needle that is inserted initially to the apex. The gutta-percha is injected into the canal as the needle is withdrawn.

This technique requires a needle large enough to nearly reach the apex. Therefore the canal must be of sufficient diameter to allow this approach. Also, the needle must be long enough to reach the apical area of an animal's canine tooth.

This procedure, which demands skillful execution, is likely to result in a poorly obturated canal without an apical seal unless used by an operator familiar with the technique and materials.

The major reason for failure of root canal procedures is inadequate apical filling of the canal. Radiographic verification of filling is essential (Fig. 6-38); if the filling is inadequate (Fig. 6-40), the gutta-percha is withdrawn (by filing if necessary) and the fill is repeated until it is correct.

▶ ENDODONTIC MANAGEMENT OF IMMATURE TEETH

The permanent teeth erupt into the mouth with root formation and length not yet complete (see p. 156). Immature teeth are weak and present problems of in-complete crown dentin development, incomplete root formation, large pulp chambers, and open apexes (Figs. 6-2 and 6-3). Immature teeth usually require endodontic attention because of trauma that results in coronal fracture and pulpal exposure.

Immature teeth with pulpal exposure are treated according to the severity and origin of the exposure. Treatment is designed to produce additional growth to the extent that maturation is possible. Those with vital pulpal tissues are treated with vital pulpotomy therapy to achieve apexogenesis, an endodontic treatment that allows the root to continue its growth to achieve a mature closed apex. Those with nonvital pulpal tissue are treated to achieve apexification. Both apexogenesis and apexification make use of the fact that calcium hydroxide raises the pH of the pulpal tissues; this alkaline environment encourages dentin and cementum formation.

Time plays a key role in these cases. A common misconception is that vital pulpotomy can be performed only in cases of recent (within a few hours) pulpal exposure or coronal fracture. The younger the tooth (and wider the root canal), the longer is the period when pulpotomy is a feasible procedure.

It is the age of the animal at the time of pulpal trauma, not the age at time of treatment, that determines canal diameter. A fractured canine tooth in a 7-year-old dog that suffered head trauma at 1 year of age will have a huge root canal and possibly an open apex, whereas the opposite, uninjured canine tooth will have a narrow root canal. To avoid surprises, the first step in endodontic treatment is to radiograph the tooth.

FIGURE 6-40
Radiographs showing inadequate root canal fill even though the access preparations on these teeth were restored. **A,** A single point has been placed to the apex but the rest of the root canal is not filled. **B,** Multiple points have been placed. This radiograph was made several months after a root canal procedure was performed without radiographic facilities. The dog is 7 years old, but the tooth was fractured several years earlier, when the root canal was much wider. **C,** Two points and an irregular mass of root canal cement, but large radiographic voids. **D** and **E,** Lower first molar tooth with a dilacerated root that was not recognized during the root canal procedure. There is (inadequate) fill of one of the distal split root canals, but the other has not been treated.

Apexogenesis

For apexogenesis to occur, vital tissue must remain in the roots (Fig. 6-41). If coronal pulp tissue has been exposed because of trauma in young animals, the pulp usually has retained its recuperative potential. The large tissue space, rich vascularity, and cellular content of young pulpal tissues greatly increase the healing potential, providing a greater potential for recovery. The sooner the pulpotomy is performed, however, the greater the success rate and the better the prospect for sustaining vitality of the radicular pulp, with subsequent normal root development. The prime concern in vital pulpotomy is to permit dentin deposition to produce a stronger root that is able to withstand future trauma. The goals of apexogenesis are as follows:

1. Sustaining a viable Hertwig's epithelial root sheath, thus allowing continued development of root length
2. Maintaining pulpal vitality, thus allowing the remaining odontoblasts to lay down dentin, producing a thicker root and decreasing the chance of root fracture
3. Promoting root end closure (apexification), thus creating a natural apical constriction for gutta-percha obturation if a future root canal is needed
4. Generating a dentinal bridge at the site of the pulpotomy (Fig. 6-42), although the bridging is not essential for the success of the procedure

Vital Pulpotomy

The goal of vital pulpotomy is to remove the coronal pulp while not damaging the remaining radicular pulp. Vital pulpotomy must be performed as a sterile procedure as far as is practical because microbial contamination of the pulp is the major danger to healing of exposed pulps. Antibiotic therapy should be used; a high blood concentration of ampicillin before pulpotomy prevents contamination of pulpal tissues during the procedure (see p. 140). Burs and instruments for placement of medications into the pulp must be sterile, the immediate environment is irrigated copiously with chlorhexidine solution before the procedure and after scaling the tooth, and sterile gloves are worn.

Technique

Access entrance is made into the exposed pulp directly in line with the root canal or along the long axis of the tooth (Fig. 6-43). This can be done with a sterile No. 2 or No. 3 round bur in a slow-speed or high-speed dental handpiece with use of copious irrigation with sterile saline solution. If canine crown height is to be reduced, a sterile tapered fissure bur (or a safe-sided diamond disk, with care) is used with water coolant to cut through the tooth, at 90 degrees to the long axis of the tooth (Fig. 6-43, *A*). The coronal 8 to 10 mm of pulp is amputated as atraumatically as possible, under sterile conditions, to remove any infected pulp and to create space for the medicaments to treat and protect the pulp (Fig. 6-43, *B*). The aim is to reach healthy pulpal tissue while minimizing damage to it. This can be achieved in one of two ways. Either a sharp, sterile spoon excavator is inserted between the pulp and the dentine wall to a depth of 8 to 10 mm; it is turned into the pulp and withdrawn with the coronal portion of pulp. Alternatively, a sharp, sterile, round bur with sterile water coolant, preferably in the high-speed handpiece, is inserted into the pulp chamber, cutting through the coronal pulp to a depth of 8 to 10 mm. At high speed a sharp bur cuts the tissue without tearing or twisting it and thus is believed to be almost as atraumatic as cutting with a dental spoon excavator. Care should be taken to avoid pushing dentine or dentinal shavings onto the pulp, which increases pulpal hemorrhage. The pulpal walls are cleansed with sterile cotton pellets. A sterile, moist cotton pellet or blunt end of a sterile paper point is placed under light pressure over the exposed pulp for 3 to 5 minutes to control hemorrhage. A pulp that continues to bleed after 5 minutes usually indicates a pulp that is inflamed and probably still contains infected tissue. Amputation of another 1 to 2 mm of pulp may be performed to reach healthier tissue, or the pulp should be removed and a conventional root canal treatment is performed. Caustic chemical agents should not be used to control hemorrhage.

Calcium hydroxide powder or calcium hydroxide powder mixed with sterile saline to a very firm paste

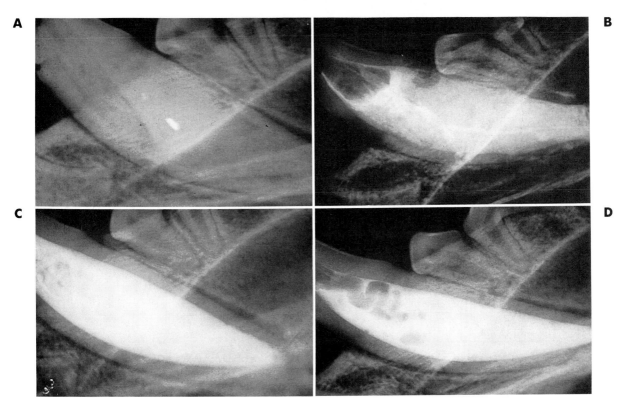

FIGURE 6-41
A-D, Radiographs showing apexogenesis; 3 to 4 months elapsed between each radiograph, with gradual lengthening of the root and apical closure.

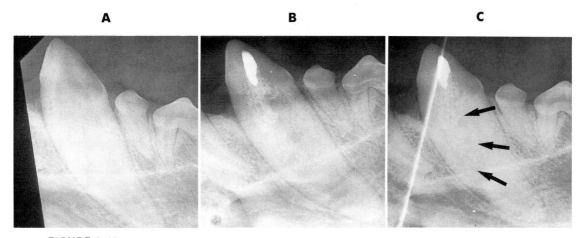

FIGURE 6-42
Dentinal bridging following pulpotomy in a fractured canine tooth. **A,** Prepulpotomy. **B,** Immediately following pulpotomy the main mass of calcium hydroxide has remained on the mesial side of the pulp chamber. **C,** After 3 months the dentinal bridge appears as an oblique radiodense line *(arrows)*.

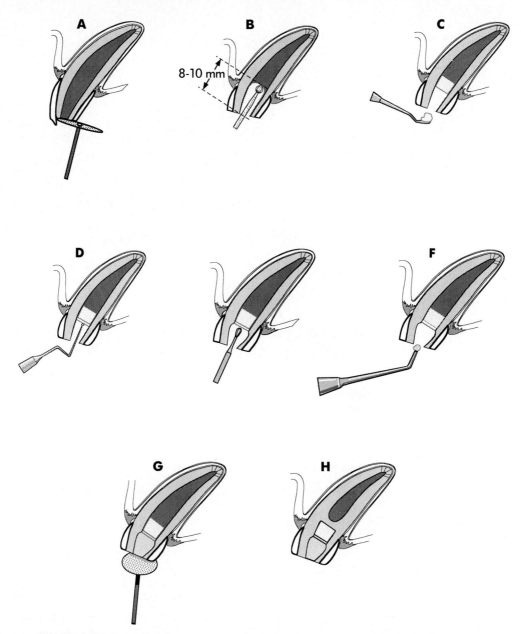

FIGURE 6-43

Vital pulpotomy: technique. **A,** The crown is transected with a sterile diamond wheel cooled with sterile saline. **B,** Approximately 8 to 10 mm of pulp tissue is removed with a sterile bur cooled with sterile saline. **C,** Calcium hydroxide powder or paste is gently packed on the pulp. **D,** A layer of hard-setting calcium hydroxide cement is placed. **E,** If composite or amalgam is to be used as the restorative material, an undercut is made with a pear bur. **F,** Restorative material is packed into the cavity. **G** and **H,** After setting, the restoration is smoothed and polished.

is placed directly onto the vital pulp with a sterile amalgam carrier and condensed under light pressure with amalgam pluggers or a plastic filling instrument to a thickness of 2 to 4 mm (Fig. 6-43, *C*). Commercial pulp capping agents such as Dycal, Life, or Pulpdent can be employed, but they are difficult to apply so that they cover the entire pulpal floor, especially in deep pulp chambers. Also because of the entrapment of air bubbles, voids can result with these fluid materials.

A calcium hydroxide cement (such as Dycal) is lightly condensed over the calcium hydroxide paste (Fig. 6-43, *D*) to provide a firm base against which to condense a permanent restorative material (Fig. 6-43, *E* to *H*; see also Chapter 7). The success of the procedure is assessed by examination of radiographs obtained at 3 to 6-month intervals (Fig. 6-44). The dentinal wall should be thicker, the apex should be closed, and a dentinal bridge should be visible. If no such changes occur, it is likely that the procedure has failed and a conventional root canal treatment is required. The apex should be examined closely to ensure that there is no apical rarefaction indicative of apical disease. Comparison with a radiograph of the contralateral normal tooth will aid radiographic interpretation.

Apexification

Apexification is endodontic therapy that involves closure of the apex by cementum formation. Apexification does not, in itself, produce any further development of the length or dentinal thickness of the root (Fig. 6-45).

Every effort should be made to attain the closure of the root apex by apexification after early pulp death. When the pulp of an immature tooth becomes necrotic, Hertwig's epithelial root sheath ceases its function of apexogenesis but can retain its function of apexification.

Immature teeth with open apex and nonvital pulp make root canal filling by conventional or surgical methods very difficult. Apexification is designed to induce apical closure by the formation of root tip osteocementum. Often the apical closure is a calcified barrier with no root lengthening. If the periapical tissue has been restored to a favorable environment,

natural root lengthening and closure by Hertwig's epithelial sheath are possible; however, further root development that takes place after pulp death is atypical and the apex tends to be shorter and less pointed (Figs. 6-41 and 6-45). Continued development depends on whether Hertwig's epithelial root sheath maintains its viability. Because the apexification procedure removes the odontoblastic layer, leaving the dental walls prone to fracture, apexogenesis or vital pulpotomy is the treatment of choice whenever possible because the added deposition of dentin in the root canal system strengthens an otherwise weak tooth.

Technique

All the necrotic contents of the immature root canal must be carefully removed to a point just short of the radiographic apex, with care taken not to disturb the root forming tissues beyond the apex. Caution should be observed in treating a young tooth because the dentinal tubules have little intratubular or peritubular calcified dentin. There is less resistance to instrumentation in treating teeth with wide canals and thin walls; it is extremely difficult to débride these root canals while still preserving enough tooth structure to support masticatory forces.

The root canal is irrigated with sodium hypochlorite to dissolve and disinfect residual necrotic tissue. Drying of the canal can be difficult because of tissue fluids escaping through the apex in the open canal. Premeasured paper points are placed to the working length and not allowed to extend beyond the apex because additional hemorrhage would occur.

A clean, sterile glass slab and spatula with no residual cement are necessary to prevent contamination of the medicament. To provide opacity and thus aid in radiographic interpretation of the extent of the calcium hydroxide paste in the root canal system, barium sulfate powder is added to the paste (one part barium sulfate to eight or ten parts of calcium hydroxide). The powder and liquid are mixed to a stiff-paste consistency that allows sufficient body for vertical condensation without needing to squeeze the material out of the canal.

The calcium hydroxide or calcium hydroxide/barium sulfate paste is placed into the root canal with a sterile amalgam carrier that is free of any retained

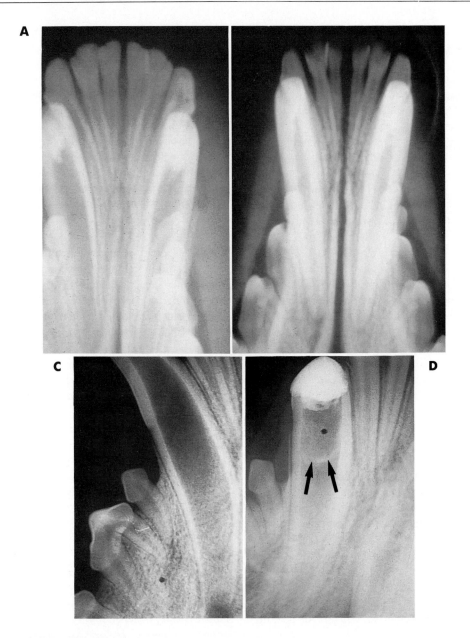

FIGURE 6-44
Vital pulpotomy: effects. **A-D,** Successful therapy. Narrowing of the root canal is evident on the 3 to 6 month postoperative radiograph. **A,** Both lower canine teeth were treated. **B,** Appearance 3 months after treatment of teeth in **A. C,** Lower canine treated. **D,** A dentinal bridge is obvious (*arrows*) 6 months later. **E-G,** Complication following pulpotomy. After the initial narrowing of the root canal (**E** and **F**) the restoration failed, leading to root canal contamination and apical abscessation, which was treated by root canal therapy (**G**).

E   F   G

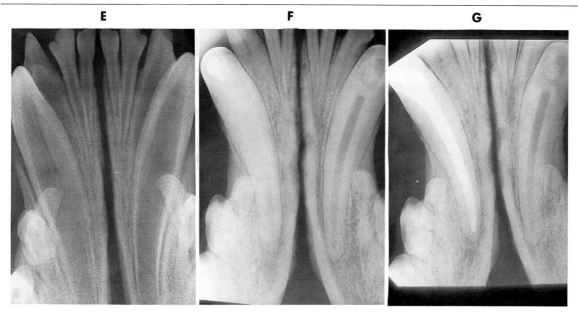

FIGURE 6-44, cont'd
For legend see opposite page.

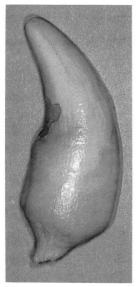

FIGURE 6-45
Canine tooth of a dog that developed distemper during a period of normally rapid growth of the length of the root. The root tip subsequently apexified. *(Courtesy of Dr. J. Arjnberg.)*

alloy particles. The paste is firmly condensed into the root canal to the periapical tissues (Fig. 6-41). For apexification to occur it is important for the calcium hydroxide to contact the periapical tissues; the apex is sufficiently open to allow this to happen if the calcium hydroxide is placed to the correct depth. Closure of the access preparation is described in Chapter 7.

The calcium hydroxide dressing should be changed every 3 to 6 months until apexification is complete; apical calcification and closure are verified radiographically (Fig. 6-41). After apexification, conventional endodontic therapy may be performed to complete treatment of nonvital pulps.

Pulp Capping

Pulp capping is the covering of an exposed (direct pulp capping) or nearly exposed (indirect pulp capping) pulp with a protective dressing to permit healing and continued function. Indications in dogs and cats are deep carious lesions, external odontoclastic resorption lesions, and elective crown height reductions.

Indirect pulp capping

Indirect pulp capping is performed when total removal of caries would result in pulpal exposure. The natural reparative mechanisms of the pulp are used. In this procedure the outer layers of carious dentin are removed. The underlying affected dentin will mineralize the odontoblasts, allowing the pulp to form reparative dentin, a therapy that avoids pulpal exposure.

The overlying surface caries is removed to the dentinoenamel junction with a large round bur. All remaining caries is removed except that just over the exposure site.

Hard-setting calcium hydroxide cement is placed over the remaining caries and areas of deep excavation close to the pulp chamber. The tooth is repaired by placing a glass ionomer cement base, followed by the final restorative of choice.

The tooth can be reentered in 3 to 6 weeks inasmuch as the primary indirect capping eventually may leak and lead to a reactivation of the carious process and pulpal involvement. The remaining caries may be carefully removed if reparative dentine has attained a sufficient depth to allow removal of the affected dentin without exposure. The tooth is restored with a hard-setting calcium hydroxide base, followed by a permanent restoration.

Direct pulp capping

Direct pulp capping is the application of a medicament to exposed pulp in an attempt to preserve tooth vitality. This differs from pulpotomy in the extent to which tissue is removed. In pulp capping only a small portion of the pulpal tissue is removed, but subsequent steps are the same as for pulpotomy procedures. Vital pulp techniques must be employed in incompletely developed permanent teeth with exposed pulp.

Pulp exposure of traumatic origin, the most common cause in dogs and cats, has a much better prognosis because it lacks the long-standing inflammation associated with dental caries seen in humans. The size of the pulpal exposure does not affect the healing potential. All pulp procedures should be performed as sterile procedures.

An injection of antibiotic may be given as soon as an accidental exposure is made. The freshly exposed pulp bleeds, which helps to flush out any con-

taminants. The cavity is flushed gently with sterile saline until all the debris is removed. Hemorrhage is controlled by gently pressing the blunt ends of large, sterile paper points onto the pulp. Continuous, gentle pressure is applied for 3 to 5 minutes to encourage clotting. Sterile cotton wool dampened with sterile saline also may be used to control hemorrhage, but care must be taken not to leave any threads of cotton wool in the canal. Caustic or thermal cautery is never used to control pulpal hemorrhage because it is far too damaging to the pulp. The cavity is dried. Calcium hydroxide powder is applied and gently pressed onto the pulp with the blunt end of a sterile paper point. The excess powder is removed with a dental spoon excavator, and the cavity is scraped clean. Hard-setting calcium hydroxide cement is mixed on a mixing pad and placed over the exposure and the adjacent dentin with a ballpoint applicator. The cement should not be spread up the sides of the cavity. After it has set hard, any excess cement is removed from the cavity walls with a dental spoon excavtor or, very carefully, with a pear-shaped bur. Calcium hydroxide powder is now in direct contact with the pulp; the cement seals the exposure and any area of thin dentin.

The cavity is lined with a glass ionomer cement to impart strength to the base of the restoration, preventing the calcium hydroxide cement from being pushed into the pulp. This also provides a further barrier between the pulp and the final filling, protecting the pulp from thermal insult and chemical leakage.

The tooth surface is prepared by exactly following the manufacturer's instructions. The material is mixed and applied to the base of the cavity over the calcium hydroxide cement and onto the surrounding dentin. Thus the base and walls of the cavity are coated with glass-ionomer, completely sealing the pulp chamber. The final filling material is applied (see Chapter 7).

After pulpal therapy the marginal or surface seal is important. Long-standing leakage of the final restoration can allow the ingress of microorganisms and contaminants into the pulpal tissues.

Crown Height Reduction ("Disarming")

Surgical crown height reduction by vital pulpotomy is a sterile procedure (described on p. 190), which should prevent infection of the pulp. The procedure usually is limited to the canine teeth of young animals, in whom it may be used to treat traumatic malocclusions (such as medially displaced lower canines impinging on the hard palate) or as a disarming technique. It should be noted, however, that shortening or extracting the canine teeth of a dog will not eliminate the danger of injury by biting (Fig. 6-46). For a dog with a mature root canal, conventional root canal therapy is recommended (see p. 165).

Obturation of Large-Diameter Canals

Total canal obturation is difficult to achieve in large-diameter canals that have undergone apexification (Fig. 6-47). After the canal is thoroughly cleaned and débrided, a root canal cement of choice, preferably a zinc oxide–eugenol type, is placed into the canal with the aid of a spiral filling instrument in a slow-speed dental handpiece. If the lumen is so large that the largest gutta-percha points will not fill the canal, bulk gutta-percha in the form of "hygienic" or "temporary stopping" can be heated and formed into large points. Preformed or handmade gutta-percha points are dipped in chloroform, a solvent for gutta-percha, to soften them. The moistened gutta-percha points are placed into the cement-filled root canal chamber and condensed laterally and apically with endodontic pluggers. Additional gutta-percha is added to the canal until the canal is filled. This modified chloropercha type of technique produces a very dense filling and appears radiographically as a complete root canal obturation.

▶ MANAGEMENT OF TEETH IN AGING ANIMALS

With aging the endodontic system goes through a continual calcification, gradually closing the lumen of the root canal to a fine diameter as it approaches the apex (see Fig. 6-2). Thus these compromised older teeth create a treatment challenge because the lumen is difficult to locate and débride. A thorough knowledge of root canal morphology, including root curvature, divergence, and direction, is essential. It is very easy to perforate these canals either laterally or through the pulpal floor in an attempt to gain access to these constricted canals. Placement of a finger in

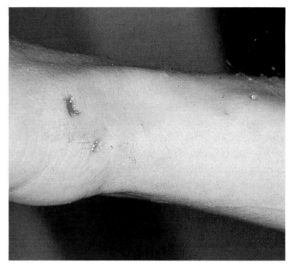

FIGURE 6-46
Wrist of a veterinary technician bitten by a dog that had been disarmed previously by extracting its canine teeth.

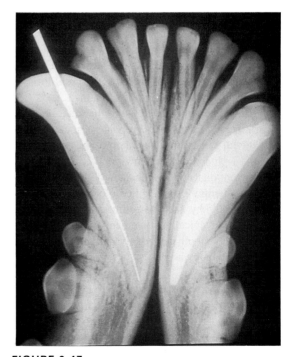

FIGURE 6-47
Radiograph showing gutta-percha filling of a very wide canal—a file is present in the contralateral canine tooth, which also was fractured.

the mucobuccal fold on the lateral aspect of each root to detect its exact angle before an attempt to gain access to the canal will help prevent mechanical root perforation. Then the operator can use a finger as a guide to follow the long axis of each root. This procedure works very well for upper fourth premolar teeth. The palatal root of the upper fourth premolar, which is the smallest in both size and root canal diameter, often is difficult to access. If it cannot be accessed, it is removed (see hemisection, p. 169), and conventional endodontics is performed on the two lateral roots (Fig. 6-18). This does not weaken the tooth to a significant extent. The furcation between the palatal root and the crown should not be entered, although it is easy to mistake the furcation for the palatal root (Fig. 6-17). Radiographs taken with endodontic files in place are essential to verify correct file position.

Older calcified root canals may not be amenable to total débridement to the apex. Normal root canal structure is elliptic, with root canal diameter narrowing toward the apex. As the root canal calcifies with age, the apical end often is difficult to access and débride to the apex. Root canal débridement is performed as far as possible apically. Some added length can be attained with continued filing with decreasingly smaller files and chelating agents (R.C. Prep, Premier Dental) that decalcify and soften dentin.

The canal is obturated to the farthermost prepared apical extent. Often radiographic verification will show the fill to be 2 to 3 mm short of the apex. These partially occluded canals show good clinical success with conventional endodontic therapy. If conventional root canal therapy of a calcified root system fails, as seen clinically by facial swelling or fistulous tract formation and apical involvement is verified radiographically, the tooth can be salvaged through surgical endodontic therapy.

▶ PERIODONTAL-ENDODONTAL RELATIONSHIPS

Periodontal disease and endodontic lesions can occur as separate or combined lesions: (1) primary endodontal, (2) primary endodontal with secondary periodontal, (3) primary periodontal, (4) primary

periodontal with secondary endodontal, and (5) true combined lesions.

1. *Primary endodontic lesions* may show mobility, fistula formation, and drainage into the mucosa or occasionally the gingival sulcus, with pulpal necrosis (Fig. 6-7). Radiographs show near-normal crestal bone length (Fig. 6-13). The lesion is resolved with conventional root canal therapy.

2. *Primary endodontic with secondary periodontal involvement* occurs as plaque accumulates along the tooth root surface with deepening pocket formation (Fig. 6-5). The tooth, if initially an endodontic lesion, will need both periodontal and endodontal therapy. The prognosis is very good, with healing of the pulpal alveolar lesion after conventional endodontic treatment and simultaneous elimination of periodontal disease by nonsurgical or surgical periodontal treatment (see Chapter 4).

3. *Primary periodontal lesions* with microbial plaque occur in association with the periodontal defect and root surface. The lesion, if allowed to progress, will cause destruction of connective tissue and loss of the tooth.

4. *Primary periodontal lesions with secondary endodontic involvement* can occur if a periodontal lesion is allowed to progress with exposure and communication via lateral canals. Exposed root surfaces free of protective cementum can allow entrance to the pulp through open dentinal tubules (Fig. 6-5). Periodontal therapy procedures themselves may lead to secondary endodontic lesions. Scaling, curettage, and flap procedures may open lateral canals or dentinal tubules, or both, to the oral environment, resulting in pulpal disease. Radiographic examination may show the primary periodontal lesion, and the secondary lesion may be difficult to diagnose. Teeth that do not respond to periodontal therapy may be endodontically involved and show pulpal necrosis that continues to express toxins into the periodontal lesion. Here, endodontic therapy must be performed to permit the periodontal therapy to resolve the periodontal disease.

5. *Combined lesions* may manifest facial swelling, lateral swelling adjacent to the apex in the mucobuccal fold, or gingival bleeding (Fig. 6-48).

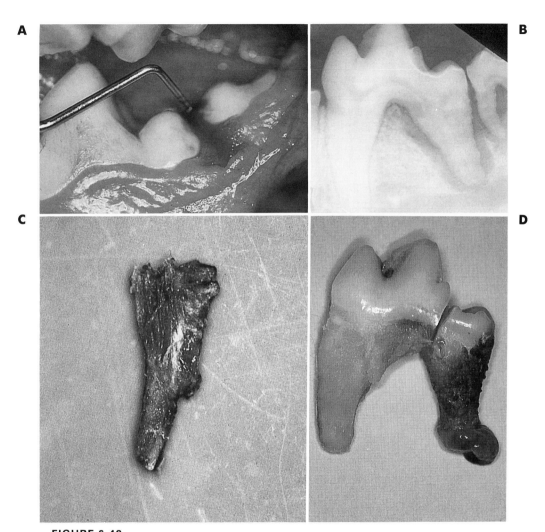

FIGURE 6-48
Periodontic-endodontic lesion of the distal root of the lower first molar tooth of a 3-year-old dog. **A,** Bleeding at the gingival margin. **B,** Radiograph shows lysis of the lamina dura and adjacent trabecular bone extending to the apex of the distal root of the first molar and mesial root of the second molar teeth. **C,** 5 to 6 mm long wood or bone foreign body found during exploration of the pocket. **D,** Extracted first molar tooth with calculus extending to the apex of the distal root and an apical granuloma on that root.

Swelling of a periodontal nature usually is coronal to the mucogingival junction, except in cases with furcation involvement or very long roots and periodontal abscessing (see Figs. A-67, A-72, and A-73, pp. 66-68). If the lesion is periodontal, a probe can be placed to the bottom of the swelling through the gingival sulcus. Endodontic swelling is not likely to reach the gingival sulcus unless it is very long-standing. Swelling can develop after root planing in cases of deep periodontal pockets if the pockets are not thoroughly irrigated after root planing.

Endodontic lesions can progress into periodontal lesions, or vice versa, through either communication via lateral canals or patent dentinal tubules that serve as portals for irritants to reach the pulp. Because dentinal tubules decrease in size as they approach the cementum, they act as a barrier to periodontal space contamination, but frequent or overzealous root planing leaves the root denuded of the nonporous protective cementum. The exposed tubule can then permit entry of bacteria into the pulp.

Prognosis of combined lesions leading to chronic endodontic-periodontic involvement is guarded. The prognosis for a periodontal lesion leading to an endodontic lesion is poor.

Treatment

Treatment of endodontic-periodontic lesions should start with antibiotic therapy if swelling is present. Endodontic treatment should be accomplished first because the lost bone resulting from endodontic lesions often will regenerate spontaneously after endodontic therapy. When the defect no longer will improve, periodontal treatment may begin. This must include prophylaxis and may require more vigorous procedures such as bone grafting therapy for pocket elimination.

A common combination lesion in dogs is seen in the upper fourth premolar tooth, in which the distal root has no bony support but the mesiobuccal and palatal roots are well supported in bone. These cases can best be treated by removal of the distal root (hemisection) and by conventional root canal therapy performed on the two rostral roots. The entrance to the pulp chamber of the retained rostral roots and crown can be restored with a composite filling material. The edges of the retained crown are rounded and planed with a No. 7802 finishing dental bur and high-speed handpiece. Prognosis and function of the retained rostral portion of the upper fourth premolar are good.

▶ COMPLICATIONS OF ENDODONTIC PROCEDURES

Most endodontic problems can be prevented if preoperative radiographs are used to determine endodontic morphology and abnormalities. Iatrogenic complications result from improper technique, instrumentation, or lack of familiarity with anatomic variations (Fig. 6-40, *D* and *E*).

The most common complications are those of technique and instrumentation (Figs. 6-17, 6-24, 6-27, and 6-40). Additional problems are restricted and occluded canals (see next section), root fractures, large immature root canals (see p. 189), lateral root canal perforations, pulpal floor perforations, and broken endodontic files lodged in the root canals (see pp. 179-180).

Occluded Canals

Occluded canals usually can be seen radiographically. They occur occasionally in dogs and cats. Success or failure of treatment is related directly to the operator's ability to débride and obturate these restricted canals to their apical extent. Radiographic examination verifies conventional endodontic failure as a result of restricted canals. In multirooted teeth, failure usually results in only one root but occasionally in two. Surgical endodontic treatment with retrograde filling of only the affected root is performed. Management of constricted canals is described on p. 198.

Root And Crown Fractures

Root and crown fractures generally result from trauma. Crowns or cusp fractures can involve the pulp or can be confined to the dentin without pulpal exposure. In immature teeth, coronal fractures into the pulp should be treated with pulpotomy, apexogenesis, or apexification procedures. Long-standing coronal fractures of mature teeth involving the pulp are treated by conventional root canal procedures.

Coronal fractures

Coronal fractures are angular, transverse, or longitudinal (along the long axis). If the fracture stops short of the crestal bone, the prognosis for longitudinal coronal fractures is good. Those incomplete fractures that extend beyond the crestal bone but do not involve the periodontium also have a good prognosis. Both types must have full-crown coverage to prevent additional cleavage (see Chapter 7). Endodontic therapy rarely is needed in supracrestal fractures that do not involve the pulp but usually is necessary in those fractures that are subcrestal, incomplete, and longitudinal. There is no hope for tooth retention after complete longitudinal fracture; extraction is indicated (see p. 253). If the coronal longitudinal fracture is in a multirooted tooth, part of the tooth can be retained with hemisection. The retained root is treated with conventional endodontic therapy, with restoration of the access opening and pulp chamber entrance from the hemisected root with a dental restorative material of choice.

Root fractures

Root fractures of a transverse or horizontal nature are divided into three divisions on the basis of anatomic position: the apical one third, middle one third, and coronal one third of the root (Fig. 6-49). These root fractures involve cementum, dentin, and pulp. They are uncommon but are seen mostly in older dogs and cats. There is usually no fracture of the crown, but slight mobility, tenderness, possible elongation, and discoloration are clinical signs. Radiographic examination is essential to confirm the diagnosis. Radiographs taken immediaely after trauma may fail to show a root fracture that may be apparent 1 to 2 weeks later.

Horizontal root fracture

Horizontal root fractures have the ability to heal themselves, provided that the fragments are in close apposition and are immobile. Most horizontal interosseous root fractures do not need endodontic treatment if there are no chronic periodontal complica-

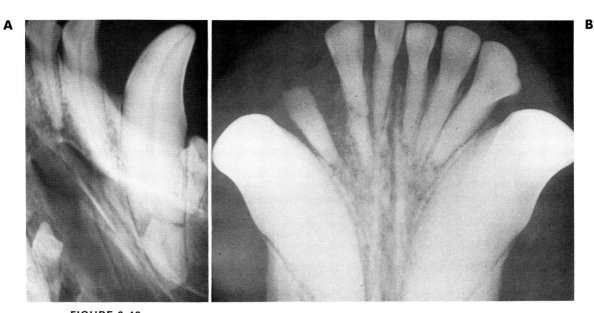

FIGURE 6-49
Radiograph demonstrates transverse root fracture of a canine tooth (**A**) and the first and second incisor teeth (**B**). A root fragment of the third incisor tooth is present in **B**.

tions. If microorganisms or epithelium invades the fracture site, prognosis is poor for the coronal segment but not necessarily the apical segment. The prognosis is most favorable for maintaining a vital pulp if the horizontal fracture is in the apical third of the root and least favorable if the fracture is in the cervical third (Fig. 6-49). Prognosis is directly proportional to the ability of the operator to stabilize interosseous horizontal root fractures. In humans no difference in prognosis exists between fractures located in the apical, middle, or coronal third of the root, provided that the teeth are immediately repositioned and firmly immobilized. In dogs, however, these fractures rarely are recognized and presented for immediate treatment, and anatomy of the teeth does not lend itself to simple, effective immobilization of single teeth (except first and second incisors). Excursions of the coronal fragment and inadequate splinting increase the frequency of pulpal necrosis. Complications usually occur within 2 months of injury. Cementum will be deposited at the fracture ends of the two segments, and the continuous deposition of cementum will join these two segments. Dentin, osteodentin, and cementum contribute to the uniting callus between the root fractures.

Injuries limited to the roots of teeth will be evident only from radiographic examination. Overexposed films increase the likelihood of diagnosis. Additional radiographs should be taken of the questionable area with a ±15-degree vertical angulation in relation to the original radiographic position. Because of partial involvement of a pulpal system in horizontal root fractures, pulp damage usually is confined to the coronal segment; the traumatic forces are unlikely to have severed the blood supply to the apical segment. Collateral circulation may be reestablished through the fracture site of the incisal segment. When the coronal segment becomes involved pulpally, only this portion requires conventional endodontic treatment. The coronal segment of the pulpal system is instrumented and treated with a calcium hydroxide base as if it were an apexification procedure (see p. 193). When a sufficient calcified callus barrier has been generated (3 to 6 months later), the calcium hydroxide should be removed and the coronal segment of the canal is obturated with gutta-percha. When both segments of the root are involved, treatment is needed for both por-

tions. When the root segments are greatly displaced, the apical segment should be removed and surgical endodontic treatment should be performed on the coronal segment if there is sufficient attachment for viability of the coronal segment. A retrograde filling is performed in the coronal segment at the fracture site immediately after a conventional endodontic procedure on the coronal segment. Splinting may be employed to aid in stabilization of an involved incisor tooth.

Lateral Root Perforations

The prognosis for a tooth with a lateral root perforation depends on the location of the perforation, the length of time the perforation is open to contamination, the possibility of sealing the perforation, and the accessibility of the main canal.

Iatrogenic root perforations usually can be managed with calcium hydroxide treatment. Location of the defect affects treatment and prognosis. If the perforation is coronal to the crestal bone, the perforation simply is restored with a restorative filling material. When the perforation is detected—usually by radiography—the calcium hydroxide paste must be placed early. This lessens the chance of periodontal complications. For calcium hydroxide therapy to be successful, the perforation has to be in an area that has osseous potential. If a large surface of the root has been destroyed, calcium hydroxide treatment would not be effective because the calcium hydroxide would be resorbed from the canal before any organized healing process could be established.

Lateral root perforation results from poor endodontic technique, particularly failure to prebend endodontic files, attempts to bypass canal obstructions, overzealous use of endodontic files, and attempts to create endodontic post space with rotary instruments. Excess gutta-percha core material should be removed with hot pluggers instead of a rotary drill (see p. 257).

Treatment

After a lateral wall perforation has been detected, the root canal is carefully instrumented to the apex, bypassing the lateral perforation. The canal is cleaned in the conventional manner and obturated with calcium hydroxide paste (calcium hydroxide and sterile saline). The paste mixture is placed in the canal with a lentulo spiral and condensed with endodontic pluggers. Calcium hydroxide will fill the lateral perforation, stimulating biologic healing. The canal may be reentered 8 months to a year later and filled with zinc oxide–eugenol and gutta-percha after the lateral perforation has closed.

Pulpal Floor Perforations

Pulpal floor perforations usually are the result of overzealous endodontic access preparation or drilling apically in an unnegotiable calcified canal with a round bur while the operator tries to locate the canal entrance. The distance from the pulpal floor to the furcation usually is less than 3 mm, making pulpal floor penetration quite easy (Fig. 6-17).

If untreated, periodontal inflammation of the furcation may rapidly produce a noncorrectable periodontal lesion. Pulpal floor perforations are best treated by placing a hard-set calcium hydroxide (Dycal) into a preparation that includes a ledge for retention just above the furcation opening. The calcium hydroxide paste stimulates biologic repair over the perforation. The root canals are obturated with zinc oxide–eugenol and gutta-percha, and a glass ionomer base is placed over the calcium hydroxide. A permanent restorative material of choice is placed over the glass ionomer base to complete the procedure.

▶ RETREATMENT AFTER FAILED CONVENTIONAL TREATMENT

Conventional root canal retreatment often can be performed in place of surgical endodontic procedures when prior conventional therapy has failed, provided that the apical tooth structures are intact. The root canal is cleared of the old gutta-percha by conventional instrumentation with use of chloroform, a solvent for gutta-percha, as the débriding agent. The canal is properly reprepared, usually to a large size, and obturated with zinc oxide–eugenol and gutta-percha.

Surgical Root Canal Therapy

The teeth most often treated with surgical or retrograde endodontic procedures are the upper fourth premolars, the upper canines, and the lower canines, in that order of frequency. The buccomesial (laterorostral) root of the upper fourth premolar most frequently is involved; root size (compared with canine tooth roots) and slight curvature of the canal make obturation difficult. Root structure and location, as well as their relationship to the adjacent structures—particularly the infraorbital vessels and nerve—must be known before treatment is commenced.

Rationale for the surgical approach

Many of the previously accepted indications for endodontic surgery no longer are valid in light of current concepts of the biologic basis for endodontic treatment. There is a high percentage of success with nonsurgical endodontic approaches with proper technique. A sound rationale for the selection of the surgical approach over the nonsurgical endodontic approach must take into account the following factors.

1. Once soft tissue flaps are reflected, they may encroach on anatomic tissue spaces, creating a potential pathway for the spread of postsurgical infection.
2. The endodontic surgical approach is not a panacea for poor nonsurgical endodontic manipulative skills or failure to understand the biologic basis for endodontic treatment.
3. The suspected presence of a periapical lesion on the basis of radiographic findings is not an indication for a surgical endodontic approach.
4. When properly prepared and obturated, the root canal and apex can be sealed adequately through the canal with reasonable assurance that the etiologic factors have been eliminated. Therefore the contention that an apical seal can be perfected only by a surgical approach also is invalid as an indication for surgery. Indeed, apical retrograde fills have been shown to be lacking in marginal adaptation and sealability.
5. The presence of overextended root canal filling material, broken instrument tips, and perforations are not necessarily valid indications in and of themselves to warrant a surgical approach. Nonsurgical treatment and observation are in order (see pp. 168, 169, 179, 180, 182, and 183).
6. When failure of nonsurgical treatment occurs,

nonsurgical retreatment generally is indicated if the cause can be identified and eliminated by that approach.

7. Surgical endodontics has not been shown to be superior to nonsurgical endodontics with regard to long-term rates of success.

In general, there are only three indications for surgery. First, if a strong possibility of failure exists with a nonsurgical approach, surgery may be indicated. Second, if a true failure exists after conventional therapy and when retreatment would not achieve a better result or is impossible, surgery may be indicated. Third, when the attempts to access the canal have failed or the canal is occluded by a broken file segment or a pulpal stone—preventing conventional access to the apex—surgery may be indicated.

The surgical flap

Principles of design

The flap is designed to permit direct access to the apex. Soft tissue flaps must be created and reflected to permit access to the surgical area, to maintain tissue integrity, and to permit proper repositioning and suturing. The following guidelines reflect these principles.

1. The maximum blood supply to the reflected tissue is essential.
2. The flap margins must be placed away from diseased tissue or the anticipated surgical defect.
3. The flap must be designed for maximal endodontic visibility, including allowing for unanticipated problems. The flap should be extended as necessary to facilitate the procedure.
4. Sharp tissue angles in the flap design should be avoided.
5. The integrity of the interdental papillae should be maintained whether or not they are to be reflected with the tissue flap.
6. Incisions should be made through the periosteum as well as the mucosa, thereby enabling reflection of the periosteum as an integral part of the flap.
7. Flap edges should not be traumatized or held with instruments or fingers. All tissue is to be retracted passively with instruments resting on bone.

8. Generally, for flaps that include the gingival margin, a minimum of one tooth on either side of the surgical site is included in the flap design.
9. Attached tissue margins should be undermined to facilitate suturing.
10. The number and placement of sutures are critical to primary healing and reduction of hemorrhage. The sutures should be placed snugly to resist residual blood flow from beneath the flap.
11. Flap design should avoid vital structures in close relationship to the tooth, such as the infraorbital artery and nerves in the infraorbital foramen during treatment of the mesial root of the upper fourth premolar tooth, and the mental vessels and nerves during treatment of the lower canine tooth (Fig. 6-50). Flap designs include semilunar, triangular, trapezoidal, or envelope.

Location for specific teeth

Upper canines. The canine eminence (juga) is palpated. The apex lies directly dorsal to the mesial root of the second premolar tooth. The flap incision can be made rostral or caudal to the canine tooth if the gingival margin is to be included, or a semilunar alveolar mucosal incision can be centered over the apex, avoiding the infraorbital nerve and vessels (Fig. 6-51).

Lower canines. The apex lies directly ventral to the mesial root of the second premolar tooth, and ventral to and just caudal to the major mental foramen. The approach can be made through the buccal mucosa ventral and caudal to the frenulum (Fig. 6-52), or it is made through a skin incision over the ventral aspect of the mandible.

Upper carnassial. The bony juga is palpated, and the center of the flap is located over the dorsal end of the juga. The infraorbital foramen is palpated to locate and avoid damage to the infraorbital nerve and vessels. The operator should take particular care in removing bone around the root apex because the infraorbital canal lies directly dorsomedial to the apex. The juga over the distal root is less prominent than that over the mesial root, and the infraorbital canal also lies directly dorsomedial to that apex. The palatal

A

Canine root relationships to first premolar roots

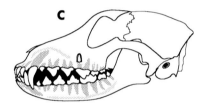

Upper   Lower

B

Lower canine root relationship to the mental foramen

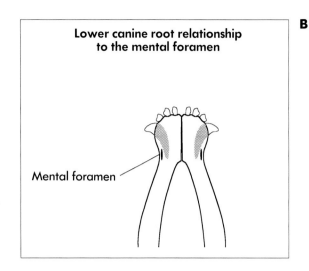

Mental foramen

C

Lateral view

FIGURE 6-50
Anatomy of root apexes. **A** and **B,** Canine teeth.
C and **D,** Upper fourth premolar teeth.

D

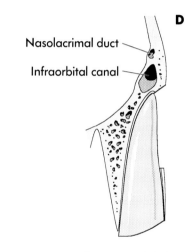

Nasolacrimal duct
Infraorbital canal

Rostrocaudal view

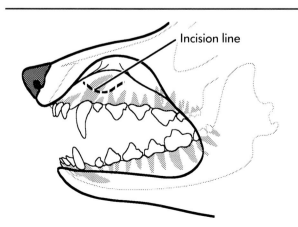

Incision line

FIGURE 6-51
Location of incision for flap exposure of the apex of
the upper canine tooth.

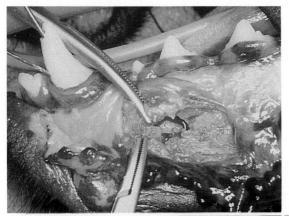

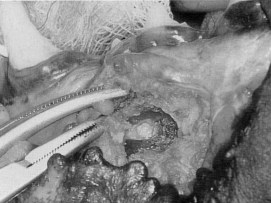

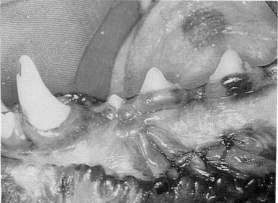

FIGURE 6-52
A, Surgical approach to the apex of the lower canine tooth. A mucosal flap has been reflected, bone has been burred away, and the tip of the root is now visible. **B,** Amalgam restoration of the apical preparation. **C,** The flap incision has been closed with interrupted sutures.

root cannot be accessed for surgical endodontic treatment.

Other teeth. Other teeth rarely require surgical endodontic treatment. The mesial and distal roots of the upper first molar tooth can be accessed with a technique similar to that for the carnassial tooth.

Surgical procedure

A full-thickness semilunar flap is raised to expose the periapical area. If additional exposure is needed, the flap should be extended. The coronal margin should be at the mucogingival line to allow the flap to be elevated instead of retracted. The flap margins are placed away from the area of disease, giving maximum visibility to the area (Fig. 6-52). If the cortical plate has already been perforated because of a periradicular pathologic process, location of the root apex

is straightforward. If perforation has not occurred, the operator must probe in the vicinity of the apex for possible bony defects. To locate the apex, a small window in the bone is made at or near the apex with a No. 4 round or No. 330 bur irrigated with sterile saline (Figs. 6-52 and 6-53, *A*). If the apex is not immediately apparent, rather than remove additional bone, an opaque object (such as a gutta-percha point) is placed in the bony preparation and a radiograph is taken with use of the opaque object as a marker to orient the approach to the apex.

After the root apex is exposed, the soft tissue is removed from around the apex and bony walls with a small curet. The apex is removed (apicoectomy) to evaluate the apical seal and to gain access to the root canal. Adequate apical root structure is removed to provide access to the root canal, to remove all acces-

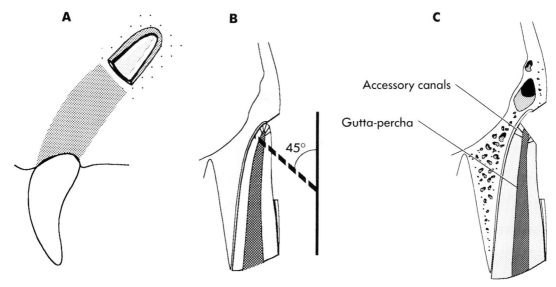

FIGURE 6-53
A, Exposure of the root apex through a window burred in the overlying bone. **B,** 45-degree angle for resection of the root apex. **C,** Resection of an inadequate length of the root, leaving part of the apical delta or lateral channels in place.

sory canals at or around the apex, and to remove the cause of disease. The apex is resected at a 45-degree angle to the lateral aspect of the face with a No. 700 or No. 701 crosscut fissure bur in a high-speed handpiece, with use of sterile saline irrigation. This angled exposure of the apex makes possible inspection and instrumentation of the apex. The resection should ensure a clean, flat root face. All root fragments apical to the resection must be removed, and the root face is inspected for accessory canals or foramina, as well as the presence of an apical seal. If accessory canals remain, the root face is further reduced to remove them (Fig. 6-53, *C*). The root canal can be prepared for a retrofill in several ways. The objective is to remove root canal contaminants and to provide access and retention for the retrofill material. The apical orifice is prepared to a depth of 2 to 3 mm into the canal and along the long axis of the root. A miniature slow-speed handpiece (see Chapter 11) and a No. 33 ½ or No. ½ round bur are preferred. Care must be exercised to avoid perforation of the root canal during the cavity preparation. A slot type of apical preparation can be made after the root is beveled for retention of a mechanical sealant such as amalgam. However, this type of preparation requires a more sensitive technique, with a greater risk of lateral root perforation, than does a simple preparation filled with a chemically bonding sealant.

Zinc-free alloy has been used to seal the apex for years, but if the root apex can be isolated from moisture during setting of the amalgam, a well-placed zinc-containing alloy may be considered. Super-EBA cement (Bosworth) is an excellent retrofill restorative. Marginal voids between the retrofill and the root structure will exist. Success depends on the depth of the restoration, the cleanliness of the canal, and the microleakage of the restoration.

Before placement of the retrofill and after the root apex has been properly prepared, the bony cavity around the root end is packed with cotton impregnated with 1:50,000 epinepherine (unless contraindicated by the anesthetic agent in use) to control hemorrhage and to prevent the spread of fragments of filling material around the bony cavity.

The restorative material is condensed or packed thoroughly to the top of the preparation (Figs. 6-52, *B* and 6-54), the excess packing material is removed, and the bony cavity is flushed with sterile saline. A radiograph is taken to verify a complete retrofill and to detect foreign bodies before suturing (Fig. 6-55). The flap is sutured with 3/0 or 4/0 absorbable material (Fig. 6-52, *C*).

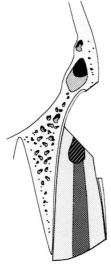

FIGURE 6-54
Restorative material has been packed into the undercut apical preparation.

► AVULSED TOOTH

Avulsion by definition is the separation of a tooth from its alveolus.

Implantation of avulsed teeth is the return into its alveolus of the tooth accidentally avulsed by trauma. Complications of reimplantation include internal and external root resorption, ankylosis, and inflammation. Inflammation in association with implantation is self-perpetuating, eventually advancing to involve the adjacent alveolar bone. The inflammatory process interferes with the elaboration of repair tissue.

Procedure for Reimplantation

The time period between avulsion and reimplantation has the greatest bearing on the success of implantation. A long, dry period causes necrosis of periodontal ligament cells. Ideally a tooth should be replanted within 30 minutes. Brief storage in saliva and milk is better than in saliva only because milk has a more suitable osmolarity for the periodontal ligament cells. Manipulation of the root physically damages the vital periodontal ligament. Root canal treatment before tooth reimplantation worsens the prognosis. Scraping or placing caustic disinfectants or other chemicals on the root is even more disastrous. Intentional removal of the periodontal ligament (to "clean" it) is followed by excessive resorption and ankylosis. Immediate implantation and postponement of pulp extirpation and canal obturation are preferred

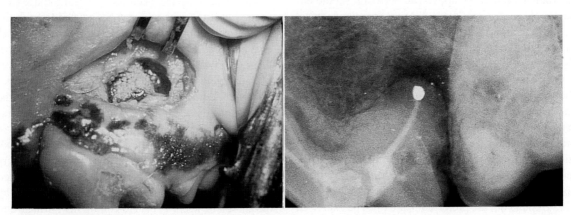

FIGURE 6-55
Surgical endodontic procedure on the distal root of the upper fourth premolar tooth. **A,** Surgical access. **B,** Radiograph of the restored apical preparation.

in treatment of avulsed teeth. Avulsed teeth are splinted to adjacent and opposing teeth with wire and acrylic (see pp. 136-137 for splint technique). The operator must make sure that the splint does not interfere with occlusion.

Root canal treatment, especially with calcium hydroxide obturation, should be performed no sooner than 2 weeks after reimplantation. A conventional root canal procedure is performed several months later. Canal fillings should be delayed until after splinting, not only to preserve the viable periodontal ligament remnants but also to maintain the maximum healing potential of the socket. Under no circumstances should retrograde fillings be used before reimplantation; invariably these reverse fillings end up as islands of foreign material in the periapical tissues and prevent the full effectiveness of calcium hydroxide that is placed 2 weeks after surgery.

In spite of excellent technique and a short period out of the mouth, avulsed canine teeth in dogs often become ankylotic, which usually is clinically evident (as fracture of the tooth) 1 to 2 years after reimplantation.

Luxation

Luxation is described as the dislocation of a tooth out of its alveolus without being totally avulsed from the mouth. Most cases of luxation are absorbed by the periodontium, without apparent long-term damage to the tooth structure. There is a distinction between a subluxated tooth and a luxated tooth. Luxation includes extrusive, intrusive, and laterally luxated teeth (Fig. 6-56). Subluxation of the tooth occurs without

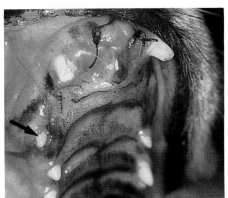
A

FIGURE 6-56
Traumatic dorsomedial luxation of a right upper canine tooth in a dog. **A,** Only the tip of the crown is visible (*arrow*) (the canine tooth on the left was fractured and extracted). **B,** Radiograph showing the intact tooth located in the nasal tissues and nasal cavity. **C,** After repositioning of the tooth, a gingival flap procedure was used to gain access to the crown of the tooth. **D,** The repositioned tooth is held in position during healing with an acrylic splint.

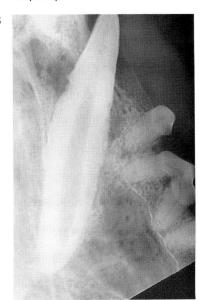
B

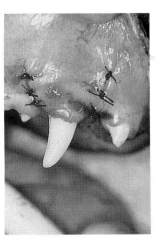
C

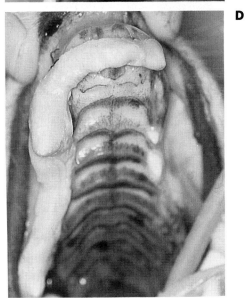
D

displacement. Luxation can result in degenerative ischemic changes. Subluxated teeth may have mobility, but usually they do not require splinting.

In luxated teeth the vascular supply to the periodontal ligament and into the root canal usually is severed. The principle of treatment for luxated teeth is the same as for avulsed teeth, except the prognosis usually is better with luxated teeth because less periodontal tissue is damaged. The likelihood of root resorption in luxated teeth is related to the severity of the luxation and the displacement. At 2 weeks the root canal is cleaned and obturated with calcium hydroxide. One year later the root canal can be obturated with zinc oxide–eugenol and gutta-percha. Both luxated and avulsed teeth show a high degree of mobility and must be stabilized by splinting for 4 to 6 weeks (Fig. 6-56, *D*; see pp. 136-137 for splinting technique).

▶ ENDODONTIC ASPECTS OF JAW FRACTURES

A long-standing axiom of jaw fracture management in humans was that teeth in the line of fracture were extracted, primarily to control infection at the fracture

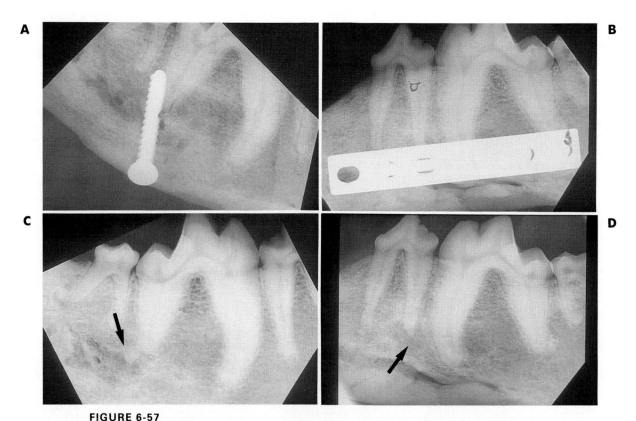

FIGURE 6-57
Bilateral mandibular fracture was treated by screw fixation on one side (**A**) and plate fixation on the other side (**B**), with impalement of tooth roots on both sides. Two months after removal of the fixation metal, a fracture of the distal root of the first molar is evident on the screw fixation side (*arrow*) (**C**) and apical lucency of the mesial root of the third premolar tooth on the plate fixation side (*arrow*) (**D**).

site. With the availability of antibiotics, advancements in endodontic therapy, and better fracture management, extraction of teeth in the line of fracture no longer is essential in every case. With the development of intraoral tooth ligation as a part of fracture fixation, teeth in the line of fracture can be used to aid in fracture management.

Teeth with long axis fracture in the direct line of the jaw fracture, fragmented teeth, coronal fractures below the crestal bone level, and transverse fractures with gross displacement of segments usually are best extracted.

Many teeth can be used to aid in fracture fixation, followed by endodontic treatment if necessary, after initial reduction has started or after removal of the orthopedic devices.

Teeth with periodontal ligament necrosis in the fracture line often result in a nonunion along the line of the necrotic periodontal ligament. The involved root can be removed (hemisection) and the necrotic bone removed, with conventional endodontic treatment of the retained root. Horizontal root fractures in the fracture line can be treated by conventional endodontic methods on the occlusal segment and surgical removal of the apical segment.

Teeth in the line of jaw fracture may require no treatment if they retain vitality throughout therapy. Postsurgical radiographic evaluation is needed to determine periapical disease.

Orthopedic fixation of jaw fracture with the use of plates, screws, intramedullary pins, osseous wires, and cross-pin or bolt systems can result in impalement of tooth roots or avulsion of the vascular supply of the root canal (Fig. 6-57). The resulting problem may not be evident until many months or even years after the bone has satisfactorily healed (see also Chapter 10).

▶ SUGGESTED READINGS

Andreason JO: Relationship between surface and inflammatory resorption and changes in the pulp after replantation of permanent incisors in monkeys, *J Endodont* 7:294, 1981.

American Association of Endodontists: An annotated glossary of terms used in endodontics, *J Endodont* 7 (special issue), 1981.

Arnall L: Some aspects of dental development in the dog. III. Some common variations in their dentition, *J Small Anim Pract* 2:195, 1961.

Bellizzi R: Veterinary endodontics, *JAVMA* 180:6, 1981.

Bellizzi R et al: Nonsurgical endodontic therapy, utilizing lingual coronal access on the mandibular canine tooth of dogs, *JAVMA* 179:370, 1981.

Bender IB, Freedland JB: Clinical considerations in the diagnosis and treatment of intra-alveolar root fractures, *JADA* 107:595, 1983.

Bergenholtz G et al: Morphometric analysis of chronic inflammatory periapical lesions in root filled teeth, *Oral Surg* 55:295, 1983.

Bhaskar SN, Rappaport HM: Histologic evaluation of endodontic procedures in dogs, *Oral Surg* 31:526, 1971.

Bigler B: Experimentelle und klinische Untersuchnugen zur Frage der aendodontischen Therapie des Hundegebisses, *Zentralbl Veterinarmed* 25:794, 1978.

Camp JH: Pulp therapy for primary and young permanent teeth, *Dent Clin North Am* 28:651, 1984.

Cohen S, Burns RC: *Pathways of the pulp*, ed 5, St Louis, 1991, Mosby–Year Book.

Colmery B: Paper presented at the meeting of the Eastern States Veterinary Association, Orlando, Fla, January 1984.

Cvek M: Clinical procedures promoting apical closure and arrest of external root resorption in non-vital permanent incisors. *Proceedings of the fifth International Conference on Endodontics*, Philadelphia, 1973, 30.

Davis MS et al: Periapical and intracanal healing following incomplete root canal fillings in dogs, *Oral Surg* 31:667, 1971.

de SonyaFillio FJ, Benatti O, de Almeda OP: Influence of the enlargement of the apical foramen in periapical repair of contaminated teeth of dogs, *Oral Surg Oral Med Oral Pathol* 64:480, 1987.

Eisenmenger E, Zetner K: Tooth fracture and alveolar fracture. In *Veterinary dentistry*, Philadelphia, 1985, Lea & Febiger.

Eisner ER: Transcoronal approach to the palatal root of the maxillary fourth premolar tooth in the dog, *J Vet Dent* 7:14, 1990.

Field EA et al: The removal of an impacted maxillary canine and associated dentigerous cyst in a chow, *J Small Anim Pract* 23:159, 1982.

Franceschini G: Traitement des fistules dentaires chez le chien par obturation des canaux, *Rec Med Vet* 8:675, 1974.

Gerstein H: *Techniques in clinical endodontics*, Philadelphia, 1983, WB Saunders Co.

Gutmann JL: Principles of endodontic surgery for the general practitioner, *Dent Clin North Am* 28:895, 1984.

Holmberg DL: Abscessation of the mandibular carnassial tooth in the dog, *J Am Anim Hosp Assoc* 15:347, 1979.

Holmstrom S: Feline endodontics, *Vet Clin North Am, Small Anim Pract* 22:1433, 1992.

Kaplan B: Root resorption of the permanent teeth of a dog, *JAVMA* 151:708, 1967.

Klein H: Schienung einer caninus Langsfrakutr beim Hund, *Kleintierpraxis* 24:144, 1979.

Kostlin R, Schebitz H: Zur endodontischen Behandlung der Zahnfraktur beim Hund, *Kleinterpraxis* 25:187, 1980.

Lane JG: Small animal dentistry, *In Pract* 3:23, 1981.

Neuman NB: Chronic oclular discharge associated with a carnassial tooth abscess, *Can Vet J* 15:128, 1974.

Okuda A, Harvey CE: Etiopathogenesis of feline dental resorptive lesions, *Vet Clin North Am, Small Anim Pract* 22:1385, 1992.

Okuda A, Harvey CE: Immunohistochemical distribution of interleukins as possible stimulators of odontoclastic resorption activity in feline dental resorption lesions, *Proc Vet Dent Forum* 6:41, 1992.

Ramy CT, Segreto VA: Apicoectomy and root canal therapy for exposed pulp canal in the dog, *JAVMA* 150:977, 1967.

Ross DL: Canine endodontic therapy, *JAVMA* 180:356, 1981.

Ross DL, Myers JW: Endodontic therapy for canine teeth in the dog, *JAVMA* 157:1713, 1970.

Rossman LE et al: The endodontic periodontic fistula, *Oral Surg Oral Med Oral Pathol* 53:78, 1982.

Seltzer S, Bender IB: *The dental pulp,* Philadelphia, 1975, JB Lippincott Co.

Sherman P: Intentional replantation of teeth in dogs and monkeys, *J Dent Res* 47:1066, 1968.

Sundquist G: Bacteriological studies of necrotic dental pulps, *Odontol Diss* 7, University of Umea, Sweden, 1976.

Sveen OB, Hawes RR: Differentiation of new odontoblasts and dentin bridge formation in rat molar teeth after tooth grinding, *Arch Oral Biol* 13:1399, 1968.

Teague HD, Tooms JP: Infraocular fistula secondary to an upper canine tooth abscess, *Feline Pract* 9:32, 1979.

Tholen M: Veterinary endodontics, *JAVMA* 180:356, 1981.

Tronstad L et al: pH changes in dental tissues after root canal filling with calcium hydroxide, *J Endodont* 7:17, 1981.

Turkey PK, Crawford LB, Carrington KW: Treatment of traumatically intruded teeth in dogs, *Angle Orthod* 57:234, 1987.

Webber RT: Traumatic injuries and the expanded endodontic role of calcium hydroxide. In Gerstein H, editor: *Techniques in clinical endodontics,* Philadelphia, 1983, WB Saunders Co.

Webber RT: Apexogenesis versus apexification, *Dent Clin North Am* 28:669, 1984.

Weine FS: *Endodontic therapy,* ed 4, St Louis, 1989, Mosby–Year Book.

Williams CA: Endodontics, *Vet Clin North Am* 16:875, 1986.

Wissdorf VH, Hettling P: Röntgenanatomische Darstellung der postnatalen Entwicklung der Incisivi und Canini beim Hund, *Waltham Rep* 30:25, 1990.

Wright JG: Some observations on dental disease in the dog, *Vet Rec* 51:409, 1939.

7

Restorative Dentistry

Restorative dentistry is the restoration of a tooth and its function as close as practical to its natural state before the occurrence of disease or trauma. Restoration of fractured teeth after root canal therapy, enamel bonding for enamel defects or erosion, the replacement of trauma-induced enamel fractures, and management of dental caries and external root resorption lesions are the primary foci of veterinary restorative dentistry.

The enamel, which is the tooth's only protection from decay, cannot be formed after eruption. Exposed root structure has no enamel covering, although cementum can regenerate if conditions are optimal.

There is a well-known human dental lesion classification system (G.V. Black's classes I to VI) based on location of lesions and type of tooth. We have elected not to use the Black system for describing dental lesions for the following reasons: differences in dental anatomy; incidence, location, and extent of disease; the absence of a classification for true root lesions in the Black system (for example, furcation involvement, midroot caries on the distal surface of a mesial root); and the confusion that results from two lesions in the same location of different teeth having different Black classifications (that is, II and III for incisors and premolars). Pending agreement by the veterinary dental community on a classification system that is relevant to canine and feline dentistry, we use the following dental lesion classification system

in this chapter, with alphabetic notation to avoid confusion with the Black system.

▶ DENTAL LESION
Classification System

Type A   Lesion confined to the crown (no involvement of the cementoenamel junction [CEJ]), with no pulpal exposure; includes most enamel hypoplasia and attrition lesions, some crown trauma and caries lesions (Fig. 7-1, *A*)

Type B   Lesion confined to the crown (no involvement of the CEJ), with clinically evident pulpal exposure; includes some crown trauma and caries lesions (Fig. 7-1, *B*)

Type C   Lesion centered on or involving the CEJ, enamel, cementum, and dentin but with no pulpal exposure; includes some feline external resorption lesions, some canine caries lesions, and occasional crown trauma with a slab that extends across the CEJ (Fig. 7-1, *C*)

Type D   Lesion centered on or involving the CEJ, involving enamel, cementum and dentin, and with pulpal exposure; includes some feline external resorption lesions, some canine caries lesions, and crown trauma with root fracture (Fig. 7-1, *D*)

Type E   Lesion confined to the root (no involvement of CEJ), including the furcation, with no evidence

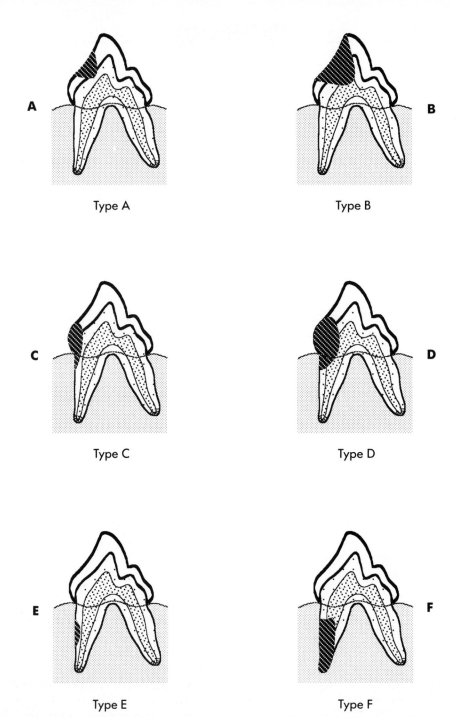

Type A

Type B

Type C

Type D

Type E

Type F

FIGURE 7-1
Lesion classification. **A,** Loss of coronal structure without endodontic involvement. **B,** Loss of coronal structure with endodontic involvement. **C,** Loss of coronal and root structure without endodontic involvement. **D,** Loss of coronal and root structure with endodontic involvement. **E,** Partial loss of root structure only without endodontic involvement. **F,** Loss of partial or total root structure with endodontic involvement.

of generalized root involvement; includes feline external resorption lesions, canine root lesions, idiopathic root fracture (Fig. 7-1, *E*)

Type F Generalized root involvement; includes some feline external and internal resorption lesions, idiopathic resorptive lesions in dogs, extensive root caries (Fig. 7-1, F)

Combination lesions are possible: a feline neck lesion that is type D on clinical examination may be type F on radiographic examination. In addition, lesions may be described by noting the tooth involved, specific location of the lesion (such as mesial, distal, buccal), and the extent or severity of the lesion (for example, a type B oblique fracture of the canine tooth with loss of one third of the crown height).

▶ INDICATIONS FOR RESTORATIVE DENTISTRY

Dental Decay (Caries)

Dental decay occurs when the oral bacteria (plaque) that cover substantial areas of the teeth feed on fermentable carbohydrates, producing organic acids (lactic, acetic, and propionic) as by-products of their metabolism. These acids diffuse into the tooth, dissolving mineral from the subsurface crystals, leading to gradual breakdown of the tooth structure. The continued process leads to cavity formation. The predominant bacteria found in association with caries in humans are *Streptococcus mutans, S. sanguis,* and lactobacilli; these organisms are not commonly a significant part of the supragingival plaque flora in dogs.

The incidence of caries in dogs varies widely in reported surveys (5% to 70% of dogs having one or more teeth with a caries lesion). The general conclusion is that, compared with humans, true caries is uncommon in carnivores. The teeth most commonly affected in dogs are the upper first molar and second molar and the lower first molar teeth (Fig. 7-2). When caries does occur in a dog, there often are multiple, advanced lesions present that affect several teeth. Primary caries is rare in cats.

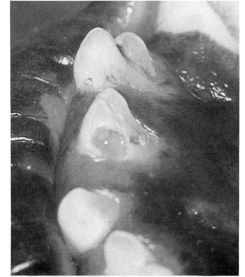

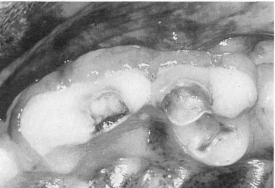

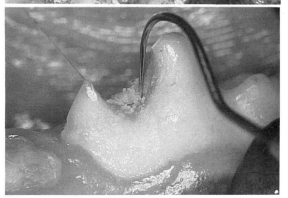

FIGURE 7-2
Clinical appearance of caries in mesial cusp of an incisor tooth (**A**), upper fourth premolar and first molar (**B**), and a lower first molar tooth (with dental explorer) (**C**).

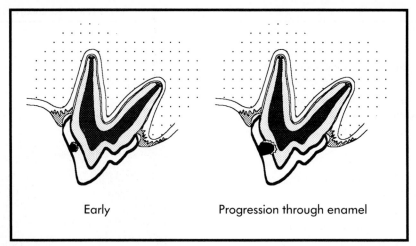

Early   Progression through enamel

FIGURE 7-3
Caries. Early lesions are confined to enamel, but progression through dentin threatens the pulp tissue.

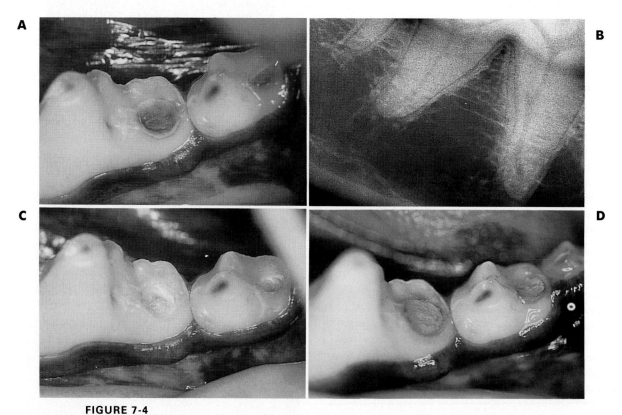

FIGURE 7-4
Treatment of caries by amalgam restoration. **A,** Caries on the distal crown cusps of the lower first and second molar teeth. **B,** Radiographs reveal normal root structure. **C,** The prepared cavities. **D,** The cavities have been filled with amalgam.

The following reasons have been suggested for this low incidence of coronal caries in carnivores: most of the teeth are nonoccluding, with sharply tapered or conical crowns that are naturally self-cleansing (compared with the occlusal-table teeth that are most commonly affected in humans); the diet of carnivores contains less fermentable carbohydrates that promote growth of *S. mutans* and other caries-producing bacteria; and salivary pH is higher (mean of 7.5 compared with 6.5 in humans), which buffers the acids produced by bacteria. An attempt to create caries in teeth of dogs by drilling defects in the enamel, inoculating lactobaccilli into the mouth, and feeding a diet high in fermentable carbohydrates failed during a 2-year study period.

Coronal caries manifests initially as a decalcified white spot that later may be stained. This small defect might be detected by a sharp explorer point. Continued decalcification results in tooth structure loss, staining, and deeper penetration into the tooth structure (Fig. 7-3). Advanced coronal caries can enter the pulpal tissues, resulting in pulpal death and abscess development.

Coronal caries is manageable with early detection. Early to advanced lesions (types A and B) can be restored with dental restorative procedures (Fig. 7-4; see also Cavity Preparation and section on restorative techniques). Type C or D caries lesions, which involve the CEJ, are more difficult to manage.

Exposed root structure is susceptible to decay (as sometimes seen in dogs). True root caries (type E lesion) can be managed by restorative procedures (a gingival flap procedure may be necessary to gain full access to the lesion) or by extraction (Fig. 7-5). Root caries follows attachment loss in some dogs with severe periodontal bone loss; it results from demineralization by acid products of bacteria, although the bacterial species causing root caries in dogs are different from those causing coronal decay in humans. External resorption, as seen in cats, has a different pathogenesis and is described next. Some lesions in dogs cannot be classified as either root caries or external resorption by clinical appearance alone (Fig. 7-6). Radiographs should be taken to ensure that the root is normal before attempting any coronal restoration.

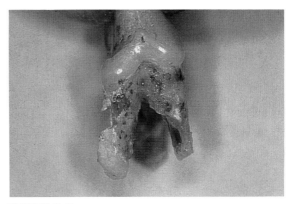

FIGURE 7-5
Cavitation (root caries?) on the root of an upper fourth premolar tooth.

External Odontoclastic Resorption (Neck Lesions, Cervical Line Lesions)

External root resorption occurs at or below the gingival margin in cats, and it usually is associated with gingival inflammation. Similar lesions occasionally are seen in dogs (Fig. 7-6). Clinically the initial resorptive lesion manifests as a slight caries-free erosion just below the crown at the CEJ (type C lesion) (Fig. 7-7). The lesion continues to erode the root tissue (Fig. 7-7, *C*), eventually invading the dental pulp (type D lesion; Fig. 7-8). When the endodontic system is involved, the tooth is not salvageable unless root canal treatment is performed at the same time. The gingiva often covers the lesion, appearing irregular, hyperplastic, and inflamed (see Figs. A-94 to A-103, pp. 73-76). Diagnosis is accomplished first with a dental explorer (see Fig. A-95, p. 74), followed by radiographic verification for the extent of external or internal resorption, or both (Fig. 7-9). One potential error that can lead to overdiagnosis of external resorptive lesions is failure to understand the root anatomy of the teeth, particularly the lower first molar tooth; the furcation of this tooth is well caudal to where it would be expected (Fig. 7-10). Occasionally, one or more teeth are extruded by the internal and external resorptive process (see Fig. A-103, p. 76). If extensive

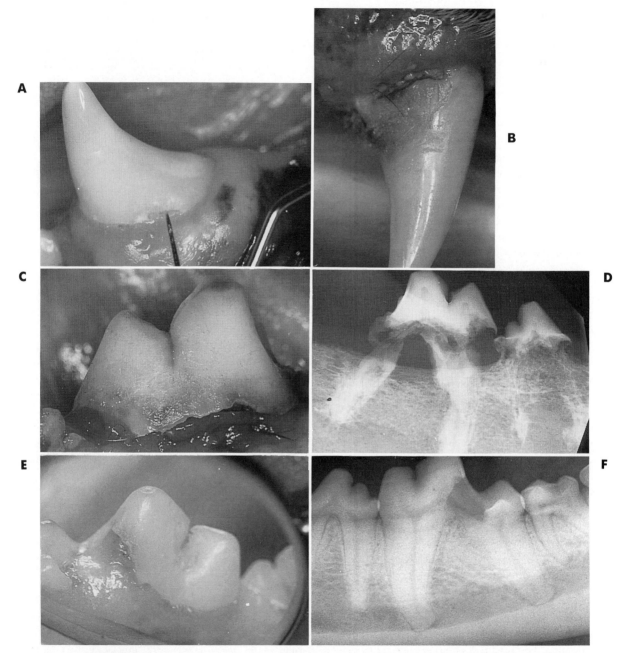

FIGURE 7-6
Tooth cavitations in dogs. **A** and **B,** Cementoenamel junction (CEJ) lesions (type C & D) in canine teeth. **C** and **D,** Clinical CEJ destruction (**C**) and extensive root destruction (type F lesion) (**D**). **E** and **F,** Type D lesion affecting the lingual side of the central cusp of the lower first molar tooth. (**E** is a reflection of the lesion in a mirror.)

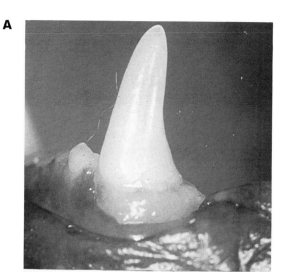

A

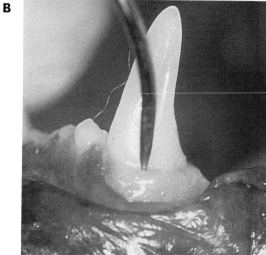

B

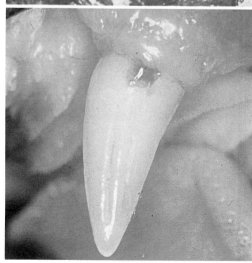

C

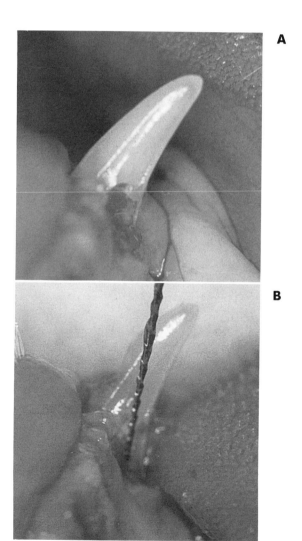

A

B

FIGURE 7-7
A and **B,** Early cementoenamel external resorptive lesion (type C) on the buccal surface of the lower canine tooth of a cat, visible only as a tiny inflammatory spot (**A**) and confirmed with a dental explorer (**B**). **C,** More obvious lesion on the buccal surface of the upper canine tooth of a cat (type C or D lesion).

FIGURE 7-8
A, Type D external resorptive lesion on the lingual surface of a lower canine tooth in a cat. **B,** A small root canal file can enter the root canal through the lesion.

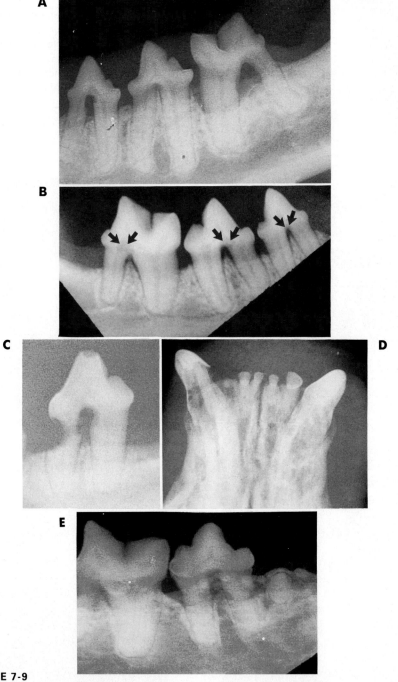

FIGURE 7-9

Radiographic features of resorptive lesions in cats. **A,** Furcation lesion (type C) and furcation bone loss affecting the third lower premolar tooth. Oblique bone loss is evident around the mesial root of the first molar tooth. **B,** Furcation lesions (type D, *arrows*) affecting the lower fourth premolar and molar teeth and possibly the third premolar tooth also (type C?). There is also bone loss. **C,** Lower fourth premolar tooth with a type D lesion on the mesial surface of the mesial root and a furcation lesion (type C). **D,** Type F lesions of both lower canine teeth. **E,** Type D lesions of the lower fourth premolar and first molar teeth and root fragment (type F) of the third premolar tooth.

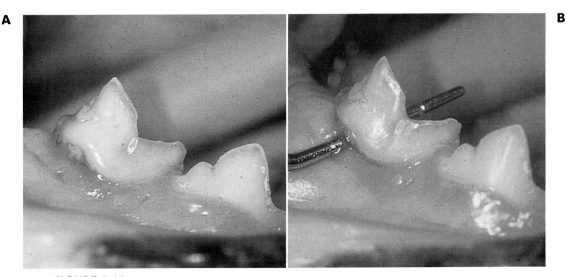

FIGURE 7-10
A, Lower first molar tooth with a possible resorptive lesion apical to the distal cusp.
B, Periodontal probe through the "lesion," which is the furcation in this tooth with periodontitis.

internal and external resorption is seen on clinical or radiographic examination (Fig. 7-9), extraction is the only practical treatment.

External root resorption is now common in domestic cats (more than 50% of cats seen for dental examination or treatment are affected, often with multiple teeth involved). Prevalence rates from several studies are summarized in Table 7-1. Examination of skulls of cats that died 30 or more years ago showed that the condition was very uncommon (approximately 1% of cats affected).

A five-step (Classes I to V) classification, based on extent of involvement only, has been proposed for neck lesions. We prefer to use the general classification of dental lesions noted at the beginning of chapter because it indicates location and extent. Further classification should be based on restorability (minor smoothing with finishing burs required; restoration required, although the lesion has not penetrated into or close to the pulp chamber or root canal; restorable but requiring root canal treatment; not restorable). Restoration of external resorptive lesions is described

later in this chapter. Usually lesions that have progressed beyond the type C lesion, often with partial or complete loss of the crown, are not salvageable. Radiographic examination helps to determine the depth of the lesion relative to the root canal and may permit identification of a clinically inapparent furcation lesion (Fig. 7-9, *A* and *B*).

Microscopic examination reveals odontoclasts in areas of active destruction (Fig. 7-11, *A*). The lesions extend into dentin, and they can extensively undermine enamel (Fig. 7-11, *B* and *C*). The destructive phase sometimes is followed by a reparative phase that produces a bonelike or cementum-like tissue that contains cells in lacunae (Fig. 7-11, *B* and *C*). The pulpal tissue is viable, and internal resorption often accompanies external resorption; this can be recognized only radiographically (Fig. 7-9).

The cause is unknown, and many theories have been proposed. Radiographic examination shows a statistically significant positive correlation between extent of tooth destruction and extent of periodontal bone loss. Currently the etiopathogenesis hypothesis

TABLE 7-1   Summary of studies of prevalence of dental resorptive lesions in cats

Author	Year reported	Country	No. of cats studied	Source of cats*	Percentage of cats having one or more lesions	Mean no. of lesions per affected cat	Age trend	Sex trend	Breed trend	Teeth most commonly affected
Schlup	1982	Switz	200	Random	28.5	2.9	Inc. w/age	None	Pure breeds	Premolars
Reichart	1984	Ger	15	Random	NR†	NR	NR	NR	NR	Premolars
Coles	1990	Aus	64	Mixed	52	3.2	Inc. w/age	None	NR‡	Premolars
Zetner	1990	Aust	24	Dental	46	NR	NR	NR	NR	NR
Remeeus	1991	NL	306	Dental	43	NR	NR	NR	Siam	NR
Crossley	1991	UK	152	Dental	57	3.5	None	None	None	NR
Present report (WEESP)	1992	NL	432	Dental	62	2.8	Inc. w/age	Inc. w/male	Siam (Asian)	Premolars
Present report (VHUP)	1992	USA	78	Dental	67§	4.1	Inc. w/age	NR	None	Premolars
Harvey	1992	USA	796	Mixed	26	2.3	Inc. w/age	NR	NR	Premolars
Dobbertin	1992	Ger	50	Mixed	20	NR	NR	NR	NR	NR

From Van Wessum et al: *Vet Clin North Am, Small Anim Pract* 22:1405, 1992.

Aus, Australia; *Aust,* Austria; *Ger,* Germany; *NL,* The Netherlands; *Switz,* Switzerland; *UK,* United Kingdom; *USA,* United States of America. *Inc. w/,* Increased with; *NR,* not recorded or reported.

*Random, Cats not selected because of oral or dental disease; *mixed,* cats seen for dental treatment and for other reasons; *dental,* cats were seen specifically for dental examination or treatment.

†Number of cats with one or more lesions was not reported as such; clinically 25% of premolars and molars had defects, percentage in canines was not reported; a higher prevalence rate (34% buccal and 29% palatal/lingual in premolars and molars, 29% buccal, and 18% palatal/lingual in canines and incisors) was found on microscopic examination.

‡Comment in text: "Three of four affected cats aged less than 6 years were Siamese."

§Prevalence based on clinical and radiologic examination.

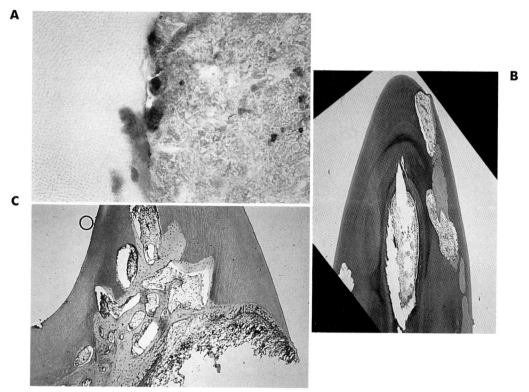

FIGURE 7-11
Destruction of coronal dentin in cat teeth. **A,** Odontoclasts actively eating away dentin in a tooth with an external resorptive lesion. **B,** Extensive undermining of the coronal dentin in a tooth with a resorptive lesion. **C,** Distal cusp of a lower first molar tooth with extensive destruction of coronal dentin. *(Courtesy of Dr. A. Okuda.)*

that seems to best fit consists of the following sequence.

1. Plaque bacteria produce an inflammatory response in the gingival tissue.
2. This results in chemotactic attraction of circulating stem cells.
3. The stem cells mature to form odontoclastic cells.
4. The initial destructive response is accompanied by immature, small-vessel granulation tissue.
5. As the granulation tissue matures, larger vessels form.
6. Remodeling with formation of bone-cementum tissue occurs in areas of adequate blood supply.

Two studies disprove the suggestion that the acid digest used to improve palatability of dry cat foods may promote the acid environment required for odontoclastic activity. Under further investigation is a possible connection between a calcium-poor diet, poor mineralization of maxillary and mandibular bone, and the presence of external resorption lesions in cats.

Treatment by restoration is confined to early lesions. If little tissue loss has occurred, smoothing the lesion with a bur and finishing stone or disk, followed by application of a fluoride varnish, is advocated. The most appropriate material for restoration of deeper lesions is a glass ionomer cement (see p. 239); in many cases, long-term results show continued de-

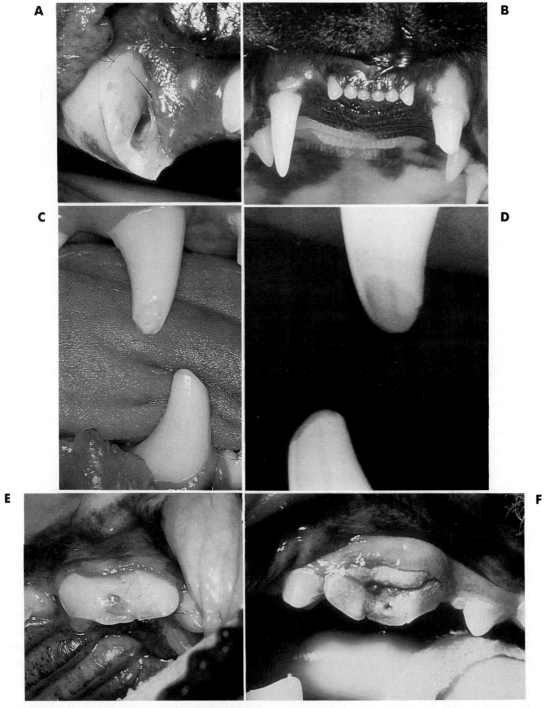

FIGURE 7-12
For legend see opposite page.

structive changes adjacent to the restoration. Prevention is difficult when the cause of the resorptive lesions is unknown. Reduction of the accompanying gingival inflammatory response, as well as plaque control by daily brushing, is recommended to control the secondary bacterial infections associated with stomatitis. Cat toothbrushes with very soft bristles are tolerated well by many cats (see Fig. 4-17, *C*). The bristles are dipped into an oral hygiene solution (see Chapter 4), and the gingival sulcus is gently stroked rather than brushed in the conventional manner. Long-term use of daily fluoride gel (0.4% stannous fluoride) may be of value in desensitizing tooth substance, remineralizing damaged enamel, and retarding accumulation of plaque.

Fracture

Coronal tooth fracture manifests as broken cusps or buccolingual/palatolingual slab fractures. Fractured crowns are common in dogs and cats, although the incidence of coronal fractures varies with the degree of activity and use by the individual animal. The teeth most commonly involved are canine (Fig. 7-12, *A* to *D*), upper fourth premolar (Fig. 7-12, *E* and *F*),

G

H

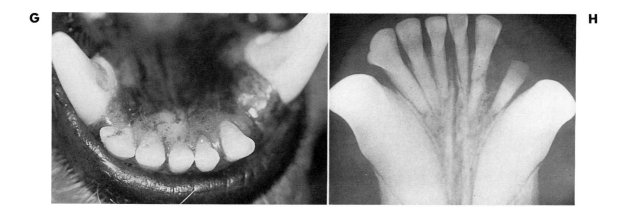

I

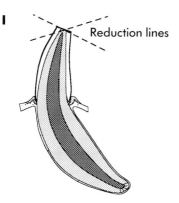

Reduction lines

Fracture does not
penetrate pulp chamber

FIGURE 7-12

Fractured teeth. **A,** Canine tooth of a dog (type D lesion). **B,** Canine tooth of a cat (type B lesion). **C,** Upper and lower canine teeth of a dog, each with type A lesions. **D,** Radiograph of teeth shown in **C** demonstrates how close the pulp chamber is to the fracture site. **E,** Slab fracture (type D) of the upper carnassial tooth of a dog. **F,** Slab fracture (type D), with the lateral slab held in place by gingival attachments. **G,** "Missing" third incisor tooth in a dog. **H,** Radiograph of **G** displays fractured root tip of third incisor and root fractures of the first and second incisors on that side. **I,** Enamel reduction lines for a type A lesion to remove unsupported enamel.

and incisor teeth (Fig. 7-12, *G* and *H*). The incidence of canine coronal fractures is high in dogs used in police or guard work.

The pulpal tissue extends most of the coronal length in young and middle aged dogs. This results in pulpal exposure with most coronal tip fractures of canines and incisors (type B lesion). The same holds true of upper fourth premolar fractures. Therefore restoration usually must be preceded by endodontic therapy. Occasionally, tip fractures do not penetrate the pulp; they require only smoothing of jagged edges (Fig. 7-12,

C and *D*) or restoration of a traumatic enamel-dentin defect (Fig. 7-13).

Unless the dog is used for guard work, simple closure of the endodontic access site after crown fracture is sufficient rebuilding of the crown; the owner, however, may wish to have a full restoration for esthetic reasons. Special attention to the replacement of the lost buccal anatomy of fourth premolars with oblique (slab) fractures (Fig. 7-14) is necessary to prevent further periodontal problems resulting from food impaction into an exposed gingival sulcus. Dogs in police

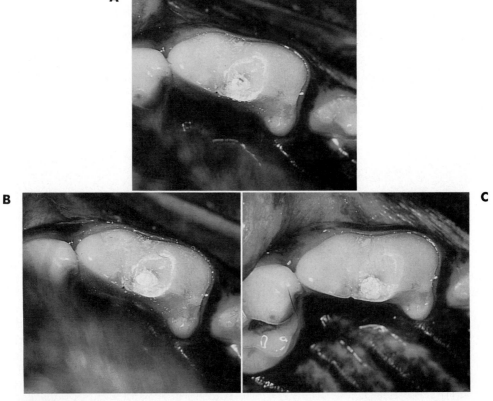

FIGURE 7-13
Amalgam restoration of a type A lesion. **A,** Fracture of the cusp tip and cavity with apparent pulp exposure in an upper fourth premolar tooth in a dog. **B,** No pulp exposure could be found, so a cavity preparation was made. **C,** The cavity is filled with amalgam.

or guard work often require full crown restoration for fractured canines and occasionally upper fourth premolars. Considerations of dental fractures in planning a restorative procedure are discussed further on p. 250.

Fractures of deciduous teeth are seen occasionally; usually extraction is the treatment of choice (Fig. 7-15), with care taken to avoid damage to the developing permanent teeth (Fig. 7-15, *B*).

Attrition

Continued grinding of teeth against any surface causes wearing away of enamel and, subsequently, dentin (Fig. 7-16). Attrition of tooth substance causes stimulation of the odontoblastic processes in the dentinal tubules. This leads to more rapid formation of new dentin on the adjacent pulp chamber surface. This new dentin ("reparative" or "tertiary" dentin) often is of a darker color than primary dentin, causing a "den-

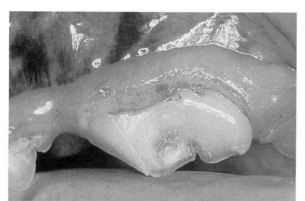

A

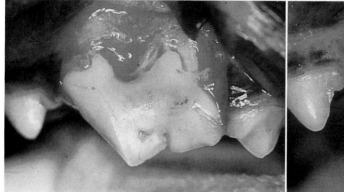

B

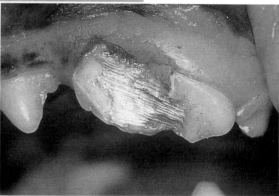

C

FIGURE 7-14
A, Slab fracture of an upper fourth premolar tooth in a dog. Gingivoplasty was performed to visualize the apical extent of the fracture line. **B,** Slab fracture of an upper fourth premolar tooth in a dog. Gingival flap surgery was performed to visualize the apical extent of the fracture line. **C,** Slab fracture of an upper fourth premolar tooth in a dog following endodontic treatment and amalgam restoration. The restoration has not restored the enamel bulge on the buccal side of the tooth, and periodontal damage is very likely to occur rapidly.

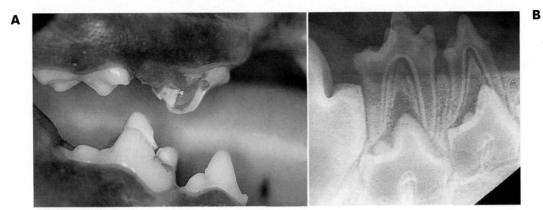

FIGURE 7-15
A, Fracture of deciduous upper and lower premolar teeth of a young dog. **B,** Radiograph shows undamaged permanent lower premolar teeth.

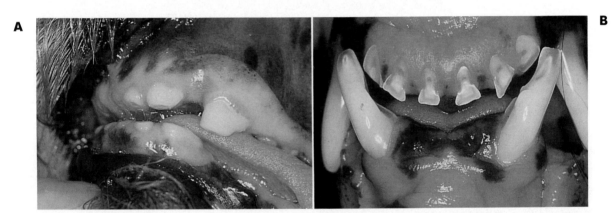

FIGURE 7-16
Dental attrition in dogs. **A,** Severe canine and incisor attrition. **B,** Severe canine and incisor attrition with dark tertiary dentinal spots visible on several teeth.

tal star" (Fig. 7-16). If the rate of attrition is slow enough so that the pulpal tissues can recede without exposure, no treatment is necessary. If, however, the rate of attrition exceeds the rate of pulpal recession, endodontic therapy may be indicated (Fig. 7-17). The decision is based on whether the dark area on the worn-down surface is firm and level with the surrounding tooth substance or whether there is a pit in the dark area that will catch the tip of a dental explorer.

Habitual chewing on cage materials, rocks, hard chew toys, and other materials (Fig. 7-18) creates excessive abrasion of tooth surfaces. Cage biters wear the distal surfaces of the canines at a rapid rate, which can result in pulpal exposure or coronal fracture (Fig. 7-19). In severe cases these teeth need full crown prosthesis to prevent fracture, although it is often possible in less severe cases to thicken the tooth at the affected area with a pin-reinforced composite dental restoration (see p. 246).

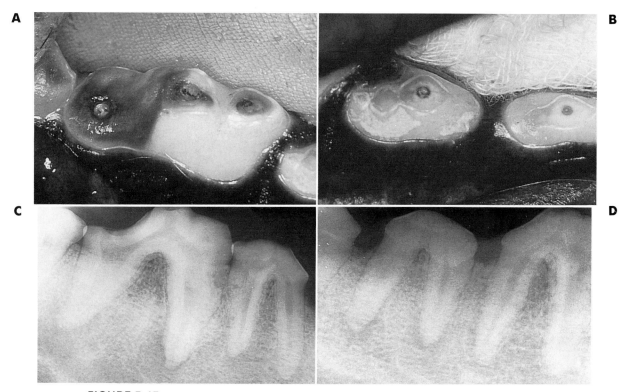

FIGURE 7-17
Rapid attrition causing endodontic lesions in a dog. **A** and **B,** Premolar and molar teeth with attrition and pulp exposures. **C** and **D,** Radiographs reveal periapical lucencies.

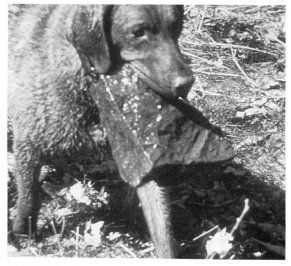

FIGURE 7-18
This dog habitually carries large rocks, risking injury to its teeth.

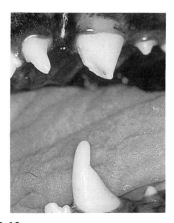

FIGURE 7-19
Fractured upper canine (type B lesion) in a dog. The lower canine has a distal coronal notch (type A lesion) resulting from chewing on metal.

Congenital and Inherited Conditions That Affect Teeth

Anomalies in the shape and number of teeth are common in dogs and cats (Fig. 7-20). These rarely are of clinical significance, and it is unethical to "alter the natural dental arcade" unless there is medical reason for doing so. These anomalies may be found in association with more obvious clinical syndromes (Fig. 7-20, *C*).

Trauma to a primary tooth can displace the developing permanent tooth bud or disrupt enamel formation, with resultant coronal or root defects, or both. One example is *dilaceration,* defined as a distorted root form (Fig. 7-20). Dilaceration can occur from any distortion of the crown relative to the root and thus may result from mechanical interference with eruption, but its usual cause is trauma to primary teeth that also displaced the permanent buds.

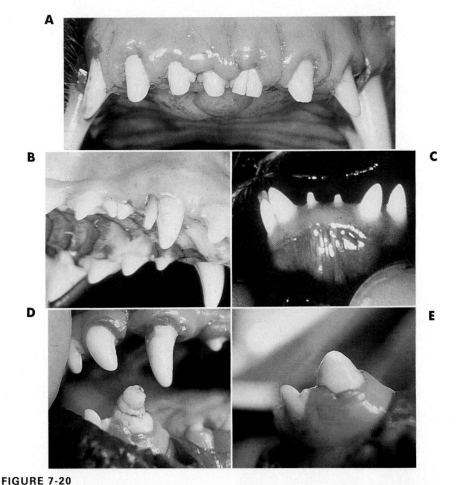

FIGURE 7-20
Dental anomalies. **A,** Conjoined or divided crown of first incisor tooth. (There are seven incisors including the abnormal tooth.). **B,** Conjoined or divided crown of a premolar tooth. (There is also a retained deciduous canine tooth.) **C,** Abnormally shaped first incisor teeth in a dog with ectodermal dysplasia. **D,** Dilaceration of the crown of a canine tooth. **E,** Composite restoration of crown in **D.**

It may be necessary to extract a severely dilacerated tooth.

Additional anomalies that affect the number of teeth or position in the jaws are described in Chapter 8.

Enamel Hypoplasia (Enamel Dysplasia, Enamel Hypocalcification)

Enamel hypoplasia can be caused by local, systemic, or hereditary factors. Local factors such as periapical inflammation or traumatic injury to a deciduous tooth may lead to hypoplasia. Febrile disorders during enamel development can interrupt the deposition of enamel, resulting in hypoplastic coronal defects. Before the common use of vaccination, distemper infection was the major cause of this condition (which is still referred to as *distemper teeth* by some dog breeders).

The condition usually affects several teeth (Fig. 7-21), although this depends on the cause of the lesion. If it is the result of local trauma or systemic pyrexia that resolves within a few days, only those areas of enamel undergoing active formation at the time will be affected. This may be seen as banding of some teeth (Fig. 7-21, *C*), with areas of normal enamel elsewhere in the tooth. Hypoplasia is more prevalent in dogs than in cats.

Amelogenesis imperfecta refers to a hereditary type of enamel hypoplasia in humans; the incidence in dogs and cats is unknown. The enamel appears as stained hypocalcified tissue that often has pits or portions of the crown missing.

Management of enamel hypoplasia usually is confined to removing sharp irregularities by burring, followed by the use of finishing stones or disks and polishing the defects (Fig. 7-22). Application of a fluoride varnish or daily application of a fluoride gel may enhance remineralization of the instrumented enamel or dentin. Occasional associated carious sites may be restored. Extensive restoration by means of acid-etch and composite resin technique (see p. 237) gives excellent immediate esthetic results, but chipping of the restoration is common within a short time. Use of mechanical retention (burring furrows into the

A 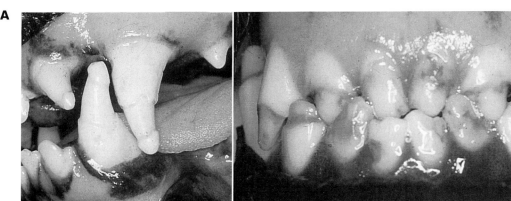 **B**

C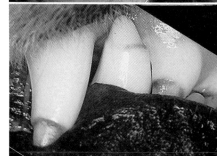

FIGURE 7-21
A, Enamel hypoplasia lesions on incisor and canine teeth of a dog. **B** and **C,** Enamel hypoplasia "bands" affecting canine and incisor teeth of a dog.

A   **B**

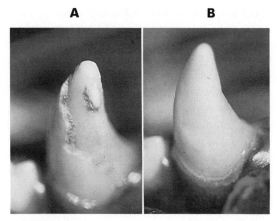

FIGURE 7-22
Enamel hypoplasia lesion on a canine tooth.
A, Before treatment. **B,** After burring smooth and
polishing remaining enamel.

enamel surface) in selected coronal sites before placing the restoration improves retention, but long-term
results are still uncertain.

▶ RESTORATIVE TECHNIQUES AND MATERIALS

Cavity Preparation

Cavity preparation is a necessary part of many restorative dental procedures. The purpose of cavity
preparation is to remove diseased material and preserve sound tooth structure. Additional removal of
tooth structure may be necessary for the convenience
of the operator or because of limitations of the restorative material to be used. There is no specific ideal
design for cavity preparation.

Principles

The operator must understand the following rules
of cavity preparation and restoration. These principles
apply to the removal of caries, treatment of external
resorption lesions, restoration of a broken crown,
or filling of access sites of an endodontically treated
tooth:

1. Removal of abnormal tooth substance without
   weakening tooth structure

2. Extension of a cavity preparation to remove all
   undermined and diseased enamel and dentin, as
   well as defects that predispose to further destruction
3. Design of cavity preparation to facilitate filling
   and finishing of the preparation to provide retention of the filling material
4. The preservation of a maximum amount of
   tooth structure to retain its inherent strength

Enamel, the inorganic component covering the
crown of the tooth, is arranged in rods running at right
angles to the tooth surface. Any unsupported enamel
at the surface of a restoration (that is, edges or portions
of unsupported or undermined enamel rods) will break
off in a short time, leaving a defect or void at the
junction of the tooth and restoration. This will trap
food and debris, leading to a breakdown of the restoration. After creation of the preparation, a simple
scraping of the cavity preparation walls with the edges
of a sharp spoon excavator will remove these unsupported enamel rods before placement of the restoration. The depth of dentin must be known while cavity
preparation is being performed. Dentin protects the
pulp from thermal shock and restorative material irritation; whenever cavity preparation, caries, or external resorptive lesion is so extensive that it encroaches on the pulp, an insulating base must be
placed over the pulpal wall to protect the pulp chamber
from irritation and eventual pulpal necrosis. Smoothness of cavity walls and margins generally is accepted
as a desirable quality. Sharp burs and diamond instruments help to prevent chipping of the enamel at
the periphery of the restoration when the bur is moved
out of the cavity preparation. Smooth margins can be
produced with twelve-bladed finishing burs (for example, No. 7901 or No. 7902). The cavity margins
can be planed or smoothed with hand instruments,
such as angle formers or gingival margin trimmers,
to remove unsupported enamel rods.

A large percentage of defects seen in veterinary
dentistry, especially in cats, occur below the CEJ (the
junction of crown and root). Without the protection
of enamel, the root surface is susceptible to decay or
external resorption. The cavity preparation is made
directly into root structure or dentin; therefore there
will be no undermined or unsupported enamel.

Technique

The following steps detail the sequence of restoration.

1. The tooth to be prepared is isolated with cotton rolls or gauze sponges to keep it free of saliva and debris. For a caries or resorptive lesion, the initial excavation can be made with a pear-shaped or round bur to the dentin at the dentinoenamel junction. For other lesions, initial excavation usually is not required.

2. The preparation is extended to the proximal, incisal, and gingival limits of the lesion to establish the general shape of the cavity. The remainder of the abnormal tooth substance is removed with a No. 1 to No. 4 round bur at slow speed (Fig. 7-23, *A* and *B*) or, if the lesion is extensive, with a hand instrument (such as a spoon excavator). The dentin may be stained by the decay, making it difficult to determine if all the decay has been removed. If the dentin has a hard, shiny appear-

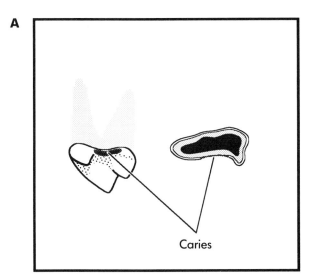

A

Caries

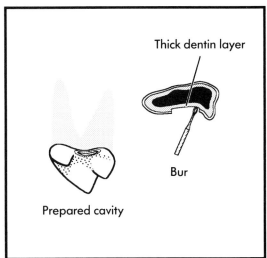

B

Thick dentin layer

Bur

Prepared cavity

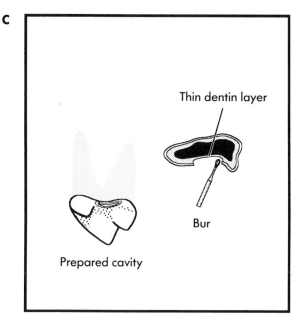

C

Thin dentin layer

Bur

Prepared cavity

FIGURE 7-23
Cavity preparation for CEJ lesions (type C). **A,** Location of the lesion. **B,** Early lesion requires minimal débridement of dentin. **C,** More advanced lesion requires deeper débridement.

A

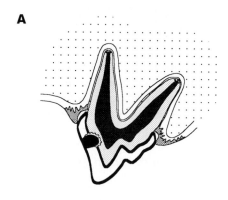

B

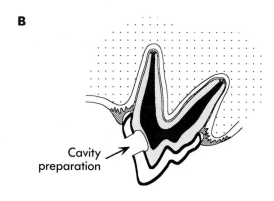

Cavity
preparation

C

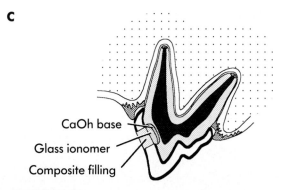

CaOh base

Glass ionomer

Composite filling

FIGURE 7-24
Cavity preparation and pulp capping. **A,** Type A lesion with deep dentinal involvement. **B,** Cavity preparation includes an undercut and has penetrated close to the pulp chamber. **C,** Restoration with composite over a calcium hydroxide pulp cap.

ance, even though it is stained and dark, it is probably healthy.

3. All unsupported enamel or dentin should be removed with a spoon excavator by lightly planing the cavity walls. Retention undercuts are placed into the dentin with a No. 1 or No. 2 round bur, pear, or inverted-cone bur if required for the restorative material to be used (see discussion of restorative material, pp. 235-237, for which materials require mechanical [undercut] retention). If the lesion has extended to or near the pulp (within 0.5 mm of the pulp) as indicated by a pink tinge or frank bleeding from the depth of the preparation (Figs. 7-23, *C* and 7-24), a medicated base of calcium hydroxide is placed over the exposed pulp before the restorative material is placed into the cavity (see following discussion of direct and indirect pulp capping). All cavity preparations should be lined or based with cavity varnish before placement of silver amalgam restorations and, within 0.5 mm of the pulp and before the final restorative material is placed (see next section), with calcium hydroxide for composite restorations. This prevents pulpal disease, sensitivity from restorative material irritation, or toxicity.

4. The final restorative material is placed (see following discussion).

Endodontic Considerations

Often deep carious lesions or fracture sites encroach on the pulp chamber, sometimes exposing it. To prevent pulpal necrosis and eventual abscessing (Fig. 7-24) the vital pulp must be protected from the external environment and from encroachment of the restorative material and resultant pulpal irritation. Currently available pulp-treatment materials may be classified as cavity varnishes, liners, and bases.

Cavity varnishes are solutions of an organic solvent and resin. Their main function is to seal the dentinal tubules. Varnishes reduce, but do not entirely prevent, penetration of acids from overlying cements into the dentinal tubules. They are ineffective in reducing thermal conductivity. Varnishes are applied with a cotton pledget in and around the cavity preparation and then air-dried. Varnishes should not be used under composite resin restorations because the organic solvent in the varnish may prevent the proper setting reaction of the resin material.

Cavity liners should be reserved for extremely thin dispersions of calcium hydroxide or zinc oxide–eugenol applied to one or more cavity walls in the proximity of the pulp. These liners are suspensions of calcium hydroxide or zinc oxide–eugenol in either a volatile organic liquid or an aqueous solution. After application, the solvents quickly evaporate, leaving a thin film of residue that is insufficient to provide a good thermal barrier. As the sole protecting medium in deep cavity preparations, cavity liners are inadequate. They should be overlaid with an appropriate base. Calcium hydroxide is the material of choice as the initial lining medium for deep pulp-capping procedures. It induces reparative dentin deposition but does not have an obtundent effect on the pulp. Because of its low compressive strength, calcium hydroxide should be overlaid with a stronger basing medium, such as reinforced zinc oxide–eugenol or zinc phosphate cement, before placement of a final restoration. Zinc oxide–eugenol probably has been used more for pulp protection and sedation than any other agent. It is considered an obtundent, capable of soothing a traumatized or slightly inflamed pulp. In deep cavity preparation with no pulp exposure, reinforced zinc oxide–eugenol is an excellent intermediary basing medium. In cases in which pulp exposures are definite or suspected, however, a liner of calcium hydroxide should precede the use of zinc oxide–eugenol. The calcium hydroxide powder mixed with sterile water is placed over the cavity wall and air dried. The zinc oxide–eugenol is placed over the calcium hydroxide, and the excess is removed from cavity walls.

Bases consist of materials such as the polycarboxylate cements, reinforced zinc oxide–eugenol cements, and glass ionomer cements. Reinforced zinc oxide—eugenol and glass ionomer cements possess greater compressive strength than the standard zinc oxide–eugenol cements. They are mixed according to manufacturers' instructions and placed over the pulpal walls (Fig. 7-24, *C*). The thickness of dentin remaining between the cutting instrument and the pulp is an important consideration; 2 mm of remaining dentin provides adequate protection for the pulp from the trauma of cavity preparation.

Indirect pulp capping

The treatment of an area of vital pulp tissue with the hope that the recuperative power of the remaining pulp is sufficient to restore it to health is referred to as *pulp capping*. When the medicaments used are applied to the pulp indirectly through a small amount of carious dentin left over a suspected pulp exposure, the procedure is referred to as *indirect pulp capping*. The objective is to arrest the carious process and to stimulate the pulp to form a barrier of reparative dentin, with remineralization of the partially decalcified dentin.

The treatment material used in indirect pulp capping is primarily calcium hydroxide followed by cavity washes, medicaments, cavity liners, and bases as already described (see also Chapter 6).

Direct pulp capping

Calcium hydroxide is the material of choice in the treatment of exposed pulp tissue (see Chapter 6). If it is used in a cavity liner form, it should be overlaid with a pressureless, thin layer of zinc oxide–eugenol and then followed by a high compressive strength cement mixed to a base consistency. This will prevent possible intrusion of the weaker underlying cavity liner into the pulp. The properly indicated restoration in the tooth is placed as soon as possible after the application of the pulpal treatment materials; this will help prevent gross contamination of the dressing and/or healing site by oral fluids. In addition, the final restoration should exhibit good marginal sealing properties and withstand the rigors of the oral environment for an extended period of time.

Amalgam

Amalgam is an alloy of silver and mercury with small amounts of other metals. Copper amalgam alloy also is available. Silver amalgam is a long-standing, excellent restorative material. Silver alloy has superior resistance to compression compared with composite filling material and is used as a filling material for retrograde endodontic therapy. Its color, however, is a disadvantage, as is the cost of additional equipment required for its use. Silver amalgam also is more difficult to place properly. Amalgam is retained in the

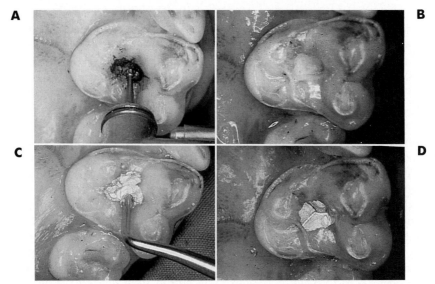

FIGURE 7-25
Amalgam restoration of a type A lesion. **A,** The lesion is prepared with a bur. **B,** The
completed preparation includes an undercut. **C,** Amalgam is packed into the cavity,
compressing from the center outward. **D,** The amalgam is carved and burnished.

tooth mechanically inasmuch as it is placed into a
cavity that has a smaller opening than the rest of the
cavity; once set, it cannot fall out. The preparation
must be undercut to ensure this mechanical retention
(Fig. 7-25). This is accomplished by angling a pear-
shaped or inverted cone bur to enlarge the floor of the
cavity without enlarging the opening (see Cavity Preparation).

Silver alloy comes in zinc and nonzinc forms. The
nonzinc form is the choice for retrograde restorations
(see discussion of apical root canal retrofill in Chapter
6) because it is unaffected by moisture and organic
materials encountered in retrograde endodontic techniques. The moisture will neither affect the setting
time nor result in expansion of the nonzinc alloy. The
alloy of choice for coronal restorative dentistry is an
alloy that contains zinc in a fine-texture form for
smoothness of carving, speed of hardening (a result
of more surface area exposed to mercury), higher copper content to resist corrosion, and ease of polishing.
Many of these "dispersed-phase" alloys are available.

Silver alloy is available in bulk, precapsulated, and
pellet forms. The precapsulated form, the easiest and
safest to use, has the silver and mercury prepackaged
in capsule form. The capsules need only to be placed
into an alloy mixing machine (amalgamator) for the
time stated by the manufacturer (see Chapter 11). The
pellet form is preferred for use with a mercury and
alloy dispenser; the mercury-alloy mixture is dis-
pensed into a capsule with a mixing pestle inside and
placed into the amalgamator. The amalgamator breaks
the pellet and mixes the silver and mercury in 9 to 20
seconds, depending on the volume of alloy to be
mixed. The silver in pellet or powder bulk form also
can be mixed by hand with the use of an amalgam
mortar and pestle. This is the least expensive way to
mix amalgam; the mixture is simply ground to the
desired consistency with the pestle. Because of the
potential toxicity of mercury vapor, amalgam should
be mixed by hand only in a well-ventilated area, and
all amalgam debris should be stored under water until
disposal.

The mixed alloy is freed from the capsule and placed in a dappen dish, then carried to the cavity preparation by means of an amalgam carrier. There it is extruded into the cavity preparation and condensed thoroughly against the lateral walls and floor of the preparation with an alloy hand condenser or plugger (Fig. 7-25, *C*). The pressure is applied from the center of the cavity outward to ensure that the undercut is filled. More alloy is placed and condensed until the cavity is filled. The excess is carved to the original anatomic shape of the tooth with an amalgam carver. After several minutes the amalgam has set to the point where it can be burnished by forcefully rubbing the surface with a smooth, round-edged instrument (Fig. 7-25, *D*).

Composite

Composite restoratives are manufactured by a number of dental manufacturing companies (see p. 378). Of the various types of composite, four types, differentiated by density or particle size, are the most practical for restorative use. These are available in chemical-cured and light-cured forms. The light-cured form is the composite of choice because it provides unlimited working time before the curing light is used to polymerize the composite. A precapsulated small-particle size, light-cured composite is ideal for bonding procedures in cases of enamel hypoplasia or erosion. These laminates are used in conjunction with an enamel acid-etching technique (see next section). Because of the capital cost of the light-curing lamp, light-cured composites are more expensive than chemical-cured composites when they are used infrequently (see Chapter 11).

Chemical-cured composite is made by a number of manufacturers (see p. 378). The manufacturer's instructions should be closely followed. This technique involves the mixing of two parts, a base and a catalyst paste, on a paper mixing pad in equal amounts. At the time of mixing, an opaque agent may be added to lighten the color of the composite. Canine teeth are whiter than the shades provided by the manufacturer for human use. The amount of the paste mix should be slightly greater than the approximate amount needed to fill the cavity preparation. The mix is placed into the cavity preparation with a plastic filling instrument (this prevents the tarnishing of some types of composite material, which could be caused by a metal instrument not designed for placement of composites). The composite is condensed ("spatulated") into the clean, thoroughly dried cavity preparation and undercuts, slightly overfilled, and allowed to set (approximately 2 to 4 minutes). After it has set, the composite is "finished" to obtain maximum smoothness. This starts with a 8- to 20-bladed finishing bur or diamond finishing bur, followed by a sandpaper disk (used on a mandrel in the contraangle attachment in the slow-speed handpiece), followed by mildly abrasive, mounted rubber points and disks.

Bonding Technique

The restoration of an eroded or hypoplastic enamel surface can be accomplished by an enamel bonding technique and use of a light-cured or chemical-cured composite system. This system also can be used for retention of orthodontic devices (see Chapter 8) and jaw fracture fixation techniques (see Chapter 10).

The entire area to be restored is first thoroughly cleaned or pumiced with a plain, nonfluoride, flour pumice (a thick paste of pumice and water is required). This is accomplished with a prophylactic handpiece and rubber prophylaxis cup in a slow-speed handpiece (Fig. 7-26, *A*). A fluoride polishing paste (as usually used for dental prophylaxis) should not be used because it interferes with etching properties of the orthophosphoric acid.

The pumiced area is thoroughly irrigated with water and dried with filtered, pressurized air or a hair dryer (on low or no-heat setting). It is important to keep the tooth surface dry and free of salivary contamination because contamination may cause the bond to fail. Acid etching agents (orthophosphoric acid) are available in gel, paste, or liquid forms. Many operators prefer the gel or paste form because it stays in position without sagging from a vertical surface. For optimal results the manufacturer's instructions should be scrupulously followed. The etchant is brushed onto the defect and surrounding sound enamel and allowed to remain in contact for 15 to 30 seconds (Fig. 7-26, *B*). A recent study suggests that a longer etching period (as much as 2 to 4 minutes) may be optimal, particularly in older dogs. The etchant should not be

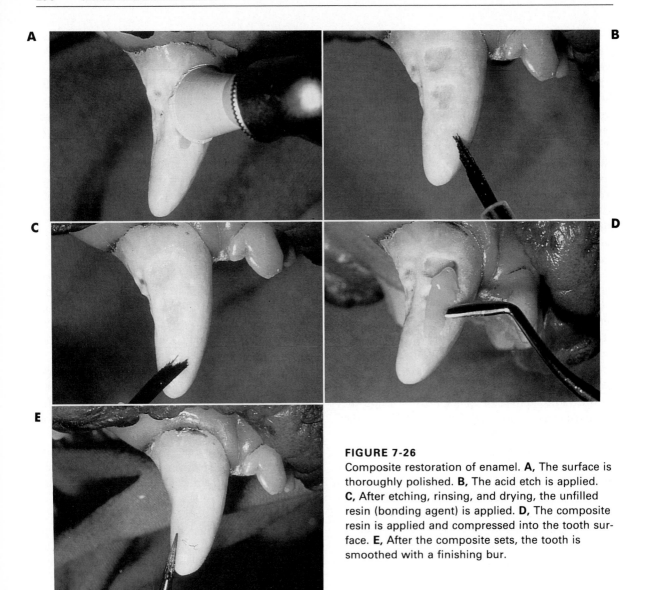

FIGURE 7-26
Composite restoration of enamel. **A,** The surface is thoroughly polished. **B,** The acid etch is applied. **C,** After etching, rinsing, and drying, the unfilled resin (bonding agent) is applied. **D,** The composite resin is applied and compressed into the tooth surface. **E,** After the composite sets, the tooth is smoothed with a finishing bur.

allowed to dry because it may cease its etching activity. The etchant is rinsed off with copious amounts of water and thoroughly dried with oil-free air. Properly etched and dried enamel has a white, frosty appearance. If this result is not obtained, the etching, rinsing, and drying steps should be repeated. Accidentally etched teeth are remineralized within 1 to 2 days after contamination by salivary fluid.

Unfilled resin ("bonding agent") (either light-cured or chemical-cured, depending on the type of composite to be used) is painted on the area to be restored with a small brush (Fig. 7-26, *C*). Excess resin is removed by blowing with oil-free air. If a light-cured system is used, the unfilled resin can be light-cured at this time before the composite is placed; however, this step is not essential.

Composite, either chemical-cured or light-cured, is placed over the area to be restored with a plastic instrument in amounts necessary to cover the entire defect and to restore the proper anatomic contours of the original tooth (Fig. 7-26, *D*). A clean mylar plastic strip ("matrix band") can be used to help establish proper coronal anatomy while compressing the composite over and into the restoration site. The mylar strip could be used on a canine tooth by wrapping the strip over the composite and around the tooth before curing.

After light-curing or chemical set, the excess composite is trimmed with 8- to 20-sided fluted finishing burs (Fig. 7-26, *E*), finishing diamond burs, and sandpaper disks and mandrel in a slow-speed dental handpiece and contraangle. To provide a polished, smooth luster, a coating of unfilled resin is placed over the finished composite (and light-cured if a light-cured system is used).

After the tooth is restored, the occlusion is checked to make sure there is no interference from opposing teeth when the mouth is closed. If interference is found, it is smoothed away until there is no interference or abnormal contact that could fracture the restoration.

Glass Ionomer Cements

Glass ionomer cements have several unique properties. (1) They effect long-term chemical bonding to enamel and dentin. Thus sound tooth structure can be preserved and normally no undercuts are necessary, which makes them ideal for external resorptive lesions in cats. (2) They can leach fluoride ions into tooth structure (cariostatic and plaque-retardant). (3) They are biologically compatible with the tooth structure and pulp; thus cavity liners are not normally necessary. (4) They possess a low thermal diffusivity, providing a long-term biologic seal with the tooth structure.

There are two forms of glass ionomers, classified as type I or type II. Type I glass ionomers, which are finely grained, are used for cementing (luting crowns, bridges, and other castings). Type II glass ionomers can be used as restorative materials because of the greater resistance to abrasion. Ketac Cem and Fuji I are examples of type I glass ionomers. The type II glass ionomers are coarser than the type I and are not as suitable for cementation purposes.

Chelon Silver, Ketac Bond, Ketac Fill, Fuji II, and ChemFil II are examples of type II glass ionomer cements that can be used as restorative materials. Ketac Bond and Chelon Silver are mixed with a spatula or glass slab, following the manufacturer's directions exactly. Ketac Fill comes in capsules and requires a special tool to break the internal separation between the liquid and powder, an amalgamator to mix the compound, and a special syringe to apply the mixture (see Chapter 11).

One problem with these compounds is their lack of durability. Chelon Silver, Ketac Silver, and Miracle Mix are examples of glass ionomers to which silver has been added. This increases the durability (abrasion resistance) of the restorative. Chelon Silver is hand mixed on a pad, then transferred to the lesion with a plastic filling instrument, slightly overfilling the lesion. Like Ketac Fill, Ketac Silver comes in capsules and requires special tools to mix and apply the mixture.

Type II glass ionomers are ideal for the repair of external resorptive lesions, as well as the filling of root canal access preparations on nonocclusal areas. They also can be used in combination with light-cure restoratives to reduce the amount of light-cure restorative required and to decrease the potential for polymerization shrinkage.

Glass ionomers bond to slightly moist dentin and enamel because, unlike composite resin systems, they are polar polymers that can compete with water for the polar enamel surface.

As with any material, glass ionomer cements must be used and stored as described by the manufacturer or they will not function properly. Glass ionomer cements are strong in compression but weak in tension and therefore should not be used in stress-bearing areas. They also are susceptible to moisture loss during setting and thus should be protected with a varnish seal during this period.

▶ SPECIFIC TECHNIQUES

Restoration of External Resorptive Lesions in Cats

Lesions often are found on several of the premolars and molars and occasionally the canines in cats; in-

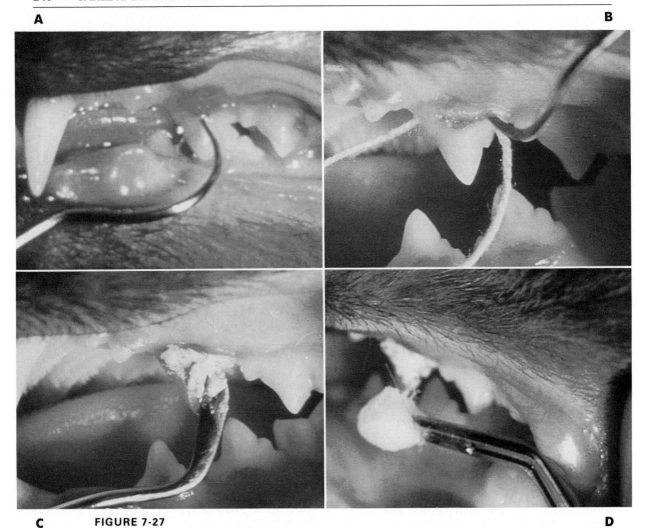

A

B

C

D

FIGURE 7-27
A, An external resorptive lesion is detected with a dental explorer. **B,** Retraction cord is applied to isolate the lesion and control hemorrhage. **C,** After preparing mechanically, if necessary, and conditioning the cavity, the glass ionomer cement is mixed and applied to the cavity. **D,** As soon as the lesion is filled, the restoration is painted with varnish to slow drying during setting.

ternal resorptive lesions are common in the roots of canine teeth. The marginal gingiva often is inflamed and hemorrhagic, complicating the restorative procedure. The lesion is detected under the gingival inflammatory tissue, which often grows into the lesion (Fig. 7-27, *A*). If excessive gingival inflammation and hemorrhage occur, it is virtually impossible to restore the lesion. The cat should be sent home for 2 weeks of thorough home care after dental prophylaxis.

At the time of restoration, gingival hemorrhage and retraction are controlled by packing a 1-cm strand of narrow-diameter gingival retraction cord into the gingival sulcus below the lesion with a retraction cord placement instrument or with the round end of the

E **F**

G

FIGURE 7-27, cont'd
E and **F,** The restoration is smoothed with a finishing bur and disk once it has set; it is then recovered with varnish. **G,** The completed restoration.

plastic filling instrument (Fig. 7-27, *B*). It is important that none of the cord impinges on the cavity. The retraction cord controls hemorrhage by retracting the gingiva. If necessary, gingival retraction liquid or a drop of dilute epinephrine can be placed onto the area for hemostasis. The gingiva must be moved apically far enough to expose the lesion. Debris is removed from the lesion with a dental spoon excavator. If retraction cord is insufficient to visualize the lesion fully

or to control hemorrhage, a flap incision is made and the gingiva is surgically treated (Fig. 7-28).

If the gingiva has invaded the pulpal tissues, prognosis is poor. Once the gingival granulation tissue has entered the pulp chamber, exposing the pulp, the tooth rarely is salvageable even with direct pulp-capping therapy. In occasional cases, tooth hemisection and root canal treatment can be performed (Fig. 7-29).

Glass ionomer cement cannot be placed directly

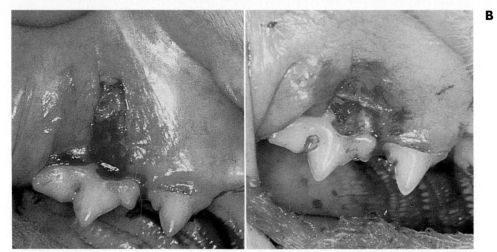

FIGURE 7-28
A, A resorptive lesion on the buccal surface of the upper fourth premolar tooth of a cat. A gingival flap has been laid back. **B,** After flap incision and dissection the lesion can be more clearly seen and evaluated.

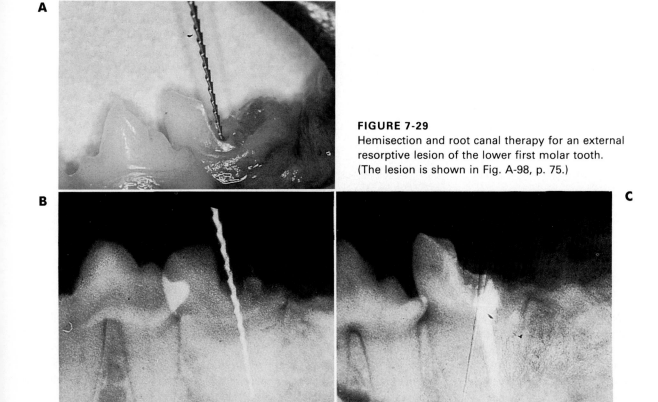

FIGURE 7-29
Hemisection and root canal therapy for an external resorptive lesion of the lower first molar tooth. (The lesion is shown in Fig. A-98, p. 75.)

over exposed pulpal tissue. Calcium hydroxide must be used over exposed or nearly exposed pulpal tissue for protection. These lesions are very sensitive, underlining the need for a calcium hydroxide base for insulation.

A hard-setting calcium hydroxide cement is mixed and placed over the thin layer of dentin covering the pulp chamber or the direct exposure (indirect or direct pulp capping) (Fig. 7-24, *C*). This is accomplished with a calcium hydroxide cement and applicator provided in kit form (such as Dycal; Kerr Dental). The manufacturer's directions provided with the calcium hydroxide kit must be followed. Excess calcium hydroxide is removed with a dental curet or a small round or pear-shaped bur, and the cavity is flushed clean.

The cavity is lightly dried with oil-free air or with cotton pellets.

The surface of the lesion is next prepared for restoration. A tooth conditioner, specific for the particular glass ionomer cement to be used, is swabbed into and over the lesion to remove loose dentin particles (smear layer) and debris, thereby opening the dentinal tubules for reception of the glass ionomer. After the recommended time (usually 10 to 15 seconds), the conditioner is thoroughly washed off. The prepared cavity is then partially dried with cotton pellets or pressurized air to leave a slight residual dampness in the cavity.

The glass ionomer cement is mixed, exactly following the manufacturer's instructions. A reinforced type II glass ionomer or silver-cermet cement is recommended. If appearance is of great importance, an esthetically acceptable, tooth-colored type II cement can be used. The mixed glass ionomer cement is placed into the cavity (Fig. 7-27, *C*). It must be condensed quickly and completely into the cavity to eliminate voids while minimizing the introduction of air bubbles. The material is pressed firmly into the cavity to fill all the recesses. The cavity is slightly overfilled. Immediately after placing the material, varnish is brushed onto the setting glass ionomer cement to protect it from dehydration (Fig. 7-27, *D*). If this is neglected, the material will crack and fail. Depending

on the type used, the glass ionomer cement is left to set for 3 to 10 minutes. Any interference during this time will interfere with the setting reaction, destroying the initial bond formation.

The restoration is finished or carved to reestablish normal tooth form (Fig. 7-27, *E* and *F*). The cement can be carved by hand with a No. 15 Bard-Parker scalpel blade or other suitable carver such as a discoid curet. The restoration can be finished to a smoother surface with the use of power equipment and dental handpieces. If a polishing cup used for dental prophylaxis is available, the restoration can be finished to a finer finish with prophylaxis paste. After finishing and contouring (Fig. 7-27, *G*), the cement is again coated with varnish or air dried to protect the restoration.

The surface of glass ionomer restorations can be strengthened by adding a layer of composite resin restorative material. The enamel (to 2 mm around the cavity margin) and glass ionomer cement are covered with etching gel and etched for a maximum of 30 seconds. The surfaces are rinsed for at least 30 seconds, then dried thoroughly with pressurized, oil-free air. It is essential that glass ionomer cement is not etched for more than 30 seconds, or its surface will be irreparably damaged. The etched surfaces must not be contaminated. The composite-bonding agent is mixed, applied to all the etched surfaces, and cured, following the manufacturer's instructions (Fig. 7-30). It is important to apply and cure the bonding agent immediately after etching; this will protect the glass ionomer from dehydration. The composite is mixed (if a chemical cure product is used) and placed in the prepared site with a plastic filling instrument. A minimum depth of 2 mm of composite is recommended. The surface is finished as for the superficial cavity.

The gingival retraction cord is removed and the whole area is rinsed and dried.

Long-term results from one series of 58 cases have been reported at the time of writing. Although most of the restorations were still present 1 year or more after placement, 72% of the restored teeth showed additional tooth substance destruction.

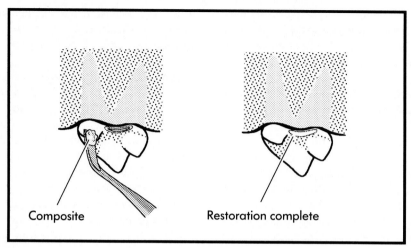

FIGURE 7-30
Following acid etching of the surface of the glass ionomer filling of a cavity, composite material is placed and finished.

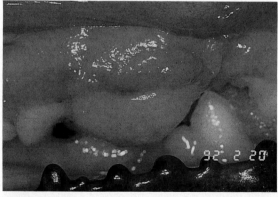

FIGURE 7-31
The buccal enamel bulge of the mesial cusp of the upper fourth premolar tooth was restored with composite and reinforced with dentinal pins 3 weeks previously. A glass ionomer restoration is in place in the distal root endodontic access site.

Reinforcement of Composite and Glass Ionomer Restorations
Pin retention

Pins for the retention and reinforcement of restorative materials to replace lost tooth structure have limited use in veterinary dentistry. Building up a tooth to original anatomic height and shape with silver alloy or composite usually is not necessary and rarely succeeds for any length of time because of the tremendous biting forces placed on materials designed for the lesser biting forces of humans (up to 1500 pounds per square inch in dogs compared to 150 pounds per square inch in humans).

Pins do not strengthen dental restorative materials; observations of failures have shown that the restorations are weaker after pin placement. However, pins do retain restorative material and will resist dislodgment resulting from the forces of mastication. In veterinary dentistry they usually are used in conjunction with endodontic post restorations or to aid in the retention of base build-up materials for full cast crown coverage. They also are used in the restoration of lost tooth structure in slab fractures (Fig. 7-31) or cage-biter lesions (see Fig. 7-34).

Pins are placed with dentin most often in vital teeth; therefore they must be sufficiently small neither to encroach on the pulp nor to come too close to the external tooth surface. To avoid perforation into the pulp or the periodontium, the veterinarian should give consideration to cavity preparation, tooth morphology, thickness of the remaining dentin, and the location of the pin channel. In relating the morphology of the teeth to pin-channel placement, a point midway between the pulp and the external surface of the tooth generally is correct. Canine and upper fourth premolar teeth usually have enough dentin for pin placement. Once the channel location is decided on, it should, when practical, be made parallel with the finished external surface of the tooth rather than perpendicular to its long axis, which often is not possible in restoring severe attrition in teeth damaged by cage biting. Only one pin per missing cusp of the tooth is used; whenever possible the pin should be placed in the area of a line angle (where the external shape of the crown changes direction). Retention is further increased if the pins are not parallel. Optimal length of the pin into the restorative material is 2 mm, as well as 2 mm into the dentin.

The self-threading pin systems consist of pins that are threaded into slightly undersized channels prepared with a drill bit custom-sized for that particular pin. Sizes available are TMS Regular–0.031-inch pin (used with 0.027-inch drill); TMS Minim–0.024-inch pin (used with 0.021-inch drill); TMS Minikin–0.021-inch pin (used with 0.017-inch drill); and TMS Minutin (Whaledent International, New York, NY; see Chapter 11). The pin kits contain the custom-sized drill bits and specific instructions for placement.

After selection of pin sites, a drill of proper size is placed into the slow-speed handpiece and a channel is drilled into the dentin to the full 2-mm length of the drill bit and then removed. The operator should avoid (1) wobbling the drill bit during drilling and (2) repeated reentry and removal of the bit, which will produce an oversized drill hole. Channels should be at least 0.5 mm from the dentinoenamel junction. Occasionally, for management of jaw fractures, for example (see Chapter 10), dentinal pins are placed through enamel. With this technique a small initial hole is drilled in the enamel with a round bur inasmuch

as drilling through enamel with the pin drill will rapidly dull the cutting edges. The proper-sized pin either is placed into the latch-type slow-speed handpiece and threaded into the channel or the pin is hand threaded with use of the hand chuck provided by manufacturer (see Fig. 7-33). The pins are engineered so that they snap off when they have reached the correct depth. The restorative material is applied over the pins and finished as previously described.

Reinforcement of Endodontically Treated Teeth

The need for reinforcement of endodontically treated teeth is directly related to the extent of tooth destruction, types of restorative materials available, the design of the cavity preparation, and the amount of retention needed for the restoration. Reinforcement of endodontically treated teeth in small animal dentistry most commonly involves (1) slab fractures of upper fourth premolars by composite or (2) pin/post-supported construction of cast restorations of upper fourth premolar and canine teeth. Although the same principles apply to all teeth, upper fourth premolars often are seen with the entire lateral surface of the tooth lost (Fig. 7-12, *E*), and the gingiva above the fracture is edematous and inflamed. The natural food-deflecting mechanism of the tooth is lost with the fractured segment, predisposing that area to rapid loss of attached gingiva.

After conventional endodontic therapy, the endodontically treated buccal root canals of the carnassial tooth—both mesial and distal—are used for retention (Figs. 7-31 and 7-32). Both roots are prepared and fitted with endodontic posts of proper width and length. Endodontic post systems, such as the Para-Post system (see Chapter 11) provide excellent instructions for placement of the posts. These systems provide reinforcement for the restorative material via the root. Caution should be exercised in the preparation and partial root obturation with pins and posts inasmuch as they increase the likelihood of fracture of the root. Posts never should be forced into the root canal. Proper post selection depends on the root canal diameter. If enough tooth structure is present to retain supplemental pins and their placement will not weaken tooth structure, self-threaded pins may be

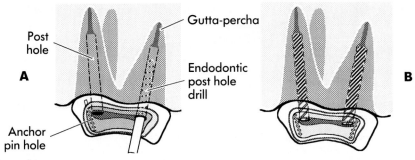

FIGURE 7-32
Endodontic post reinforcement of a crown restoration of an upper fourth premolar tooth. **A,** Both major roots are prepared for endodontic posts. **B,** The posts are cemented into the preparation.

used with the endodontic post system for added retention.

The endodontic post system kit typically contains several different diameters of posts, with a post hole drill for each size (see Chapter 11). After size selection has been determined on the basis of root canal diameter, the mesial and distal canals are prepared with the proper size drill in a slow-speed handpiece to a depth that will ensure that at least half the length of the post will be embedded in the root (Fig. 7-32). The post may need to be shortened to provide this correct ratio while not extending beyond the residual crown height. Drilling of the canal is accomplished along the same pathway as the endodontic root system.

The drill can remove the core gutta-percha to the desired depth; however, total gutta-percha removal may occur, particularly with freshly seated gutta-percha. Lateral root wall perforation also may occur. These complications can be avoided if endodontic treatment for slab fracture and restoration with posts are performed at the same appointment. After selection of the gutta-percha point is made and test-seated for tug-back (see Chapter 6) during endodontic therapy, the apical one third of the master gutta-percha point is cut off. The root canal is filled with cement, and the excised tip of gutta-percha is inserted into the canal. The tip is guided into place with the use of an endodontic plugger of proper size and seated firmly into position in the apex. The thermoplastic quality

of gutta-percha can be activated with a heated instrument (see Chapter 6). Apical seal is confirmed radiographically. An adequate apical seal will leave the coronal two thirds of the root canal clear for preparation, placement, and cementation of the endodontic post without fear of removing the entire pulpal contents. For a large, functionally important tooth, a cast crown and custom post will provide the greatest likelihood of retention of the restoration.

After post-hole preparations in both canals are complete, the endodontic posts are fitted and seated with cement, such as a type I glass ionomer cement (Figs. 7-32 and 7-33). To avoid air entrapment the cement is placed into the post holes with a spiral filling bur or endodontic file. After cementation, threaded pins can be placed into sound dentin (if present) to supplement retention (Fig. 7-33, *A*). After the cemented posts are stable, glass ionomer or composite restorative material is placed around the posts and pins (Fig. 7-33, *B*). If composite is used, it is light cured or placed in controllable amounts if chemically cured; the composite is slightly overfilled beyond the proper coronal anatomy. Then the restoration is finished with finishing burs and sandpaper disks to the correct coronal contour. The natural cervical bulge must be recreated to deflect food from the gingival sulcus during mastication (Fig. 7-31). A final polish with a flexible rubber polishing disk and cup completes the restoration. If glass ionomer material is employed as a core,

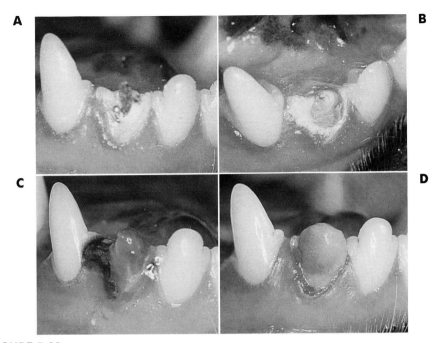

FIGURE 7-33
Endodontic post and dentinal pin reinforcement of an incisor tooth restoration. **A,** The endodontic post has been cemented in place, and two dentinal pins have been placed. **B,** A core of glass ionomer material is built up over the post and pins. **C,** The silver–glass ionomer surface is acid-etched. **D,** Composite is placed over the core. The layer of composite used in this case is too thin and the crown is too high. The darker core is visible through it, and it chipped soon after placement.

the chemical bond of glass ionomer to dentin can be used to advantage. The completed core preparation can be acid etched (Fig. 7-33) and covered with composite resin; then a composite cap is placed (Fig. 7-33, *E*). The cap must be more than 2 mm in thickness for long-term successful function.

Restorative material should not be placed beyond the coronal length of the natural tooth or adjacent teeth. Restorative material that extends beyond the existing natural tooth structure will fracture readily, often taking part of the needed labial surface composite with it.

Use of a post and composite or glass ionomer core as a crown-lengthening procedure is described on pp. 253-256.

Restoration of Distal Canine Tooth Crown Attrition *("Cage-biter Teeth")*

Canine teeth worn on the distal aspect through cage biting need some form of restoration to prevent coronal fracture from continued abrasion. The ideal restoration is full crown coverage with stainless steel; the bulk of steel placed into the defect will provide long-standing resistance to abrasion.

The distal surface of worn canines can be restored with pin-supported composite material, although composite will not provide the wear resistance or retention of full-crown restoration.

The technique makes use of several threaded pins (Whaledent; Fig. 7-34) for retention of the composite material. It must be remembered that pins are placed

A **B** **C**

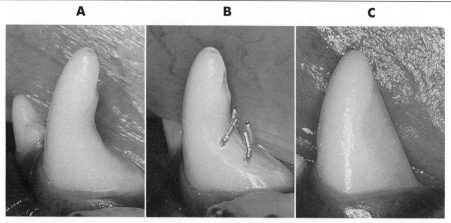

FIGURE 7-34
Composite pin restoration of "cage-biter" teeth. **A,** The worn distal surface of the canine tooth. **B,** Four dentinal pins have been placed and bent to conform to the shape of the restoration. **C,** Composite is added until the tooth is substantially thicker to slow down subsequent wear.

into the tooth for one function only: retention of the restorative material. They do not lend strength to the restoration or the tooth but weaken both to a degree. Retentive plans are placed at the corners of the defect into the dentine (but not into enamel if enamel is still present). Ideally the pins are placed just central to the dentinoenamel junction, carefully avoiding the pulp (Fig. 7-34, *B*). After the pins are in place, a dentinal adhesive is placed on the exposed dentinal surface, and the surrounding enamel is acid etched for additional retention and composite seal. Light-cured or chemically cured composite can be used (see p. 237). If the restoration is to be thicker than 2 mm, light-cured composite must be placed and cured in layers. A mylar strip can be used as a matrix form; it is tightened around the tooth and restorative material with finger pressure to compress the composite to anatomic form. The composite is held in place until set in the case of chemically cured composite, or it is light cured with the mylar strip in place. The restoration is shaped and finished with sanding disks and mounted rubber wheels. The restoration must be checked for occlusal interference and adjusted if necessary by trimming excess material. A coating of light-cured or chemically cured bond is placed over the final restoration for a high-gloss finish and seal. The

distal aspect of the tooth can be "thickened" beyond its normal contour to provide additional restorative material for continued wear (Fig. 7-34, *C*).

▶ METAL CROWN RESTORATIONS

In restorative dentistry a crown is "a restoration that covers all or part of the clinical crown of a tooth; its retention is normally derived from the preparation of the surface of the tooth." Crowns are termed *extracoronal restorations* because they cover all or most of the coronal portion of the tooth and gain their support and retention primarily from this outer surface of the tooth.

Retention, or resistance to dislodgment, is developed between the inner surface of the casting and the external surfaces of the prepared tooth. A portion of the tooth surface is uninvolved in some crown preparations. To compensate for this reduction in coverage, retentive crowns or boxes may be cut into the tooth; however, they usually are not necessary.

The crown is used primarily to restore fractured teeth, extensively decayed teeth, or otherwise compromised teeth that could not withstand normal wear and tear. The purpose of crown restoration is to prevent further breakdown of the remaining tooth struc-

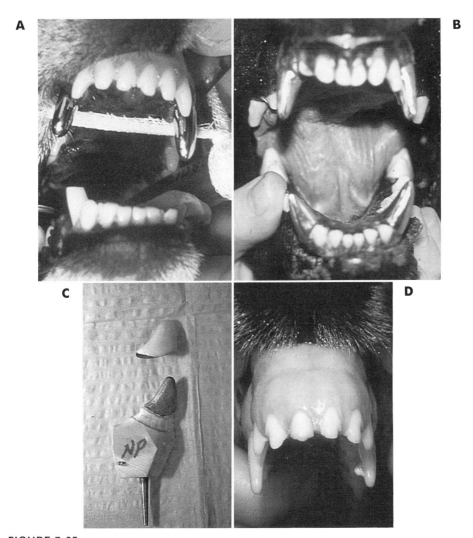

FIGURE 7-35
A, Two gold upper canine crowns in a dog. **B,** Four steel alloy canine crowns in a dog.
C, Porcelain-fused-to-metal crown and core preparation on a stone model. **D,** Porcelain-metal crown on an incisor tooth; which one is it?

ture, to restore normal function to the tooth, and, in some instances, to create a normal esthetic appearance.

A crown can consist of a cap placed over the remaining crown substance (or over a built-up crown core of glass ionomer or composite material), or it can be made as a combined crown and endodontic post prosthesis.

In veterinary dental work, crowns most often are made for canine and, less often, for incisor teeth. This section describes techniques for these simple, single-rooted teeth. Considerations specific to premolar and molar teeth are described separately (see p. 262).

Crown Materials

Highly glazed porcelain is the best material that can be used in contact with oral tissues, but it is vulnerable to cracking and breaking. Second in order of tissue compatibility is a highly polished, nontarnishing, metallic alloy such as gold or chrome-cobalt steel alloy. Third are the resins, which tend to absorb fluids, become discolored, and change shape over time.

Gold is considered too soft for most veterinary dental crowns, but sometimes it is used at the request of owners (Fig. 7-35, *A*). Some veterinary dentists occasionally use gold alloys, but most choose the more serviceable steel alloys (Fig. 7-35, *B*).

If esthetics are a concern, then a porcelain-fused-to-metal crown is chosen (Fig. 7-35, *C* and *D*). Full porcelain crowns (or jackets) are too fragile for veterinary dentistry. Acrylic jackets are used primarily as temporary crowns. Light box–cured composite crowns, which are currently being investigated, may be appropriate for some circumstances. An advantage is that the procedure can be completed during one anesthetic episode.

Treatment Planning: Evaluation of Dental Fractures

The apical end of the fracture must be known to properly restore the tooth. At least 6 to 8 mm of healthy tooth "skirt" length should be covered by the finished crown. This eliminates excessive pressure on the post if an endodontic post build-up is first placed in the fractured crown. A short skirt of enamel and

an endodontic post could fracture the root and dislodge the crown.

Fractured crown

Dental fractures are summarized in Fig. 7-36. The following characteristics are grouped according to the classification outlined earlier.

A. Normal coronal length is present, with no tooth structure loss.

B1. Mild loss of coronal structure (60% to 80% of original crown length remaining) occurs, and pulp is exposed. This type requires endodontic treatment, with conservative crown restoration after trimming of exposed enamel (B2).

B3. Regaining some of the lost crown height requires crown preparation and coverage; usually only reduction of rostrogingival enamel is necessary to provide for placement of the cast crown. Crown reduction is kept to minimum, thus preserving crown strength while reducing the likelihood of coronal fracture. To reduce the likelihood of fracture as a result of leverage force, the cast crown is no more than two thrids of the original crown length *when completed*. The crown shoulder is finished above the gingiva. This can be accomplished because sufficient crown structure is left to provide retention of the cast crown. The crown margin (shoulder) is more easily cleansed if it is supragingival, reducing the likelihood of periodontal disease.

C. Moderate to advanced crown loss (45% to 60%) occurs. In many cases an endodontic post build up is needed to increase crown length. There is little or no need for crown reduction as part of the preparation. The finish line may be placed into the gingival sulcus to gain needed crown skirt length for retention of the cast crown (C2). Cast crown coverage with the finish line of the shoulder below the marginal gingiva is necessary for added retention. Good long-term oral hygiene is needed to prevent periodontal involvement resulting from subgingival shoulder placement.

D1. There is severe loss of crown structure (60% to 100%). After endodontic therapy, sufficient skirt length (minimum 6 to 8 mm) for cast crown retention must be created. This is gained by

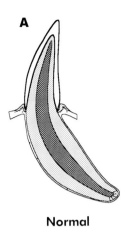

A

Normal

FIGURE 7-36
Coronal fractures. Considerations for crown restoration.

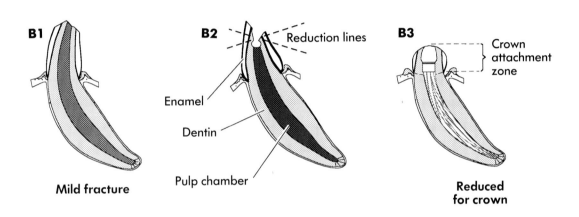

B1

Mild fracture

B2

Reduction lines

Enamel

Dentin

Pulp chamber

B3

Crown attachment zone

Reduced for crown

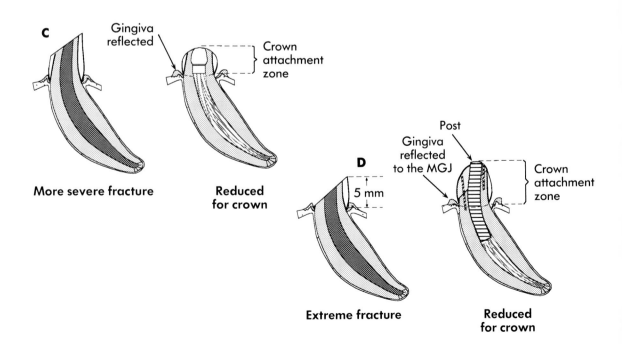

C

Gingiva reflected

Crown attachment zone

More severe fracture

Reduced for crown

D

5 mm

Extreme fracture

Post

Gingiva reflected to the MGJ

Crown attachment zone

Reduced for crown

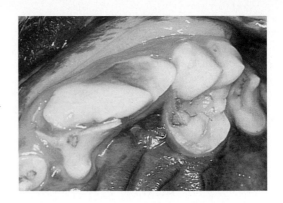

FIGURE 7-37
Fracture through the crown and furcation of an upper fourth premolar tooth in a dog.

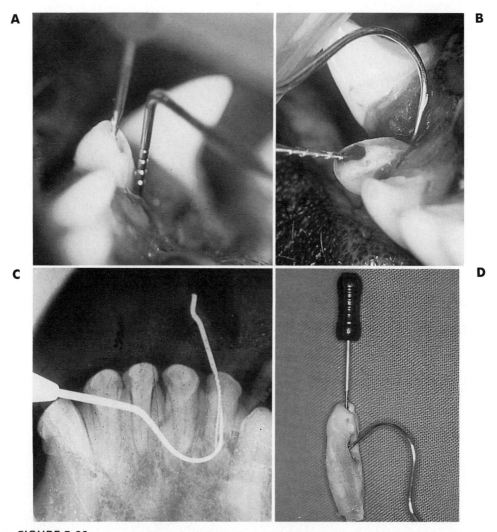

FIGURE 7-38
A, Fractured incisor tooth (with endodontic file in place) and periodontal probe indicating a deep pocket. **B,** A dental explorer finds a defect in the root. **C,** The dental explorer tip enters the root canal. **D,** The extracted tooth. A linear slab of the root had fractured in addition to the coronal fracture.

placement of an endodontic post and core build-up or by crown-lengthening surgery (see pp. 253-256).

Fractured roots

Teeth with vertical fractures extending more than one half the length of the root or involving more than one third of the width of the tooth, or both, should be extracted (Figs. 7-37 and 7-38). Teeth fractured horizontally more than one third the length of the tooth subgingivally also should be extracted (Fig. 7-12, *H*). Radiographic evaluation may determine long axis fractures, but long axis fractures in a mesial/distal direction are difficult to see radiographically. They must be diagnosed clinically with dental explorers and digital manipulation. The application of iodine to the crown will stain the fracture line. Endodontically compromised teeth must be treated before crown restoration. A crown fracture that extends subgingivally can be investigated by inspection after gingival flap surgery (Fig. 7-14, *B*).

Preparation for Crown Restoration
Crown-lengthening procedures

Crown lengthening permits clarification of the extent of a fracture and provides needed tooth structure to restore an otherwise unsalvageable tooth.

Gingivoplasty can be used when the fracture does not extend beneath the alveolar crest (Figs. 7-14, *A*, and 7-40). When the fracture does extend below the alveolar crest, a mucoperiosteal flap with osteoplasty can be used. The flaps are reflected away from the tooth with a periosteal elevator to expose the crestal bone (Figs. 7-41 and 7-42). The crestal bone is removed with rongeurs or saline-cooled burs to a depth of 3 to 4 mm below the apical extent of the fractured crown (Fig. 7-41, *A*). The buccolingual palato-gingival flaps are sutured in place with simple interrupted sutures over the reduced crestal bone to create the new attachment level (Figs. 7-41, *B* and 7-42, *B*). The exposed "crown" should have at least 6 to 8 mm of skirt length to ensure retention of a cast crown following crown lengthening.

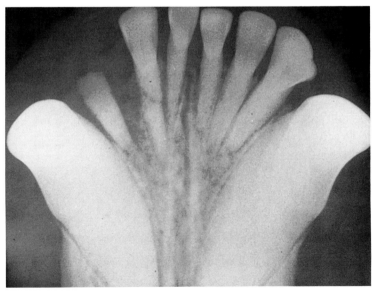

FIGURE 7-39
Incisor teeth with fractured roots.

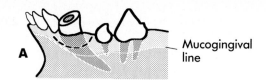

Mucogingival line

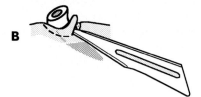

Gingivectomy, lateral to medial, adds 4 to 5 mm to crown length

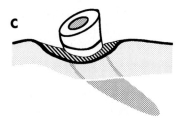

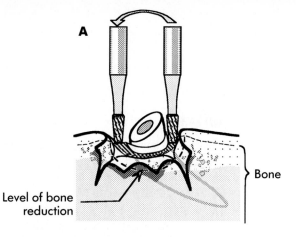

Bone

Level of bone reduction

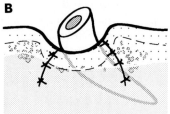

Bone removed and gingival flaps replaced

FIGURE 7-40
Crown lengthening by gingivoplasty. **A,** Incision line for gingivoplasty. **B,** The gingiva is incised at an angle to produce a beveled edge. **C,** The crown now has sufficient length for restoration.

FIGURE 7-41
Crown lengthening by osteoplasty. **A,** Following dissection and retraction of gingival flaps, bone is burred away to expose several millimeters of root, if necessary. **B,** Gingival flaps are replaced to just cover the new bony margin.

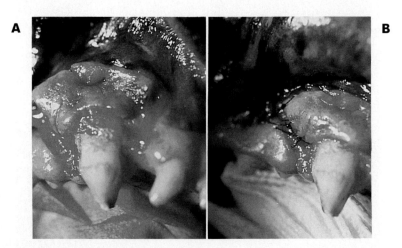

FIGURE 7-42
A, The gingival flap is retracted to expose bone for osteoplasty. **B,** The flaps are sutured to restore gingival margins.

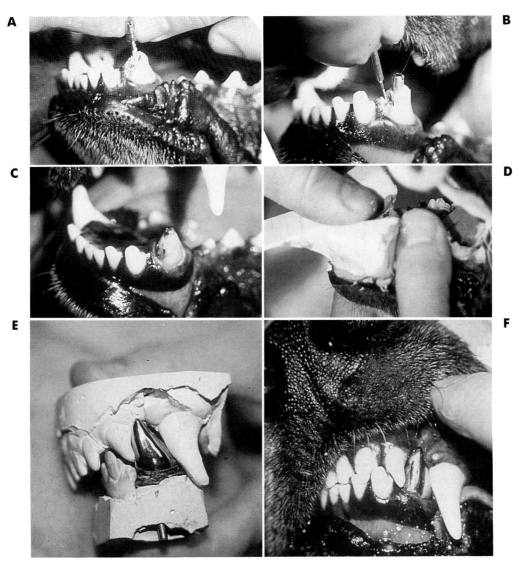

FIGURE 7-43
Endodontic post and core buildup for crown fabrication. **A,** The post is seated in the prepared root canal. **B,** Dentinal pins are added to resist rotation of the crown. **C,** Glass ionomer cement is built up around the post and pins to form a core. **D,** Impressions are made of the crown preparation. **E,** The crown on the laboratory model. **F,** The crown cemented in place.

Crown lengthening also can be attained with an endodontic post and core build-up (Fig. 7-43). The preparation for seating the post is as described for postreinforcement of a carnassial tooth slab fracture (see p. 245). The root canal is prepared to a depth that provides a ratio of 1:1 or 2:1 of post depth to exposed post length. The endodontic post is shaped to conform to the root canal and coronal anatomy (Fig. 7-43, *A*). The top of the post should extend to just below the desired height of the final crown build-up. The post is adjusted (cut off) to meet these dimensions and seated with suitable crown and bridge cement: zinc oxyphosphate, glass ionomer, or composite cement). Additional retention of core build-up material can be obtained with the use of supplemental threaded pins (Fig. 7-43, *B*; see also p. 245). A composite, glass ionomer, acrylic, or cement build-up is placed around the post and supplemental pin(s) and shaped with finishing burs, stones, and disks before an impression is taken (Fig. 7-43, *C* and *D*). The shoulder of the cast crown is placed subgingivally for added retention (see later discussion). Although the crown shoulder is more easily kept clean when placed above the gingival margin, subgingival placement often is required for added retention. This is not a problem when daily oral hygiene care is excellent (Fig. 7-43, *E* and *F*).

Margin preparation

In dental terms a *margin* is any surface junction between tooth and restorative material. The term applies specifically to the finish line developed in the preparation of the tooth, as well as to the termination of the restoration that fits this finish line.

Margins are the most critical portion of any restoration for two reasons. First, they seal the breach in the tooth surface created by the preparation. Second, the margin should be placed beneath or above, but not at, the crest of the gingival tissue surrounding the tooth. Any errors in the marginal fit of the casting will leave a discrepancy in normal contour and will cause surface roughness. This promotes collection of debris and bacteria, resulting in irritation of the adjacent tissue. Thus poor-fitting "restorations" can be a major contributing factor to periodontal disease.

Types of margins. The four basic types of margins (Fig. 7-44) are as follows:

1. *Feathered margin*. This type of margin is created by slicing off the side of the tooth to produce a flat surface (Fig. 7-44, *A*). The advantages are ease of preparation and conservation of tooth structure.

2. *Shoulder* (butt joint). This margin is a ledge or shoulder above or below the gingival portion of the prepared tooth (Fig. 7-44, *B*). It requires more removal of crown substance than for other techniques. It is not recommended for cast crowns but is the margin of choice for porcelain and acrylic or composite jacket crowns and porcelain-fused-to-metal crowns. These materials are very weak in cross-section and require greater thickness at their margins to provide sufficient edge strength.

3. *Beveled shoulder*. This is a shoulder margin that is beveled along the marginal angle. This modification of the shoulder margin is preferred in forming a metal margin. The premise here is that the crown, even if inadequately compensated in casting and too small to seat completely, will seal against the tooth at the marginal area as a result of the beveled marginal contact.

4. *Chamfer*. As used in dentistry, chamfer means a curved bevel (Fig. 7-44, *C*). Varying degrees of chamfer may be produced, ranging from the near feathered margin to the almost shouldered margin. These variations are referred to as light, medium, and heavy chamfer. Because of the varying contour of a tooth, certain areas or surfaces tend to be feathered whereas others are shouldered. The skilled veterinary dentist takes advantage of these features to give greater versatility and better fit.

The taper of the prepared surface of a tooth permits withdrawal of a wax pattern (in the dental laboratory) and subsequent seating and withdrawal of the casting (crown). Retention of the crown is theoretically enhanced by designing it with parallel sides. However, absolute parallelism is impractical in dental preparations. It is difficult to draw (ease off) the wax model from the parallel walls for creation of the metal crown. Thus some taper of the walls is necessary. Ideally, this taper should be 2 to 5 degrees from parallel for

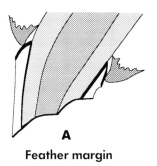

A
Feather margin

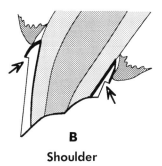

B
Shoulder

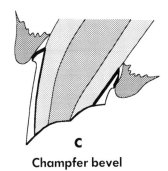

C
Champfer bevel

FIGURE 7-44
Types of crown margin.

each surface, or 5 to 10 degrees overall (Fig. 7-44).

Isolated defects, such as voids created in a surface by removal of decay or old restorative material, may be eliminated by filling them with cements before the impression is made. Accidentally created undercuts also must be "blocked out" with undercut wax or other suitable materials.

Tooth reduction must be kept to a minimum. Most canine teeth are preshaped naturally for crown coverage. Reduction of tooth surface only weakens the tooth. The main consideration is to provide just enough clearance for the tooth to function properly against the opposing arch. Crown reduction in humans is performed on all exposed tooth surfaces to provide space for the prosthetic crown in an arch arrangement where the teeth are in proximal and occlusal contact. Also, the crowns of human molar teeth are bell shaped. The lateral and medial surfaces created by this bell shape must have the gingival/coronal undercuts reduced to allow a rigid crown to fit over the entire coronal surface. Dogs and cats do not have a bell-shaped canine crown, and there is no occlusal or cusp-tip contact with the opposing arch for most teeth. In addition, carnivores are not capable of mandibular protrusive and lateral movement. Finished cast crown length should never exceed about two thirds the original crown length because of the strong leverage forces placed on the crown in function, especially by working dogs.

Preparation for a Custom Post and Crown

The endodontic space that will accommodate the post is prepared by removing endodontic filling material with a hot plugger or careful use of long diamond burs. The angulation of the post preparation must be carefully designed, particularly if a combined post and crown casting is to be used; the casting must be able to fit into the post preparation and over the remaining crown substance to the correct external margin preparation. An alternative is to make separate post/core and crown castings (Fig. 7-45). As for the crown preparation, the sides of the post preparation should be 5% to 10% from parallel. The impression that is taken for manufacture of the post and crown must include the post preparation. Impression material is placed carefully into the post preparation, and a reinforcing structure (such as a tooth pick or discarded endodontic file) is inserted into the preparation and then covered with additional impression material before the main mass of impression material is pressed into place (Fig. 7-45, *B*). The finished post should include a groove to permit extrusion of excess cement (Fig. 7-45, *C*). The post preparation is filled with temporary filling material (for example, Cavit).

Impressions for Crown Construction

An impression is taken of the prepared tooth (and post if one is used). If all aspects of the finish line

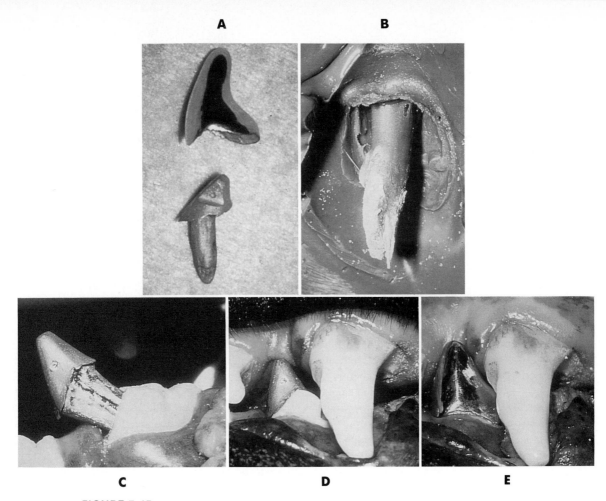

FIGURE 7-45

Custom post, core, and crown restoration. **A,** The custom post and core *(below)* and crown *(above).* **B,** Rubber impression of the endodontic post preparation. **C,** The post and core preparation is ready for trial fitting in the tooth. Note the groove on the side of the post to permit escape of excess cement. **D,** The post and core are cemented in place. **E,** The crown is cemented on the core.

FIGURE 7-46

Impression tray in place for lower incisor and canine teeth.

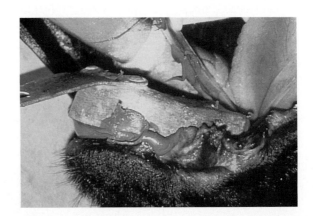

are not easily visualized, a retraction cord is used to distend the gingival sulcus before impressions are made so that the finish line can be recorded. A rubber or silicone impression material is used to outline the crown preparation exactly so that the laboratory can make an exact fit for the crown (Fig. 7-46).

Crown restorations require three impressions: an upper or lower arch impression, including the crown preparation; an upper/lower lateral impression in occlusion; and a bite registration for correct articulation. These impressions and registration allow the laboratory to articulate the stone models of the arcades into the exact occlusion present in the patient. The cast crown then can be fabricated to permit enough clearance to avoid striking the opposing teeth. Many crown and bridge laboratories prefer to pour their own models into the rubber impressions. These rubber impressions usually are submitted in their trays with no further preparation.

Attention to detail is imperative to ensure accurate reproductions. If the impressions are not exact, the finished restorations will not seat well onto the actual dentition. A weakened adhesive bond between the appliance and prepared tooth will result in eventual failure.

Impression trays

The first step in producing accurate impressions is the choice of suitable trays to hold the impression materials until they harden. Desirable trays have the following features:

1. Rigid construction to minimize distortion
2. An obstruction-free fit for the arcade or area of interest, which requires availability of a variety of sizes and shapes
3. Walls of sufficient depth to contain a proper depth of impression material to cover the entire crown of canine teeth
4. Easy removal of the finished impression and stone cast
5. Reusable, with residual impression material and stone easy to remove

Prefabricated veterinary impression trays are available (see Chapter 11).

Some practitioners prefer custom-made trays, especially desirable to obtain impressions of individual

teeth (as for crowns) or to reproduce specific areas of an arcade. Two methods are satisfactory in these situations.

Individual teeth. These "trays" can be made from plastic hypodermic syringe tubing of a size that will fit comfortably around the prepared tooth. Syringe barrels can be cut off in 1-inch lengths with a hacksaw. When filled with impression material, the tube can be placed over any individual tooth with minimal waste.

Sections of a quadrant. Kerr's Form-A-Tray is a two-part, liquid and powder mix that begins as puttylike substance and can be molded to individual needs. The material hardens rapidly to become a permanent form. The advantages are many: it is inexpensive, simple to form to any desired shape, and can be used many times. Detailed mixing instructions are included with the material. During the "putty" stage, it tends to stick to one's hands. A little petroleum jelly on the palms will solve this problem. The fumes from this material are very strong as the chemical reaction takes place and thus should be mixed in a well-ventilated area. Because the tray material is almost impossible to clean from such containers as metal pans, a disposable paper container should be used for the mixing process. Paper cups work well, as do wooden spatulas (tongue depressors). A long, narrow tray can be formed around the clinician's finger, resulting in an efficient mold for partial arch impressions.

Use of soft-walled trays, such as surgical gauze, bottoms of Styrofoam cups, or thin-walled plastic bottles are likely to result in distortion and thus an inaccurate impression.

Making impressions

Alginate materials. These make the most common and least expensive impressions. Fast-setting alginate is measured and mixed according to the manufacturer's recommendations (three scoops for each impression or two scoops for cats and small dogs). The alginate must be spatulated rapidly to form a smooth consistency (45 seconds for fast-set and 60 seconds for regular-set material). Immediately after mixing is completed, the tray is filled, some alginate is smeared onto the teeth, and the tray is applied firmly in the mouth. To prevent slumping of the material and an inaccurate impression, the mouth and tray are held parallel to the ground. Trays with perforations to retain the alginate are particularly good. Once the teeth are set into the impression material, the tray must be held steady for about 2 to 3 minutes while the alginate sets (Fig. 7-47, *A*). The tray and alginate are then removed with one brisk movement in a direction that will allow the canine teeth to slide out of the impression without tearing it (Fig. 7-47, *B*). If the stone models are not poured up immediately, a water-saturated paper towel should be placed over the impression to help prevent shrinking and distortion of its shape; the impression is then wrapped in a plastic sandwich bag or used surgical gloves. Alginate impressions that are kept moist are accurate for approximately 6 hours.

"Rubber" impressions. These materials, polyether elastomer (for example, Impregum; Premier,) or a variety of polysiloxanes (see Chapter 11), are used for individual tooth impressions. These materials provide the exact details required for crown and bridge fabrication.

The materials usually are contained in tubes. Equal lengths of base and catalyst are placed side by side on a paper mixing pad. Then these lines are rapidly spatulated together into a homogeneous mixture. After mixing, the material is placed into a small individual tray, precoated on the inside surface with adhesive, and placed over the prewetted tooth. The usual set time is approximately 2 to 2½ minutes if accelerator was not added to the mix. The removed impression is rinsed with water and set aside for the crown laboratory. Unlike alginate, this material will not distort for a few days; consequently it does not require keeping damp or immediate stone casting.

Carding wax. This wax comes as individual sheets. The red or yellow types are common, and either type is satisfactory. These sheets are used for "bite registrations." Rubber material can be used for this purpose, but it is an expensive and unnecessary waste of the material. Wax is not only satisfactory but inexpensive and simple to use.

A wax sheet is immersed into a bowl of hot water. The wax rapidly becomes soft and pliable. The endotracheal tube is removed, and the tongue of the patient is pushed caudally. The softened wax sheet is placed over the lower incisors and canines, and the mouth is closed (Fig. 7-47, *C*). A flow of cool water

is directed over the wax, which will rapidly regain its original rigidity.

For crowns on canine teeth, a bite registration and impressions from first premolar to first premolar usually are adequate.

Stone casts

Stone casts are made from impressions by pouring powdered stone mixed with water into the impression. For manufacture of a full crown, most dental laboratories prefer to make their own casts from the impressions supplied by the clinician. The laboratory makes a wax crown on the cast that will accommodate occlusion of the other teeth (thus the need for both upper and lower jaw impressions and the bite registration). The wax tooth is then invested, heated to melt the wax, and spun to expel the wax; then the tooth-shaped void in the investment material is filled with liquid metal.

To make a cast the clinician follows these steps:

1. Blow or shake excess moisture (do not dessicate) from the impression.
2. Spatulate small amount (about one-half cup) of powdered stone with gypsum hardener until it is of the consistency of toothpaste (the solution should not flow from the spatula until it is vibrated).
3. While holding the impression and tray on the vibrator in one hand, scoop a small amount of stone/gypsum with the spatula and touch it to the impression (starting with the back teeth) until a small amount flows into the tooth impressions.
4. Tilt the tray forward to allow the stone to flow, and repeat the procedure until each tooth impression is slowly filled.
5. Continue to vibrate the tray until all evidence of air bubbles is gone.
6. Add remaining stone/gypsum and vibrate for a few more seconds.
7. Mix more stone/gypsum, but this time make it a little thicker.
8. Turn the tray stone-side down onto a paper towel, and allow it to dry for a minimum of 4 to 5 minutes for fast-set stone or a 6-hour minimum for regular set stone.

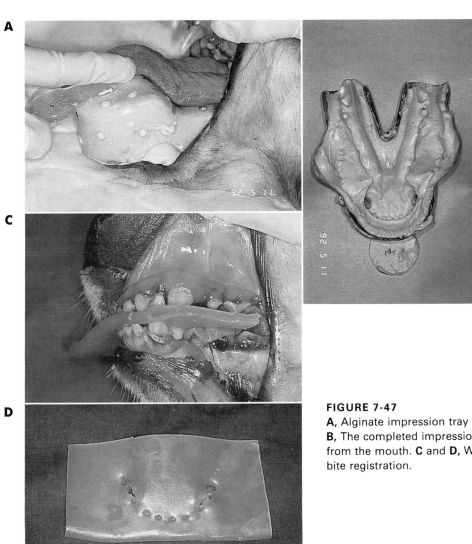

FIGURE 7-47
A, Alginate impression tray in place in the mouth.
B, The completed impression following removal
from the mouth. **C** and **D,** Wax plate used to form a
bite registration.

9. When set, pull the cast slowly from the alginate, or lift the alginate from the tray and carefully cut away from the model.

10. Mount the casts on an articulator to demonstrate the bite relationships; trimming the edges with a Model Trimmer is optional. If crowns are inadvertently broken from the cast, *carefully* replace in proper alignment and readhere with cyanoacrylate cement.

Cementing the Crown

The crown must be checked in the mouth to ensure that it seats fully to the finish line and that the occlusion is correct. The prepared tooth must be clean and dry before the crown is cemented. A slurry of pumice and water is used with a prophylaxis cup, and the tooth is rinsed and air dried.

Several different types of cement are available. Zinc phosphate cement and composite cement both have strong resistance to crushing and work well for cementing crowns in working dogs. Glass ionomer cements and carboxylate cements also have their advocates.

The new composite cements require an acid-etched tooth and a metal-etched internal crown surface. These chemically cured cements provide excellent retention; etching of endodontically treated teeth is not harmful. Vital teeth, however, should not be acid etched before crown cementation; the force used in seating the crown could cause the cement to penetrate the dentinal tubules and irritate the pulp. As with any dental material, the manufacturer's instructions for use should be carefully followed.

The crown is filled with the prepared cement, pressed into place, and held firmly in place for 1 minute. Once the cementation process is complete, the restored tooth margins should be cleaned and polished to remove any residual cement. The sulcus should be explored and flushed free of any debris. The occlusion is rechecked (Figs. 7-35 and 7-45).

Multiple Tooth Prosthesis

When several teeth are replaced by the same prosthesis, technical errors are more likely to occur. Teeth splinted to implants and/or other teeth by crowns that are joined must all have the same path of insertion. The longer the splint, the more likely that the prosthesis will fracture under stress.

Adjusting the prosthesis to the proper occlusion and repairing it when several replacement teeth are involved is more difficult. Until the veterinary dentist has extensive experience in crown construction and excellent laboratory support, multiple tooth prostheses should be avoided.

Crown Coverage of Caudal Dentition

With rare exceptions the only caudal crowns used in veterinary dentistry are for the upper fourth premolar and (occasional) lower first molar teeth in dogs.

Although most fourth premolar teeth can be restored with pin-reinforced composite techniques, full crown coverage is practical. It requires much more sensitive technique than does canine tooth crown coverage. To avoid abnormal contact with the opposing molar tooth, special consideration must be given to reduction of occlusal contact areas to allow for the bulk of metal coverage. The distal wall contact with the upper first molar must be reduced to provide room for the cast crown. All existing gingival line undercuts also must be reduced, providing slightly tapered walls that converge from the gingiva to the occlusal surface (Fig. 7-48). The cast crown should be designed to be reduced in height from its original height.

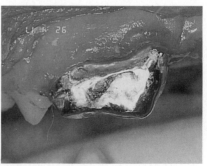

FIGURE 7-48
Metal crown on an upper fourth premolar tooth.

Care of Restored Teeth

The pet owner should be counseled about the possible problems that led to the initial fracture and initiate an oral hygiene program that will protect the restoration and prevent further damage to the teeth.

▶ TOOTH IMPLANTS

Titanium implants are commercially produced for humans to replace teeth that have been removed or lost. A core of vital bone is able to grow through a hollow titanium cylinder inserted in the jaw. Implants must be placed atraumatically and aseptically so that the bone that supports them does not undergo necrosis. The placement requires specialized insertion instruments, sterile technique, and understanding of the proper path of insertion and the physiology of bone.

Technique

The gingiva and underlying bone must be healthy. Extraction sites must be healed, with radiographic verification of good-quality trabecular bone. A mucoperiosteal flap is elevated to allow for trephining a core from the alveolar bone. To prevent thermal necrosis the procedure is carried out at low speed with an internally irrigated drill. The implant is placed in the receptor site and buried to within 1 mm of the crest of the alveolar ridge (Fig. 7-49). Careful planning is necessary at this point to ensure the proper path of insertion for the anticipated post and pontic. After replacing and suturing the mucoperiosteal flap, a 3- to 6-month period of "osteointegration" is allowed. Osseous integration is checked radiographically to determine the best time for placement of the post and crown. The implant is then uncovered, and a prepared post with the appropriate crown (pontic) is cemented in place (Fig. 7-49, *B*). Implants that fail should be removed and the jaw allowed to heal for 3 to 6 months before the procedure is repeated.

Post and core implants are very expensive at this time and offer few advantages for the veterinary dentist. As the technology progresses and the operator becomes familiar with dental procedures, implantology will become a more valuable tool. Numerous problems relative to the animal's habits are associated with keeping an appliance in its mouth. Because carnivores are by nature orally oriented, they tend to chew on whatever is present at the moment. Clients must fully understand this and be prepared to remove sources of chewing trauma other than food and to maintain daily oral hygiene by brushing and flushing the appliance.

Allogenic tooth transplantation as a potential restorative implant technique has been studied in dogs. Root resorption, evident by 24 months, was associated with fracture and loss of the crown.

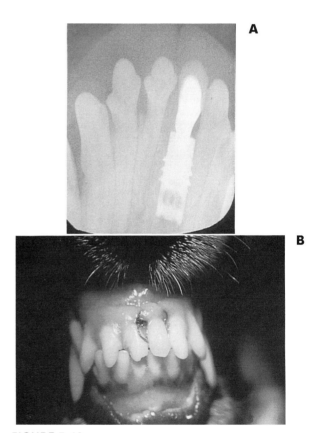

FIGURE 7-49
Implant restoration. **A,** The implant device is set into the bone of the jaw. **B,** The completed implant with crown.

▶ SUGGESTED READINGS

Arnjberg J: Schmelz- und Wurzelhypoplasien nach Staupe, *Kleintierpraxis* 31:313, 1986.

Arther A, Camy G: L'etching onmordancage de l'email: un necessité en dentistere veterinaire, *Point Vet* 21:256, 1989.

Ashton AP, Howard D: Repair technique for dental abrasion in the dog, *Vet Rec* 101:372, 1977.

Baraban DJ: The restoration of pulpless teeth, *Dent Clin North Am* 12:105, 1967.

Bedford PGC, Heaton MG: A repair technique for dental abrasion in the dog, *Vet Rec* 101:327, 1977.

Bender IB, Freedland JB: Clinical considerations in the diagnosis and treatment of intra-alveolar root fractures, *JADA* 107:595, 1983.

Bennet I, Law D: Incorporation of tetracycline in developing dog enamel and dentin, *J Dent Res* 44:788, 1965.

Bieniek KW, Kupper H: H-Ceram: ein neues Verfahren zur prosthetichien Rehab von Hundezahnen, *Kleintierpraxis* 33:93, 1988.

Bodingbauer J: Hochgradige Zahnunterzahl (aplasie) biem Hunde, *Wien Tierarzt Monaschr* 61:301, 1974.

Bodingbauer J: Milchzahnpersistenz beim Hund, *Kleintier Praxis* 23:339, 1978.

Caputo AA, Standlee JP: Pins and posts: why, when, and how, *Dent Clin North Am* 20:299, 1976.

Caputo AA et al: The mechanics of load transfer by retentive pins, *J Prosthet Dent* 29:442, 1973.

Coles S: The prevalence of buccal cervical root resorptions in Australian cats, *J Vet Dent* 7:14, 1990.

Colyer F: *Variations and diseases of the teeth in animals,* London, 1936, John Bale.

Dicks F, Zollner W: Glas-ionomer-zement fur einen praktikablen Einsatz in der Tierzahnheilkunde, *Prakt Tierarzt* 11:32, 1988.

Dilts WE, Coury TL: A conservative approach to the placement of retentive pins, *Dent Clin North Am* 20:397, 1976.

Dorn AS: Crown restoration of canine teeth with composite bonding, Proceedings of the ACVS, 1983.

Dubielzig RR: Effect of canine distemper virus on ameloblastic layer of developing tooth, *Vet Pathol* 16:268, 1979.

Eisenmenger E: Konservierende Behandlung von Zahnfrakturen des Hundes, *Wien Tierarzt Monaschr* 58:30, 1970.

Eisenmenger E, Zetner K: *Veterinary dentistry,* Philadelphia, 1985, Lea & Febiger.

Field EA et al: The removal of an impacted maxillary canine and associated dentigerous cyst in a chow, *J Small Anim Pract* 23:159, 1982.

Gardner AF et al: Dental caries in domesticated dogs, *JAVMA* 140:433, 1962.

Golden AL, Marretta SM: The use of espe ketac-bond aplicap for the restoration of cervical lesions, *J Vet Dent* 6(2):5, 1989.

Golden AM et al: Survey of oral and dental disease in dogs anesthetized at a veterinary hospital, *JAAHA* 18:891, 1982.

Grancher D et al: Fluorose beim Hund, *Kleintierpraxis* 33:203, 1988.

Grove TK: Functional and esthetic crowns for dogs and cats, *Vet Med Rep* 2:409, 1990.

Hamilton CJ, Ridgway RL: Dowel and core preparation, and full gold coverage of maxillary canine teeth in a German shepherd, *Vet Med/Small Anim Clinician,* 71:176, 1976.

Hamp SE et al: A macroscopic and radiologic investigation of dental diseases of the dog, *Vet Radiol* 25:86, 1984.

Hanson EC, Caputo AA: Cementing mediums and retentive characteristics of dowels, *J Prosthet Dent* 32:551, 1974.

Harvey CE, Alston W: Dental disease in cat skulls acquired before 1960, *Proc Vet Dent Forum* 4:41, 1990.

Hobday F: A case of canine dentistry, *J Comp Pathol Ther* 10:362, 1897.

Holmstrom SE: Endodontics illustrated: the practitioner's guide to root canal therapy, *Calif Vet* 40:18, 1986.

Holmstrom SE: Restorative materials, *Vet Focus* 2:9, 1990.

Jirava E et al: Uber die Behandlung von Frakturierten zahnen bei Hunden, *Berl Munch Tierarztl Wochenschr* 12:235, 1966.

Klein H: Schienung einer Caninus langsfraktur beim Hund, *Kleintierpraxis* 24:144, 1979.

Klein H: Vergleich verschiedener uber Kronung-stechniken am kunstlich frakturierten Caninus des Hundes, *Diss Tierarztl Hochscule Hannover* 1:88, 1979.

Kornfeld M: *Mouth rehabilitation,* ed 2, St Louis, 1974, Mosby–Year Book.

Kupper H, Bieniek KW: Die transdentale Fixation bei der Kronenversorgung von Hundegebissen, *Prakt Tierartzl* 9:28, 1987.

Lane JG: Small animal dentistry, *In Pract* 3:23, 1981.

Lewis TM: Resistance of dogs to dental caries: a two-year study, *J Dent Res* 44:1254, 1965.

Lyon K: Subgingival odontoclastic resorptive lesions: classification, treatment, and results in 58 cats, *Vet Clin North Am, Small Anim Pract* 22:1417, 1992.

Markley RL: Pin reinforcement and retention of amalgam foundations and restoration, *JADA* 56:675, 1958.

Marvich JM: Repair of enamel hypoplasia in the dog, *Vet Med/Small Anim Clinician* 70:697, 1975.

McLean JW: The science and art of dental ceramics, vol 1, *Nature of dental ceramics and their clinical use,* Lombard, Ill, 1979, Quintessence Publishing Co.

Metrick L: Canal obliteration with a post crown, *J Can Dent Assoc* 1961.

Miranda FJ et al: Diagnosis and treatment of pulpal distress, *Dent Clin North Am* 20:290, 1976.

Moffa JP: *Physical and mechanical properties of gold and cast metal alloys; alternatives to gold in dentistry,* Department of Health, Education and Welfare Pub No NIH 77-1227, Washington, DC, 1977, US Government Printing Office, 1977.

Moffa JP et al: Pins: a comparison of their retentive properties, *JADA* 78:5229, 1969.

Neagley RL: The effect of dowel preparation on the apical seal of endodontically treated teeth, *Oral Surg* 28:739, 1969.

Neumann W: Rekonstruktion frakturierter Zahne beim Hund mit verschiedenen Kunststoffmaterialien, *Praktische Tierarzt* 11:26, 1988.

Okuda A, Harvey CE: Etiopathogenesis of feline dental resorptive lesions, *Vet Clin North Am, Small Anim Pract* 22:1385, 1992.

Okuda A, Harvey CE: Immunohistochemical distribution of interleukins as possible stimulators of odontoclastic resorption activity in feline dental resorption lesions, *Proc Vet Dent Forum* 6:41, 1992.

Peterson RN, Wightman JR: Aesthetic restoration of a fractured anterior tooth in a dog, *Vet Med/Small Anim Clinician* 74:683, 1979.

Phillips RW: Dental materials, *Dent Clin North Am* 27:643, 1983.

Reichart PA et al: Periodontal disease in the domestic cat: a histopathologic study, *J Periodont Res* 19:67, 1984.

Runyon CL et al: Allogenic tooth transplantation in the dog, *JAVMA* 188:713, 1986.

Scheffler VKH: Restitution des dens Caninus beim Dientshund, *Munch Vet Med* 34:504, 1979.

Schneck GW: Caries in the dog, *JAVMA* 150:1142, 1967.

Schneck GW: A case of enamel pearls in a dog, *Vet Rec* 92:115, 1973.

Schneck GW, Osborn JW: Neck lesions in the teeth of cats, *Vet Rec* 99:100, 1976.

Stanley HR: Pulpal response to dental techniques and materials, *Dent Clin North Am* 15:115, 1971.

Van Wessum R, Harvey CE, Hennet P: Feline dental resorptive lesions: prevalence patterns, *Vet Clin North Am, Small Anim Pract* 22:1405, 1992.

Winkler S: Resins in dentistry, *Dent Clin North Am* 19:211, 1975.

Wright JG: Some observations on dental disease in the dog, *Vet Rec* 51:409, 1939.

Zetner K: Die prosthetische Versorgung von Zahn-frankturen mit Adhesivkunstoffen, *Kleintierpraxis* 21:271, 1976.

8

Occlusion, Occlusive Abnormalities, and Orthodontic Treatment

A relationship between oral anatomic form and physiologic function is apparent in all animals. In some species, humans have selectively bred animals in ways that have distorted the natural occlusion for that species; this is most dramatically true of the dog.

Attempts to correct malaligned teeth in animals have been made by owners and breeders of animals since the nineteenth century and possibly before. Tooth extraction to relieve crowding, rubber ligatures, finger pressure, and wires were used on dogs and occasionally cats. Only in the last 30 years have veterinarians and dentists begun to use orthodontic appliances and surgery to correct malocclusions in companion animals by addressing dental occlusion rather than tooth alignment alone.

▶ OCCLUSION

Normal Occlusion

Normal canid occlusion can be traced to ancestral dogs. The established occlusal pattern is the result of repeated breeding of phenotypes, with a functional occlusal relationship. This bite pattern, known as *scissors* bite, is still found in wild canids such as wolves,

hyenas, coyotes, and foxes, as well as in many domestic dogs.

The upper arch in mesocephalic dogs, viewed from an occlusal aspect, is a sigmoid curve. The lower arch, quite different from the upper arch, is a flat-sided blunt wedge. The line of occlusion in a dog with a mesocephalic skull is a smooth sigmoid curve passing through the central fossa of each molar, across the mesiodistal length of the premolars and canines and through the cingulum of the upper incisors (Fig. 8-1). The same line runs along the buccal cusps and incisal edges of the lower teeth, thus specifying the occlusal, as well as interarch relationships, once the molar position is established.

Classification

The human dental arch form is a rather uniform curve of matching upper and lower arches. A system of classifying human malocclusions based on the position of the upper first molar teeth compared with the lower first molar (the Angle class I, II, and III system), used in human dentistry for many years, has been applied to dogs and cats.

The length of the upper and lower arches varies

within breeds and types of dog and cat. Because of the brachycephalic head types, classification of canine occlusion on the basis of upper and lower molar relationships is impractical. Malocclusions that involve the entire arch relationship are brachygnathia, prognathism, and wry bite. Those involving individual teeth or quadrants are rostral (anterior) cross-bite, caudal (posterior) cross-bite, base-narrow canines, or teeth that individually cause soft tissue trauma (rotated or tipped teeth). The system for classification of canine and feline occlusion used in this text is shown in the box below, with examples in Fig. 8-2.

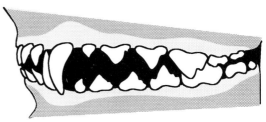

Mucogingival line

FIGURE 8-1
Lateral view of the normal occlusion of a dog.

Classification of Dental Occlusion—Carnivores

Type 0: Normal Occlusion

Upper and lower canines and upper third incisors appear in evenly spaced "scissor" occlusion. The upper and lower incisor edges overlap slightly so that the incisal edges of the lower incisors occlude on the cingulum of the upper incisor. The upper premolar crowns interdigitate with the lower premolars so that the lower premolar occludes rostral to its upper counterpart. The upper fourth premolar and lower first molar teeth form a sectorial set. The crowns of the upper and lower molar teeth occlude with each other (except in cats, which have no lower grinding occlusal tables).

Type 1 Malocclusion

The overall canine and incisor relationship is normal, with the following characteristics:
A. The *upper* premolar teeth are occluding rostral to the normal position in terms of the upper-lower premolar position.
B. The *lower* premolar teeth are occluding rostral to the normal position in terms of the upper-lower premolar position.
C. One or more teeth are in abnormal alignment (tipped or rotated).
D. Open-bite occlusion is seen; when the animal's jaws are closed to the extent that it is possible, the upper and lower incisor teeth do not overlap and dorsoventral space appears between them.

Type 2 Malocclusion

The *upper* incisor and canine occlusal line is rostral to the lower incisor–canine occlusal line, with the following characteristics:
A. The *upper* premolar teeth are occluding rostral to the normal position in terms of the upper-lower premolar position.
B. The *lower* premolar teeth are occluding rostral to the normal position in terms of the upper-lower premolar position.
C. One or more teeth are in abnormal alignment (tipped or rotated).
D. Open bite occlusion is seen; when the animal's jaws are closed to the extent that it is possible, the upper and lower incisor teeth do not overlap and dorsoventral space appears between them.

Type 3 Malocclusion

The *lower* incisor and canine occlusal line is rostral to the upper incisor–canine occlusal line, with the following characteristics:
A. The *upper* premolar teeth are occluding rostral to the normal position in terms of the upper-lower premolar position.
B. The *lower* premolar teeth are occluding rostral to the normal position in terms of the upper-lower premolar position.
C. One or more teeth are in abnormal alignment (tipped or rotated).
D. Open-bite occlusion is seen; when the animal's jaws are closed to the extent that it is possible, the upper and lower incisor teeth do not overlap and dorsoventral space appears between them.

NOTE: Combination abnormalities are possible (for example, type 2 A, C).

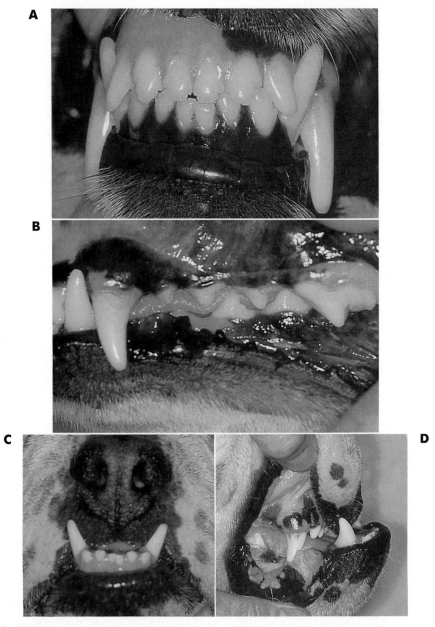

FIGURE 8-2
Examples of canine and feline occlusion. **A** and **B,** Normal canine occlusion. **C** and **D,**
Bulldog (maxillary brachygnathia). **E,** Dolichocephalic dog (scissors bite but with large
interdental spaces). **F,** Brachygnathic dog (mandible is short; maxilla is normal length).
The lower canine tooth is level with (and lingual to) the upper canine tooth. **G,** Wry
mouth causing open incisor bite on the left side. **H** and **I,** Normal occlusion in a cat.

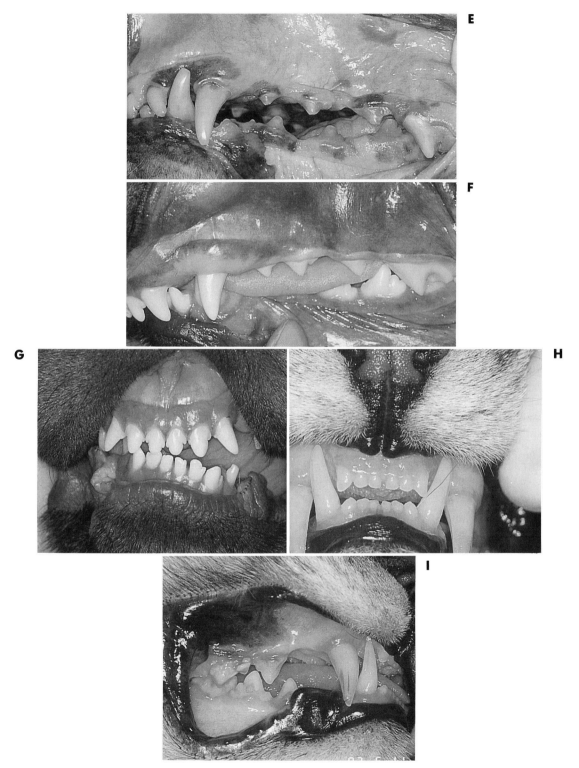

FIGURE 8-2, cont'd
For legend see opposite page.

The selective breeding of dogs for show purposes has contributed greatly to the incidence and severity of malocclusions. Often phenotypes are created with severe genetic malocclusions. This is particularly true if abnormal occlusion is either expected or not regarded as a major fault in the conformation standard. Nomenclature for occlusions often has been misinterpreted, resulting in some common but incorrect descriptions. Correct definitions of some commonly used terms are as follows:

Brachygnathia—excessive shortness of one or both jaws

Brachycephaly—short, broad skull

Prognathism—abnormal protrusion of one or both jaws

Thus bull dogs, which have a brachycephalic skull, often are described as prognathous even though the mandibule is normal (as shown by lack of rotation of teeth or abnormal interdental spaces in the mandible [Fig. 8-2, *C*]). This combination of brachycephaly and normal mandible can be referred to as *relative prognathism*.

Dolichocephalic dogs may have abnormally long jaws (as evidenced by abnormally large interdental spaces) but a normal scissors bite if the extent of abnormality is approximately equal in the upper and lower jaws (Fig. 8-2, *E*).

The lay term *overshot* indicates that the lower jaw is significantly shorter than the upper jaw. Similarly, the term *undershot* indicates that the lower jaw is significantly longer than the upper jaw. Neither term necessarily implies that *either* jaw is normal.

► MALOCCLUSION

Inherited or Acquired Etiologic Factors

Malocclusion is primarily the result of inherited dentofacial proportions governed by breeding the dog or cat for a desired head shape or size. These problems become established phenotypes as a result of line- and in-breeding practices. They may be altered somewhat by trauma (for example, a blow to one side of the face may slow growth on that side, producing a wrymouth; Fig. 8-3) or altered function. Slowed growth

as a result of illness during a period of normally rapid jaw development may cause malocclusion.

Certain types of malocclusion are present with certain breeds and head types. The short, broad maxilla of the brachycephalic breeds is an obvious example. The pertinent factor in establishing the cause of malocclusion is not whether there are inherited influences on the jaws and teeth (because obviously there are) but whether malocclusion is caused by inherited characteristics or some other cause.

Malocclusion could be produced by inheritance in two possible ways. The first is an inherited disproportion between the size of the teeth and the size of the jaws, which produces crowding or abnormal spacing of the teeth. The second possibility is an inherited disproportion between size or shape of the upper and lower jaws, which would cause improper occlusal relationships (Fig. 8-4). The more independently these characteristics are determined, the more likely that disproportions could be inherited. Large teeth but small jaws could be inherited, for instance, or a long

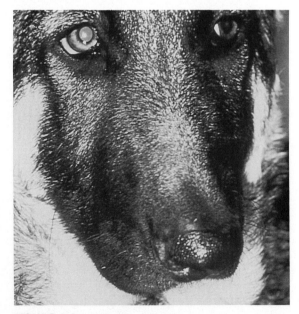

FIGURE 8-3
Asymmetry of the maxilla caused by traumatic slowing of growth on one side in a young dog.

A

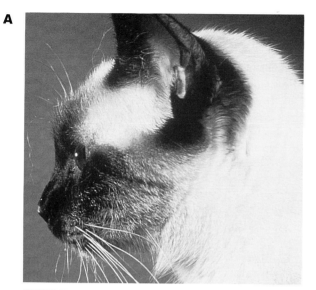

B

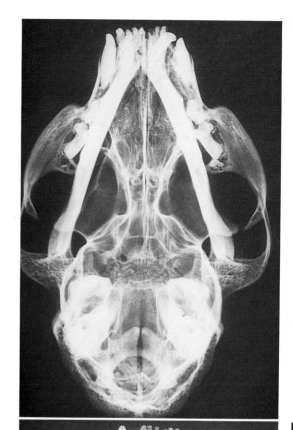

FIGURE 8-4
Face and radiographs of the head of a normal cat
(**A** and **B**) and of a cat with inherited mucopolysac-
charidosis (**C** and **D**).

C

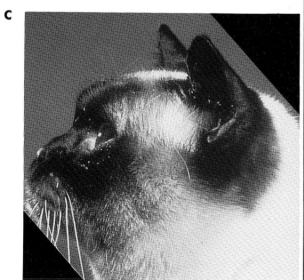

D

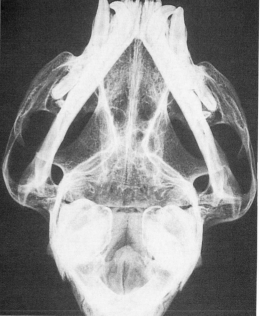

upper jaw and a short lower one. Conversely, if dentofacial characteristics tended to be linked, an inherited mismatch would be unlikely.

Present-day dogs come in a variety of breeds and sizes. Genetic isolation and uniformity, as seen in wild dogs, produce rare instances of malocclusion. When all animals in a group carry the same genetic information for tooth size and jaw size, there would be little possibility of animals inheriting discordant characteristics. Genes that introduced disturbances into the masticatory system would tend to be eliminated from the population. In many breeds the "typical" specimen has normal scissors occlusion, tooth size–jaw size discrepancies are infrequent, and each specimen tends to have the same jaw relationship. When outbreeding between originally distinct breeds occurs, malocclusions may develop. This view of malocclusion as primarily a genetic problem was demonstrated by Stockard, who methodically cross-bred dogs and recorded the effects on body structure. Stockard believed that dramatic malocclusions occurred in cross-bred dogs — more from jaw length or width discrepancies than from tooth size–jaw size imbalances. However, he did not examine nonbrachycephalic miniature breeds in which tooth size–jaw size abnormalities are common. His research confirmed that "independent inheritance of facial characteristics is a major cause of malocclusion and that the rapid increase in malocclusion accompanying urbanization was probably the result of increased outbreeding" (that is, breeding among dissimilar stock; in Stockard's studies he bred basset hounds with English bulldogs, for example).

Many small and medium-sized breeds carry the gene for achondroplasia, a deficient growth of cartilage resulting in short legs and an underdeveloped midface. Most terriers, bulldogs, and other breeds carry this gene. Achrondoplasia is an autosomal dominant trait with variable penetrance; therefore the trait will be expressed more dramatically in some breeds or individuals than in others. Stockard explained that some malocclusions were based not on inherited jaw size but by the extent to which achondroplasia was expressed in that animal and that severe malocclusions could be developed by crossing morphologically different breeds.

Orthodontic research has shown that the simple belief that malocclusion is the result of independent inheritance of dental and facial characteristics is not completely correct. The precise role of heredity as an etiologic agent for malocclusion has not been clarified. Certain inherited metabolic abnormalities produce consistent occlusal problems (for example, hypothyroid cretinism).

Cephalometric evaluation of cranial and facial development enabled human orthodontists to measure the changes in tooth and jaw positions produced by growth and treatment. Although extensively employed in human orthodontics, its use in canine orthodontics has yet to be developed. Different breed types have different "normals." Which breeds are to be studied, how many cephalometric evaluations are necessary for each, what planes must be included or excluded, and where and what to measure have yet to be decided. Significant cephalometric differences have been demonstrated for cats and dogs with mucopolysaccharidosis compared with skeletally normal animals (Fig. 8-4).

A severe malocclusion may compromise oral function. There may be difficulty in mastication if only a few teeth meet, and jaw discrepancies may force adaptive alterations in swallowing. Malocclusion may contribute to both dental decay and periodontal disease. Plaque and food are retained in areas that are out of normal function, making it harder for the animal or owner to care for the teeth. Fortunately, because the food of companion animals is provided in a form controlled by the owner, functional impairment of occlusion is not of great clinical significance.

Ethical Considerations

Crowded, malaligned teeth and jaw size discrepancies are the most common malocclusions seen in dogs and cats. The goal of canine and feline orthodontics is to relieve soft tissue or hard tissue trauma resulting from malocclusion, while remaining aware of restrictions imposed by ethical and legal issues. Specific limitations must be addressed in veterinary orthodontics, as delineated by two major professional organizations:

■ *American Veterinary Medical Association.* Its Principles of Professional Ethics states that it is unethical to perform a procedure for the purpose of concealing a congenital or inherited abnormality that sets the animal apart from the normal as described in the standard for the breed. Specifically, for dogs and cats, any procedure that will alter the natural dental arcade is unethical. Should the health or welfare of the individual patient require correction of such genetic defects, it is recommended that the patient be rendered incapable of reproduction.

- *American Kennel Club.* Its dog show rules state that altering the natural appearance of a dog for the purposes of correcting an abnormality is cause for disqualification of that animal.

A system for occlusal examination that assigns scores to particular abnormalities in dogs has been proposed as a way of indicating whether an occlusal abnormality is inherited or not. No evidence, however, indicates that the proposed criteria can differentiate between inherited and noninherited causes.

Clinically Obvious Malocclusions
Base-narrow canines

Base-narrow canines generally are considered to be genetic in origin. The lower canine teeth may hit the palate, the gingival margin of the upper third incisor, or the upper canine tooth (Figs. 8-5 and A-109, p. 76). They can result from an extreme retrognathic mandible (more caudal than normal location of the mandible), brachygnathous mandible, excessive anisognathism (uneven jaw size), or retained deciduous canines that have directed the lower canines into a more lingual than normal base narrow position. All these conditions are considered to be genetically linked. Treatment is described on p. 285.

Rostrally displaced canine teeth

Rostrally displaced canine teeth, a genetic condition, is most common in Shetland sheepdogs in whom it is referred to as *lance canine,* but it also is seen in Scotties and other medium or small breeds. The upper canine tooth is severly displaced rostrally, hitting the upper third incisor tooth (Fig. 8-6). If left unattended, periodontal disease and upper lip ulceration can result. The best treatment is to extract the abnormally positioned canine or to shorten the crown by vital amputation (which still leaves a pathologic periodontal problem because of its abnormal position and difficulty in cleansing the gingival sulcus in the mesial aspect of the tooth). The condition can be treated orthodontically (see p. 293). The dog should be neu-

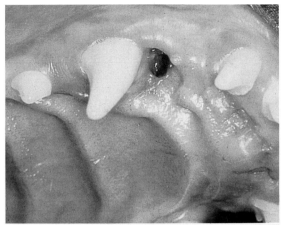

A

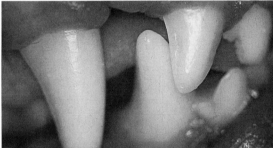

B

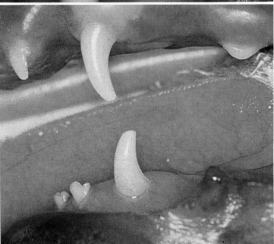

C

FIGURE 8-5
Base-narrow mandibular canine teeth causing occlusal damage to the palate. **A,** Ulceration in the palate. **B,** Occlusion, showing abnormal scissors bite. **C,** Puppy with base-narrow deciduous canine.

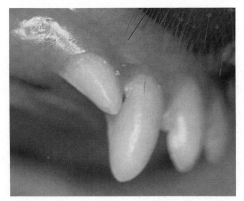

FIGURE 8-6
Rostrally displaced upper canine teeth in a Shetland sheepdog.

A

B

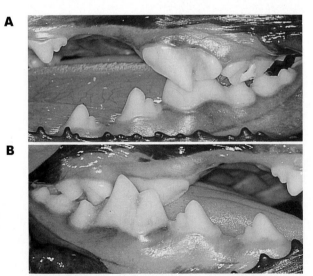

FIGURE 8-7
Unilateral caudal (posterior) crossbite in a collie. **A,** Normal side (upper third premolar tooth is missing). **B,** Crossbite side (upper third premolar tooth is missing).

tered. This condition occurs occasionally in cats (see Fig. 8-27).

Crossbite

Caudal (posterior) crossbite. Caudal crossbite occurs when the line of occlusion of the premolar/molar teeth is incorrect buccolingually, so upper premolar or molar teeth are positioned lingual to the lower premolars or molar teeth. This condition, which also is called *lingual crossbite,* is seen most often in dolichocephalic, narrow-nosed dogs, such as the borzoi (Fig. 8-7). More extreme malocclusions of the premolar and molar segments are very unusual. Orthodontic correction of posterior crossbite has been attempted with very little success. If periodontal tissues are severely compromised, the most severely malpositioned tooth should be extracted. This condition is presumed to be inherited.

Rostral (anterior) crossbite. A rostral crossbite is common in domestic dogs. One or more upper incisors are displaced lingual to the lower incisors when the teeth are in occlusion (Fig. 8-8), or lower incisor(s) are displaced buccally to the upper incisors. Anterior crossbite can reflect a jaw discrepancy but usually results in dogs from retained primary incisors. Both of these causative conditions are likely to be inherited. The permanent incisors erupt lingual to the primary incisors; prolonged retention of the primary incisors can deflect the permanent incisors lingually. Lingual displacement can arise by tipping of the incisors by the occluding teeth as they erupt. This abnormality occurs in a wide variety of head shapes and sizes. Treatment is usually not necessary unless severe peridontal involvement results from the crossbite.

Crowding

Incisor crowding is common in dogs with small jaws; it is presumed to be an inherited condition. Typically the second incisor on both sides in the mandible will be displaced buccally or lingually out of the normal incisor curve (see Fig. A-79, p. 69). If the crowding results in significant compromise of periodontal tissue, extraction of one or more crowded incisors is indicated.

Premolar and molar crowding is common in brachycephalic dogs. Typically the premolar teeth

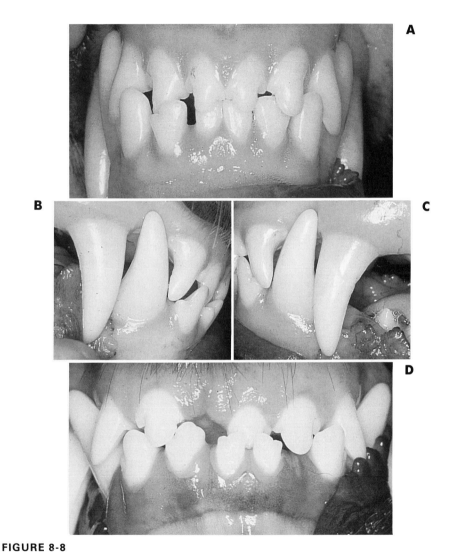

FIGURE 8-8
A-C, Rostral (anterior) crossbite in a dog (lower third incisors on both sides and right lower second incisor). **D,** Rostral (anterior) crossbite in a dog. Orthodontic treatment had been attempted and had resulted in loss of one of the upper first incisor teeth. The crossbite is still present.

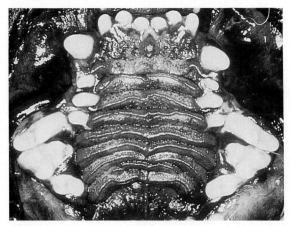

FIGURE 8-9
Maxillary premolar crowding and rotation in a Pekinese.

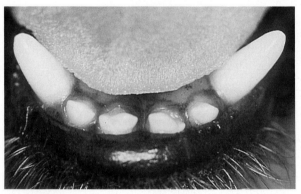

FIGURE 8-10
Hypodontia in a dog (only four incisor teeth are present).

have a normal shape but are rotated relative to the long axis of the jaw, or they overlap each other (Fig. 8-9). The affected teeth are predisposed to periodontal disease.

Absence of teeth

Absence of teeth in dogs and cats can be an inherited abnormality or can result from disturbances during the initial stages of formation of a tooth. The following terms apply to this condition.

Anodontia, the total absence of teeth, is the extreme form.

Oligodontia is the congenital absence of many but not all teeth.

Hypodontia is the absence of only a few teeth (Fig. 8-10).

Inasmuch as the primary teeth give rise to the permanent tooth buds (for those permanent teeth with a deciduous predecessor), there will be no permanent tooth if the primary predecessor was missing. It is possible, however, for a primary tooth to be present and the permanent counterpart to be absent. Anodontia or oligodontia in humans usually is associated with an infrequent but mild systemic abnormality—ectodermal dysplasia—although this is only a rare occurrence in dogs and cats (see Fig. 7-20). Occasionally, oligondontia occurs in a patient with no apparent systemic problem or congenital syndrome.

Anodontia and oligodontia are rare, but hypodontia is a relatively common finding in dogs, especially purebred and line-bred dogs in whom the genetic fault has been perpetuated. It is most common in small-breed dogs but occurs in larger breeds also; in the Doberman breed it is cause for disqualification in the show ring. Congenital absence of one or more teeth is uncommon in cats. The premolar teeth are the most commonly missing, usually the second premolar. Rarely are the carnassial or canine teeth missing.

Eruption sometimes is delayed—up to 2 years in occasional cases (Fig. 8-11); a radiograph must be obtained before a definitive diagnosis of absence of a tooth can be made. Familial delayed eruption occurs in Tibetan and wheaten terriers and probably in other breeds as well.

Supernumerary teeth

Supernumerary teeth result from a genetic defect or from disturbances during dental development. They may disrupt normal occlusal development and can contribute to periodontal disease. Supernumerary teeth, sclerotic bone, and heavy fibrous gingiva also can interfere with eruption. The general rule is to extract only those supernumerary teeth that may contribute to malocclusion or crowding. If there is room for an extra tooth and its position does not predispose the animal to periodontal disease or occlusal attrition, it should not be extracted. Dolichocephalic head types can accommodate extra premolars without crowding or occlusal disturbances (Fig. 8-12). Additional in-

cisor teeth are common in brachycephalic dogs; 25% of bulldogs in one survey had seven or more incisor teeth (see Fig. 7-20, *A*). Supernumerary teeth are common in cats, usually an additional second upper premolar.

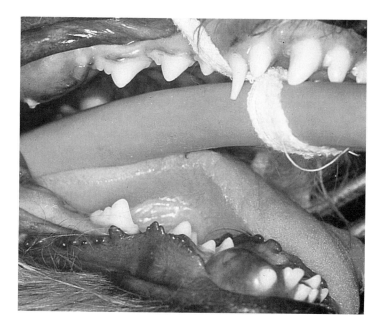

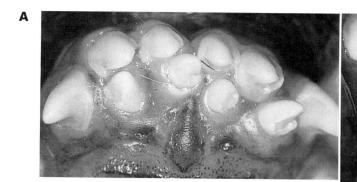

FIGURE 8-11
Delayed eruption of teeth in an 8-month-old Wheaten terrier. The lower canine has only just emerged from the gingiva, and several deciduous teeth are still present.

FIGURE 8-12
Supernumerary incisor (**A**) and premolar (**B**) teeth in a dog. The shape and size of the crowns suggest they are not retained deciduous teeth. There is also rotation of the premolar teeth.

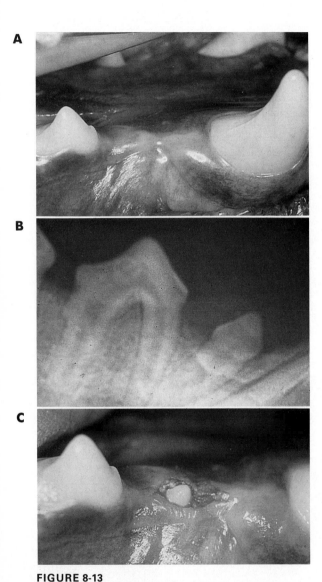

FIGURE 8-13
Partially impacted lower first premolar tooth in a mature dog. **A,** The gingiva is intact but inflamed in the area of the tooth. **B,** Radiograph of the impacted tooth. **C,** The crown of the tooth is uncovered by operculectomy.

Malformed teeth

Malformed teeth are not as prevalent as supernumerary teeth. These abnormalities in tooth size or shape, which result from disturbances during tooth development, are described in Chapter 7.

Impacted teeth

A tooth is impacted when its path of eruption is prevented by an abnormal tissue or a structure lying in the normal path of eruption or by abnormal angulation of the tooth that brings it into contact with an adjacent tooth.

Although theoretically any teeth can be impacted or incompletely erupted, the tooth most often affected is the upper canine, although even this is uncommon in dogs and almost never seen in cats. Impaction, which can occur in all breeds, is more prevalent among the toy breeds. The canine is either impacted into the palate or laterally impacted in the nasal cavity. The cause of impacted teeth is not known, but genetic displacement of the tooth bud is a logical theory. Diagnosis is by radiography.

Fully impacted (bone-encased) teeth are poor candidates for orthodontic treatment. They are very rigid in their position, and they do not affect the masticatory capacity of the animal. If infection or cyst formation is present around an impacted tooth, it should be surgically extracted.

Partially impacted teeth. Partially impacted teeth are those that have part or all of the coronal aspect of the tooth in soft tissue and the root portion in bone. Partially impacted teeth can create a problem if the tissue-covered crown is cystic or in the line of occlusion. This can result in tissue trauma during mastication. These teeth are best treated by operculectomy, the surgical removal of covering tissue to expose the crown (Fig. 8-13). Operculectomy can in some cases stimulate further eruption while relieving soft tissue trauma.

Retention of deciduous teeth

Retention of deciduous teeth is common in toy-breed dogs. The small bone size may result in orientation of the permanent tooth bud relative to the deciduous tooth in a direction that causes it to grow parallel to rather than directly beneath the deciduous tooth. Displacement of teeth becomes important when it results in occlusal trauma and tooth attrition or soft tissue damage. The retention of the deciduous tooth for as short a period as 2 weeks after eruption of the permanent tooth can produce occlusal defects in the permanent dentition. Malocclusion will produce early wearing of the teeth (attrition), rotation and crowding of the teeth that results in periodontal disease, and soft tissue trauma in many instances; occasionally it will prevent the mouth from closing completely.

In the absence of any specific genetic studies proving otherwise, the pattern of occurrence of retained deciduous teeth in certain breeds or head types (Yorkshire terrier, miniature poodle, Pomeranian) strongly suggests that this condition is inherited. It should not be called a *developmental abnormality* if to do so deflects consideration of need for genetic counseling and ethical considerations regarding treatment.

The mechanism governing resorption of the root structure of the deciduous teeth is not fully understood. Although the presence of the developing permanent tooth bud stimulates the resorptive process, it is not the sole governing factor. When deciduous teeth are retained, it is the permanent tooth that deviates from its normal eruptive pathway and comes into the dental arch in an unnatural position. Changes are produced in the soft tissue when the permanent tooth erupts next to the deciduous tooth that can be as harmful as those changes caused by the malocclusion itself. The permanent tooth surface in contact with the deciduous tooth often is deprived of normal periodontal tissues, and even a slight periodontal defect can persist after the loss or extraction of the deciduous tooth, or both. Once a periodontal lesion is established, gradual progression over a period of years is likely.

The permanent teeth have a characteristic eruption pathway when the deciduous teeth are retained. The lower incisors and canines erupt lingual to the deciduous teeth (Fig. 8-14). The permanent lower canines are "base narrow" and tend to damage the tissues of the hard palate as they erupt. Frequently the mandibular canines will not fully erupt upon striking the palate. If the condition is not corrected before root apexification takes place, the full root length will not develop. The maxillary permanent canines erupt rostral (mesial) to the deciduous canines, closing the interdental space between the lateral incisors and the canines (Fig. 8-14). The resulting occlusal defect is seen in the lower dentition. The lower canines are forced forward rostrally and lingually to maintain their position rostral to the maxillary canines. The resultant crowding of the rostral arch tends to move the lower incisors forward to produce an abnormal occlusion that resembles prognathism. Rostral (anterior) crossbite also is produced as the lower incisors rotate and displace in their eruptive efforts. Sometimes the mandibular third incisors are impacted and fail to erupt at all. In addition, the attrition produced as a result of the mandibular canines striking the maxillary lateral incisors can lead to destruction of both teeth over a period of time.

Retention of deciduous premolar teeth is much less common. Retained deciduous teeth are seen occasionally in medium- or large-size dogs and are rare in cats (see Fig. 8-28).

Interceptive orthodontics. It is obvious from the nature of the displacement caused by retained deciduous teeth that the best time to extract is *immediately.* The following advice is a good guide: "Never allow a deciduous tooth to remain in the mouth once there is any evidence of eruption of the crown of the permanent tooth in that location." Thus the clinician should not wait for the deciduous teeth to "fall out" even though the crowns may be loose. It is the root of the tooth that is directing the eruption path of the permanent tooth, and it must be extracted in a timely manner.

In cases of minor jaw length differences in the young puppy, often it is beneficial to extract the deciduous incisors or canines, or both. By doing this, the full genetic growth potential of the inadequate jaw can be expressed (although the inherited nature of the condition that causes the malposition of the deciduous teeth must be considered in terms of the ethics of correcting abnormalities in puppies). In selecting teeth for extraction, the guiding principle should be to remove those teeth that would interfere with the forward growth of the short jaw and, if possible, to leave those teeth that would tend to stop growth when the desired length has been achieved. This problem is referred to as *adverse dental interlock* and can be seen when a growth spurt allows the mandible or maxilla to tem-

FIGURE 8-14
For legend see opposite page.

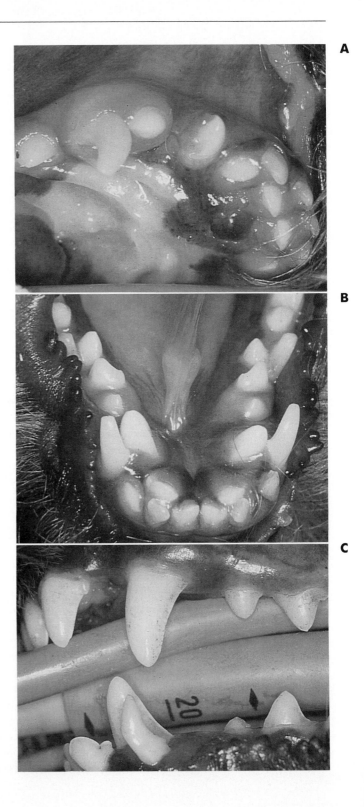

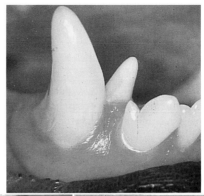

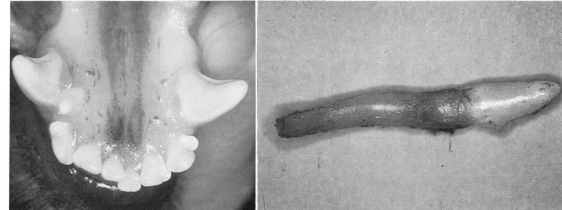

FIGURE 8-14
Retained deciduous incisor and canine teeth in dogs. **A-C,** These retained deciduous
teeth are in the usual position for retained teeth. **D-F,** Apparent retained deciduous
lower canine tooth in abnormal position in a dog. The size and shape of the extracted
tooth suggest it is a deciduous tooth rather than an anomalous tooth.

porarily move ahead of the coordinated growth pattern. If, for instance, the mandibular canine teeth are positioned caudal to the maxillary canines, the growth that results in lengthening the mandible will proceed, but the mandible will tend to "bow" ventrally. If the lower canines are not "released" by extraction, an "overshot" condition will result. Similarly, if there is an adverse interlock of the maxillary incisors caudal to the mandibular ones, extraction of the upper deciduous incisors will permit the eruption of the permanent incisors into their correct position, rostral to the lower incisors if the maxilla meanwhile grows to its correct relative length. Leaving the lower incisors in place forces the permanent dentition to assume its normal position lingual to the upper incisors.

With timely extraction the hope is to correct a possible mechanical dental interlock of the incisors or to intercept a developing malocclusion. The theory is that the removal of incisors before their normal time of exfoliation will allow the erupting permanent incisors to advance more rapidly forward to catch up with the advanced counterpart. This procedure has limited merit. True brachygnathous or prognathous occlusion cannot be prevented by this procedure.

The extraction of primary canines to prevent a developing problem has merit. As already indicated, the permanent lower canines erupt medial to the primary canines, whereas the permanent upper canines erupt rostral to the primary canines. Prolonged retention of the primary canines forces the permanent canines into malocclusion (Fig. 8-14). The lower permanent canines assume a "base-narrow" position, striking the palate on closure, instead of occupying their normal position lateral to the maxilla, whereas the upper permanent canines will be displaced rostrally. This prevents the lower canine from assuming its normal position. Management of established base-narrow lower canine teeth is described on p. 285.

Asymmetry of jaws and tooth location

Wry bite. Wry bite is the result of unequal arch development (Fig. 8-2, *G*). In severe cases one side of the head can show overdevelopment or underdevelopment while the other side remains normal (Fig. 8-3). However, the wry malocclusion may affect the dental arch only and may be slight. The occlusal malalignment can be detected by tracing the midline of the head from the top forward: down the nose and between the teeth. The lines between the central incisors on the top and the bottom will not match. In uncertain cases an occlusal radiograph in exact symmetric position can be obtained of the upper rostral arch. Wry bite caused by mandibular asymmetry also is possible. Wry bite often results from trauma that arrests development of one jaw segment temporarily very early in life (before weaning in many cases), although inherited wry bite abnormalities also occur.

Open bite. Open bite occurs when an abnormality of a tooth or jaw prevents normal full closure of the jaws. Various factors can cause this condition, including abnormal tooth shape, size or location, improperly performed dental work, or congenital and acquired abnormalities of the jaws or temporomandibular joints. Thorough examination is essential.

Acquired abnormalities. Dental trauma can lead to the development of malocclusion. Damage to permanent tooth buds from an injury to primary teeth, drift of permanent teeth after premature loss of primary teeth, and direct injury to permanent teeth are primary causes. Jaw trauma and presence of a mass are other causes of acquired malocclusion.

▶ ORTHODONTIC TREATMENT
Principles

The movement of teeth has three basic prerequisites: sufficient space, adequate pressure, and anchorage. Orthodontic movement of teeth can be described as prolonged application of pressure to a tooth. Movement occurs as the bone around the tooth remodels; bone is resorbed by osteoclasts in areas of compressive pressure and is remodeled by osteoblasts at the opposite (tension) side. The tooth moves through the bone, carrying its attachment apparatus with it, as the socket of the tooth migrates. If the orthodontic pressure is too great, periodontal necrosis and eventual ankylosis and tooth fracture will accompany tooth movement. The gingival fiber networks also are disturbed by orthodontic tooth movement and must remodel to accommodate the new tooth positions. Collagenous fiber networks within the gingiva normally complete their reorganization rapidly, but the elastic supracrestal fibers remodel much more slowly. Therefore it is possible for a tooth to return part or all of the way to its original position several weeks or even months after relocation. The gingival fiber networks must be allowed to remodel to accommodate to the new tooth positions by holding the tooth in that position *(retention)*.

Teeth are moved primarily as a result of one or a combination of the following forces: tipping force, bodily force, and rotating force.

Tipping force

Tipping is the movement of the crown without changing the position of the root apex. Most veterinary orthodontic techniques result in tipping. This form of orthodontic movement is the easiest and quickest to accomplish but is also the most likely to result in structural damage because of excessive pressure or prolonged application of pressure. The application of a constant pressure to the crown of a tooth will cause it to change position if the applied force is of sufficient duration and intensity and the path ahead is not blocked by another tooth. Tipping, with an average orthodontic force, occurs with the fulcrum at about one third of the root length from the apex. If forces are light enough, the fulcrum is at or close to the apex. Excessive force moves the fulcrum coronally. Because most veterinary orthodontic patients undergo therapy during a period of prolific jaw or root growth, therapy is superimposed on normal growth processes.

Bodily force

In the correction of many malocclusions, teeth must be moved bodily; that is, the root of the tooth is moved along the same plane as the crown. Both the root and the crown must be changed in position to achieve adequate correction of the abnormality. This results in a much more stable tooth when the movement is complete, because the pressures applied to the tooth are absorbed along the natural planes of oral structure. Bodily movement can be accomplished, in most instances, by application of force at more than one point on the surface of a tooth. Overall, there is resorption along the entire compression surface and bone deposition along the tension surface; however, it is probable that a tooth moves bodily in a series of "wiggling" movements toward its new position because of a certain amount of "give" in all appliances. This wiggling allows both resorption and deposition to occur on the same surfaces to keep the tooth from becoming excessively mobile, stabilizing its position and preventing traumatic injury to the delicate structures at the apex of the tooth. Greater force is required for bodily movement, and evidence of root resorption is observed more frequently than with tipping procedures. Root resorption is more likely if the orthodontic pressure is high or applied for a long period.

Rotating force

The reaction of a tooth to a rotating force is more complex than tipping or bodily movement in one direction. Theoretically it is a bodily movement in one place; actually it usually is a combined tipping and rotational action. Because the root is seldom perfectly round, areas of compression and tension will occur on various portions of the root, periodontal ligament, and alveolar bone. The reorganization of the principal periodontal fibers that run from the root surface to the bone surface proceeds fairly rapidly. A retention period of 28 days prevents relapse in dogs. Failure to observe this retentive period usually results in a relapse toward the original malposition. If the tooth movement is performed quite early, just as the per-

manent teeth are beginning to erupt and while the periodontal tissue is actively growing, retention of rotated teeth may be more successful because of the formation of new fiber bundles in the apical region, which assist in maintaining the corrected position.

The most frequently encountered rotational displacement in dogs is seen in the premolar region of the maxillary arch. These teeth, when compared with the width of the teeth that have to occupy the space, rotate because of a lack of arch length. This is quite common in brachycephalic breeds; usually the second and always the third upper premolars are rotated (Fig. 8-9). Because crowding is the problem, correction necessitates the movement of adjacent teeth to make room for the rotated tooth to move into proper position. Extraction is probably the best treatment to improve the overall periodontal health of the patient.

Optimal orthodontic force

The optimal orthodontic force is the force that is required for physiologic movement. According to orthodontists, this would be equivalent to the capillary pulse pressure or about 25 g/cm^2 of root surface. In actual practice, with current orthodontic appliances few teeth are moved with such light forces. Bodily tooth movement within the 50- to 200-g range does not ordinarily cause radiographically perceptible apical root resorption. The measurement of forces employed in human dentistry is not particularly accurate at present and is nonexistent in veterinary dentistry. Tooth size, root shape, functional forces, point of application, and type of force all influence the net amount of force reaching a particular area of root surface. Equally important are direction of force, duration of force, distance through which the force is operating, and continuity of the force. Patient age, individual tissue reaction, and metabolic and endocrinologic balance also make a difference. The optimal force should be one that moves the tooth most rapidly in the desired attitude and direction with the least tissue damage and the slightest amount of pain or discomfort. In veterinary orthodontics, with the current lack of information and equipment to measure these forces, we must rely on our powers of observation, particularly close clinical and radiographic monitoring, to obtain the desired results.

Heavy continuous force is damaging to both the

teeth and periodontal tissue and should not be used; damage may be irreparable. A good example of this type of pressure is the overly enthusiastic owner who decides to place an elastic band on a tooth or teeth to reposition them. Once the resistance of the alveolar bone is breeched, the movement of the tooth becomes rapid and predictable—it comes out.

An alternative to the dangerous heavy continuous force is to use heavy forces through very short distances by periodic intermittent applications that allow for tissue repair between adjustments. A good example of this technique is the use of an expansion screw device to load the appliance on a weekly basis instead of elastics that place lighter but continuous pressure on the tooth.

Light continuous force will move the teeth primarily by frontal assault, with little necrosis of periodontal tissue at the point of greatest pressure. With less tissue damage during treatment, because of the light forces involved, less permanent damage will occur. With gentle, continuous forces, teeth appear to move more rapidly and with less pain to the patient.

Duration and intensity must be considered. If an appliance is left on the teeth for a long period of time, root resorption may occur as a result of repeated pressure. There is little tendency toward root resorption within a reasonable period of time (8 to 9 months), provided that conventional forces have been used and systemic predisposing factors are not present.

Anchorage

Teeth move when subjected to pressure. Depending on the kind of pressure, the manner in which it is applied, the type of attachment to the tooth, the distance through which the force is active, and the time that the pressure is applied, the tooth will move in a certain direction at a certain speed and assume a certain position with respect to adjacent structures. However, a tooth does not move by itself. Depending on how the force is applied, different teeth have different resistances to tooth movement. Recognizing this, the veterinary dentist can use certain teeth for "anchorage" to move other teeth into a more desirable position. The term *anchorage* in orthodontics refers to the resistance to displacement offered by an anatomic unit used to effect tooth movement.

Teeth are the most frequent anatomic units used for anchorage. The important factor in assessing resistance of a potential anchor is the part of the tooth anchored in alveolar bone. The number of roots and the size, shape, and length of each root are vitally important. Another way to express this is the total root surface area. A tooth with a large surface area is more resistant to displacement than one with a smaller surface area. A multirooted tooth is more resistant to displacement than is a single-rooted tooth; a longer rooted tooth is more difficult to move than is a shorter-rooted tooth; and a triangular-shaped root offers more resistance than does a conical one. Other factors that also must be considered are the relationship of adjacent teeth, the forces of occlusion, the age of the patient, and individual tissue response variables. Anchorage teeth that have more surface area than the tooth to be moved should be selected; in some instances it may be necessary to include more than one tooth as the anchorage unit. A good example of this is moving a rostrally displaced maxillary canine tooth by anchoring the elastics to the upper fourth premolar and the lower first molar. The more apically the anchor is placed on the crown, the greater is its resistance. Anchorage is only relative; anchor teeth move as well as the target teeth. Anchorage reinforcement may not always be necessary, but it is a consideration in developing an orthodontic treatment plan for any patient.

Light prolonged forces in the natural environment (forces from the lips, cheeks, or tongue resting against the teeth) have the same potential as orthodontic forces to cause the teeth to move to a different location.

The behavior of orthodontic materials and mechanical factors must be considered in the design of an orthodontic appliance that can deliver ideal light forces.

Treatment

Certain malocclusions or individual tooth problems can be corrected orthodontically to the betterment of the animal. A treatment plan must take into consideration the functional need and ethics. This may dictate the judicious use of dental extraction (see Chapter 10) or pulpotomy (see Chapter 6) rather than orthodontics to relieve soft tissue trauma.

Rostral (anterior) crossbite

Although many different systems have been described for orthodontic movement of incisor teeth in dogs, anterior crossbites usually do not cause functional problems. Dogs and cats have a simple hinge type of jaw movement; lateral and protrusive movements seen in human jaw function may be affected by anterior crossbites. Anterior crossbite in dogs may cause periodontal problems because of the malalignment or crowding; this can be prevented by proper oral hygiene or extraction. Orthodontic treatment of anterior crossbite rarely is indicated except for correction of a cosmetic defect, which is unethical.

Caudal (posterior) crossbite

Posterior crossbites need not be corrected. They do not severely affect function. In addition, they are extremely difficult to correct and can result in disastrous complications. If periodontal tissues are at risk because of the abnormal location, angulation, or juxtaposition of teeth, the affected teeth should be extracted.

Base-narrow canines

Base-narrow canines, the most common abnormality in the dog for which orthodontic movement is indicated, can be treated by several methods. Extraction of the lower canine that is striking the palate will relieve the tissue damage. However, the lower canine tooth is important esthetically because it helps to keep the tongue in place in the mouth and because it is visible when the mouth is open, for example, during panting. If the upper canine tooth is extracted and the lateral alveolar bone and attached gingiva is resected, space is available for the full height of the lower canine (Fig. 8-15). Unless the upper lip is lifted, the upper canine tooth is not externally visible.

Second, canine length can be reduced so that soft tissue trauma to the palate can be relieved. This can be accomplished by vital pulpotomy (Fig. 8-16; see Chapter 6). If the extent of malocclusion is mild, burring and smoothing of enamel and dentin without pulpotomy may be sufficient (Fig. 8-17).

The third technique is orthodontic movement. If sufficient lateral space is available, the lower canine or canines can be moved into normal position by constructing an acrylic or composite palatal bite plane either directly or indirectly (Figs. 8-18 to 8-20). The orthodontic force is provided naturally by the animal when it closes its mouth: the tip of the abnormally located tooth is forced in the desired direction.

An indirect bite plane is made by a dental laboratory from an impression and cast, and it is cemented in place at a second appointment. (Making dental impressions and casts is described in Chapter 7.) Use of an indirect bite plane made on an oral cast prevents thermal damage to the oral tissues during the curing phase, which produces an exothermic reaction in most acrylics. Indirect bite planes usually are not as stable as direct appliances. Another alternative is use of an acid-etched composite bite plane; in creating the device, a space can be left between the device and the gingival margin for improved oral hygiene while the device is in place (Fig. 8-20). If orthodontic correction is performed using any technique, the animal should be neutered.

Orthodontic acrylic. Orthodontic acrylic is a polyethyl methacrylate used to form an active appliance or a retainer. It is supplied as a polymer (a powder in various colors) and a monomer (a liquid). The two are mixed as directed by the manufacturer and harden within minutes to form the appliance. Acrylic devices are very versatile. Thickness and form can be altered by adding more liquid or powder, or both, or by removing portions that are too thick with an acrylic bur. Holes can be drilled or wires can be embedded for attachment, and pressure-producing units such as expansion or retraction screws or memory finger wires can be attached or embedded. Certain acrylics produce less exothermic reaction—for example, Merdon 7 (Caulk Dental Co., New York, NY); these can be used safely for direct application in the mouth.

Direct bite plane

Technique. A thorough dental prophylaxis is performed with use of a slurry mixture of flour pumice and water as the final polishing material. Fluorides added to pumice interfere with adhesion of composite resins. Wax strips are used to make a dam or outline the area of application of acrylic (Fig. 8-18, *B*). The acrylic should encompass the lingual aspect of the incisors, extending just beyond the distal margin of

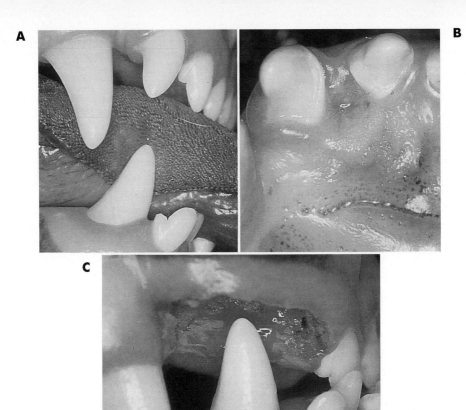

FIGURE 8-15
Extraction, gingivoplasty, and osteoplasty for maloccluded canine tooth. **A** and **B,** The lower canine tooth is base-narrow and prognathic (or the upper jaw is brachygnathic) causing impaction of the lower canine into the palate with ulceration adjacent to the upper third incisor tooth. **C,** The upper third incisor tooth has been extracted, and the lateral alveolar plate and gingiva have been resected to provide room for the lower canine tooth.

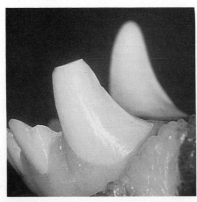

FIGURE 8-16
Pulpotomy for treatment of a palatal soft tissue impaction caused by a base-narrow canine tooth.

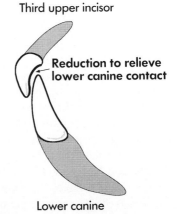

FIGURE 8-17
Smoothing off abnormal contacts to relieve malocclusion.

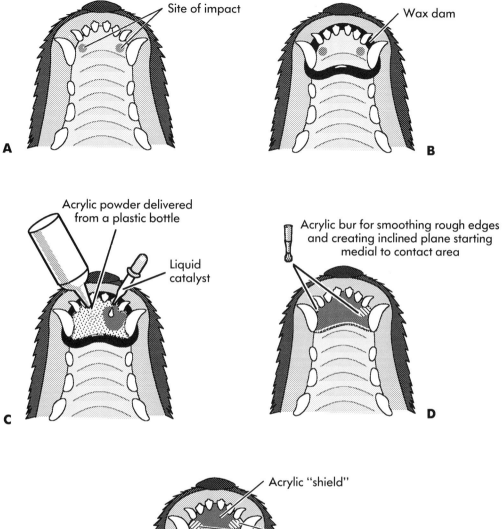

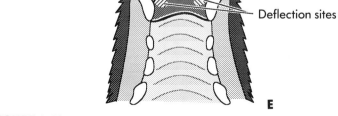

FIGURE 8-18
A, Palatal defects resulting from bilateral base-narrow canine occlusion. **B,** Wax strip placed to form a dam around the upper canine and incisor teeth. **C,** Acrylic powder and liquid is mixed in the dammed area. **D,** Once set, the acrylic is burred to form the deflecting inclined plane. **E,** The completed device.

the maxillary canines. A figure-of-8 wire snugly fitting around the canine teeth will help hold the acrylic to the teeth. This wire (usually a 20 to 24 gauge stainless steel) is embedded in the acrylic as it is formed. The acrylic powder and liquid (preferably nonexothermic crown and bridge acrylic such as Merdon 7) are added slowly and carefully to cover the entire area encompassed by the wax dam (Fig. 8-18, *C*). Initially it is very soft; overspills can be removed with a plastic spatula or a gauze sponge. To determine the exact contact point of the crown tip of the mandibular canine tooth, the clinician must extubate the patient, retract its tongue, and close its mouth. If this is done while the acrylic is still soft, the teeth will make an impression into the acrylic and a groove or inclined plane can be impressed into the soft material to guide the teeth into proper position. After the acrylic has set and is hard, additional shaping of the material can be

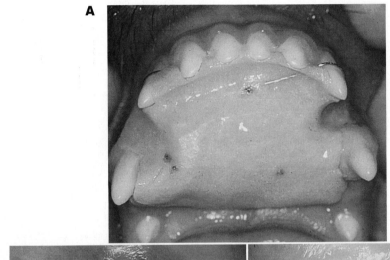

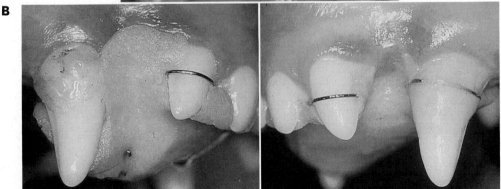

FIGURE 8-19
Acrylic device for movement of a unilateral base-narrow lower canine tooth. The device includes a space shaped to ensure retention of the contralateral lower canine tooth in its normal position. **A,** Palatal view. **B,** Buccal view, base-narrow side. **C,** Buccal view, normal position side.

accomplished with an acrylic bur (for example, Goldie acrylic bur; see Chapter 11) after the utility wax dam has been removed (Fig. 8-18, *D* and *E*).

Some forward (rostral) movement of the displaced canines can be accommodated by grooving the acrylic in a rostral/labial direction to curve around the mesial margin of the maxillary canines. These two-direction movement procedures obviously are limited in scope and take more treatment time than the simpler one-direction movement technique. This technique is satisfactory only if there is space into which the tooth can be moved. Lower canine teeth that are trapped directly medial (lingual) to the upper canine teeth cannot be moved successfully by this technique. The time required for movement with this technique is from 2 to 6 weeks. The earlier it is performed, the faster the movement; however, during the time of rapid growth spurt, while the canine teeth are erupting rapidly, con-

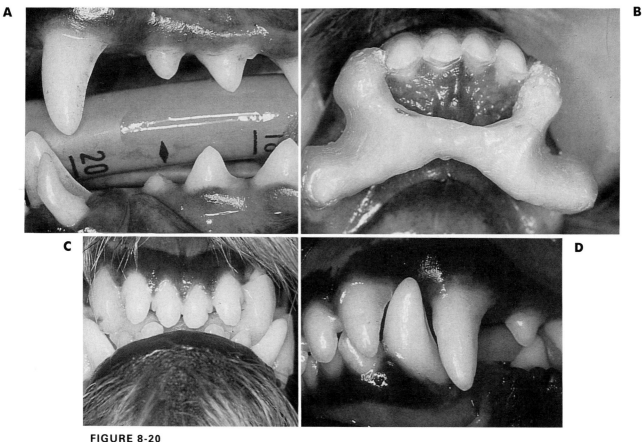

FIGURE 8-20
Composite inclined plane for movement of base-narrow lower canine teeth in a dog. **A,** Retained lower canine deciduous tooth and base-narrow permanent lower canine tooth. **B,** Occlusal view of the composite device attached to the canine and third incisor teeth. **C,** Rostral view of the device showing the lower canine teeth impacting the device at an angle. **D,** Normal occlusion following removal of the device.

striction of the growth of the maxillary arch by the acrylic plate could lead to serious complications for the adult animal. The device can be made as right and left sections connected by a telescoping bar to permit growth in palatal width while the device is in place. Usually it is best to wait until the teeth have fully erupted, although some soft tissue damage in the hard palate will be evident. This damage, if not allowed to persist for too long, is reversible and is less traumatic than constricting the growth of the maxilla.

Complete cooperation of the owner in instituting and maintaining rigid home care instructions (daily toothbrushing and flushing with chlorhexidine solution, soft food, no chew toys or bones) is absolutely essential for the successful outcome of procedures that require placement of orthodontic devices in the mouths of dogs or cats. Once the mandibular canines have been repositioned in the interdental space between the upper lateral incisors and the maxillary canine teeth for several days, the appliance can be removed because the maxilla continues to act as a natural retainer.

If only one tooth is affected, the appliance should be formed to retain the normal tooth in its correct position (Fig. 8-19). Forming the appliance to move

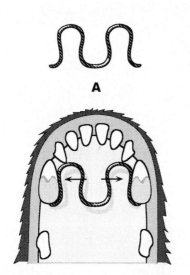

A

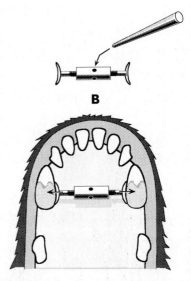

B

C

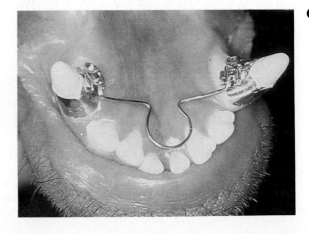

FIGURE 8-21
Alternative treatment techniques for bilateral base-narrow lower canine teeth. **A,** Activated orthodontic wire. **B,** Screw thread–activated expansion bar. Both devices are attached to the lower canine teeth with composite cement reinforced with additional composite built around the attachment point. **C,** Activated wire in place in a dog.

one tooth without stabilizing the other canine will cause the jaw to rotate, in addition to causing movement of the target tooth.

Expansion devices. A fourth technique for relocation of medially displaced lower canine teeth is to apply the orthodontic force to the tooth with an expansion device cemented directly to the tooth (Fig. 8-21). This technique results in equal pressure being ordered against both lower canine teeth; thus it is not appropriate when the condition is not symmetric. Success depends on selection of the correct force by the veterinarian (extent of activation of a wire or frequency of adjustment of an expansion screw). Because of the uncertainty of calculation of the correct force and contraindication in animals with asymmetric malocclusion, the bite plane technique is preferred to the expansion device technique.

Rostrally displaced upper canine teeth

Treatment options for rostrally displaced upper canine teeth are extraction (Fig. 8-22) or orthodontic movement (Figs. 8-23 and 8-24).

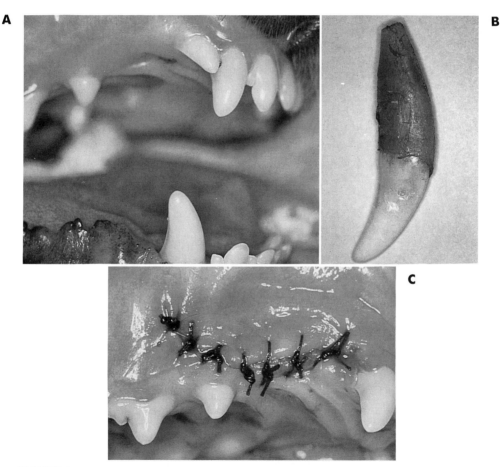

FIGURE 8-22
Extraction of rostrally displaced upper canine teeth. **A,** The tooth before treatment occluding against the upper third incisor tooth. **B,** The extracted tooth. **C,** Extraction site with flap incision sutured closed over the alveolectomy site.

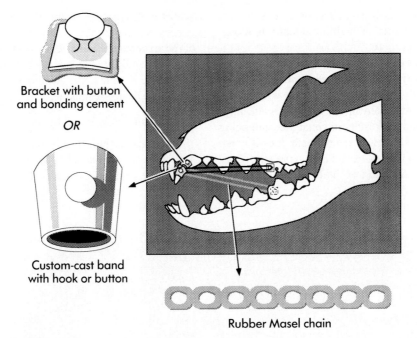

FIGURE 8-23
Orthodontic treatment of rostrally displaced upper canine tooth in a dog.

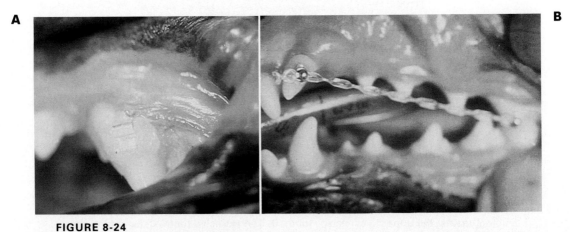

FIGURE 8-24
A, Button bracket on the buccal surface of the upper fourth premolar (anchor) tooth.
B, Masel chain in place.

To move a rostrally displaced maxillary canine tooth, the clinician places an orthodontic bracket or button on the labial and lingual surfaces of the canine tooth. A similar bracket is adhered to the upper fourth premolar and, in some cases, the lower first molar, both of which are used as the anchor teeth (Fig. 8-24, *A*). Adherent elastics placed on each side of the canine tooth produce an even retraction without rotation. If there is not enough open contact on the lower first molar tooth to prevent striking by the upper fourth premolar when the mouth is closed, the bracket can be placed on the lingual surface of the molar. Orthodontic elastics or *Masel chain* ("power chain") are used to provide the orthodontic force (Fig. 8-24, *B*). If orthodontic correction of this abnormality is performed, the dog should be neutered.

Bonding of orthodontic appliances to the teeth requires a mechanical locking of an adhesive to irregularities in the enamel surface of the tooth that is produced by acid-etching technique. Careful attention to the components of the bonding system, acid-etch technique, bracket size and design, and tooth surface preparation ensure retention of bonded appliances. Proper position for the attachment or bracket is predetermined. Because the working time with use of bonding cements is short, the attachment must be carried to place rapidly and accurately.

Technique. The clinician cleans the teeth, finally polishing with a slurry of flour pumice and water. Fluoride prophylaxis paste is not used. Copious rinsing with water and air drying the tooth follow. The teeth to be used are etched with a phosphoric acid etching gel for 30 to 60 seconds and then rinsed thoroughly with water. When properly etched, the tooth appears chalky white. If this does not occur, the etching process is repeated. Etching is described in more detail in Chapter 7.

The buttons or brackets selected are rinsed thoroughly and air dried. Several types of cement are available; for purposes of attaching orthodontic brackets, Panavia or Resiment composite cement provide excellent results. The cement is mixed exactly according to the manufacturer's directions and applied to the tooth surface and bonding surface of the bracket or button; then the device is promptly placed and held firmly for several seconds. After setting occurs, rough edges of cement are burred smooth.

The Masel chain is used free of tension, and the number of loops from bracket to bracket are counted. Approximately 75% of this length is then stretched and attached to the brackets. For instance, if the at-rest length covers 10 loops, then the elastic under tension should be only 7 loops. The chain from the canine to the lower first molar should be measured with the mouth moderately (about halfway) open to allow for stretching on full opening of the mouth.

The chain or elastics (2-ounce orthodontic elastics, one-eighth to three-sixteenths inches) should be changed at weekly intervals inasmuch as the elasticity usually is gone by this time. At the same time the teeth and oral tissues should be checked for complications. The owner must adhere to a rigid program of oral hygiene (daily brushing and flushing with chlorhexidine solution) and examination of the appliance on a daily basis.

It takes approximately 2 weeks for the elastics to overcome the natural resistance of the alveolar bone to movement of the tooth. After this time period the pressure can be changed by changing the number of loops in the elastic chain. Overcorrection usually is not a problem; however, tooth extrusion can occur if the tooth is not closely monitored. Correction usually will take from 8 to 12 weeks, depending on the size and age of the dog. Retention with ligature wires or an acrylic splint is suggested for at least 4 weeks to allow the bone and tissue to reorganize.

This same procedure can be used to replace a rostrally displaced mandibular canine tooth, but it is accomplished much more slowly because of the denser mandibular bone structure.

Study casts made from dental impressions are very useful. They are essential for indirect applications of orthodontic appliances for fabrication of the appliance. They also provide an accurate way of comparing the extent of change as the treatment is applied. Impression techniques are described in Chapter 7, and preparation of stone casts are described on p. 260.

Complications of orthodontic appliances

Soft tissue trauma results from pressure of the device or the exothermic reaction of direct acrylic technique. Good oral hygiene is essential; the procedure should not be initiated unless the owner is willing to commit to performing daily care while an orthodontic device is in the animal's mouth. Other complications result from poor tolerance of the device (generally because it is poorly designed, for example, rough edges, obstruction of the tongue), fracture of a poorly designed device, and overcorrection or undercorrection of the abnormality.

▶ FELINE MALOCCLUSION

The classification of feline occlusion (see box, p. 267), causes, and genetic considerations are the same as for dogs.

The most common malocclusions are seen in the flat-nosed breeds. The pattern is typically a wry malocclusion with one lower canine protruding in an exaggerated unilateral mandibular prognathous position (Fig. 8-25). The canine often is outside the upper lip when the mouth is closed. This can result in tissue trauma to the upper lip either externally or internally in the contact area (Fig. 8-25, A). Simple relief of trauma is by coronal amputation and vital pulpotomy of the prognathous canine (Fig. 8-25, B). The canine tooth can be orthodontically repositioned; an elastic or power chain is attached to the canine by a band and secured to a bonded bracket on the lower molar with a technique similar to that described for rostrally displaced canines in dogs (Fig. 8-26).

Rostrally displaced upper canine teeth are seen occasionally in cats (Fig. 8-27); treatment options are as described for the dog.

Retained deciduous teeth (Fig. 8-28) and supernumerary teeth occur in cats less commonly than in dogs.

Acquired occlusal abnormalities can result from external trauma such as mandibular fracture or temporomandibular joint injury or electric cord injury (Fig. 8-29).

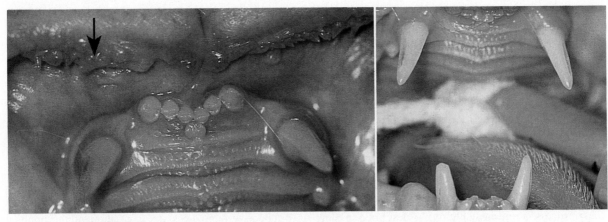

FIGURE 8-25
Protruding lower canine teeth in a cat with brachycephaly. **A,** Upper lip granulation and hyperplasia *(arrow).* **B,** Pulpotomy to shorten lower canine tooth.

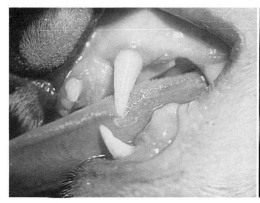 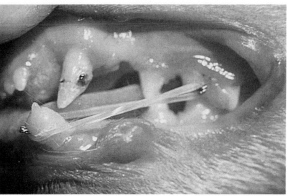

FIGURE 8-26
A, Rostrally displaced lower canine tooth in a cat. **B,** Button and orthodontic elastic in place.

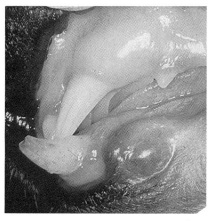

FIGURE 8-27
Rostrally displaced upper canine tooth in a cat with dolichocephaly.

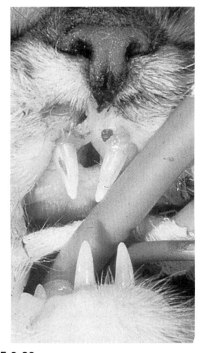

FIGURE 8-29
Medial collapse of the upper and lower canine teeth in a cat caused by loss of palatal and mandibular bone as a result of an electric cord injury.

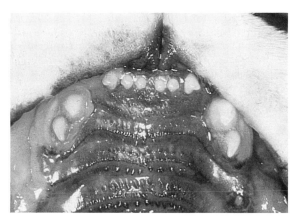

FIGURE 8-28
Retained deciduous canine tooth in a 12-year-old cat.

▶ SUGGESTED READINGS

Aller S: Retained deciduous teeth and delayed development of dentition of Tibetan terriers, *Proc Vet Dent Forum* 4:75, 1990.

Andrews AH: A case of partial anodontia in a dog, *Vet Rec* 90:144, 1972.

Aitchison J: Changing incisor dentition of bull dogs, *Vet Rec* 75:153, 1963.

American Kennel Club: Dog show rules (available from American Kennel Club, 51 Madison Ave, New York, NY 10010).

Arnall L: Some aspects of dental development in the dog. Some common variations in dentition, *J Small Anim Pract* 2:195, 1961.

AVMA Council Report: Unacceptable surgical procedures applicable to domestic animals, *JAVMA* 168:947, 1976.

Baker LW: The influence of the forces of occlusion on the development of the bones of the skull, *Int J Orthod Oral Surg Radiogr* 8:259, 1922.

Beard GB: Anterior crossbite: interceptive orthodontics for prevention, Maryland bridges for correction, *J Vet Dent* 6(2):14, 1989.

Bell AF: Dental disease in the dog, *J Small Anim Pract* 6:421, 1965.

Bodingbauer J: Retention of teeth in dogs as a sequel to distemper infection, *Vet Rec* 72:636, 1960.

Brass W: Zur korrecktur von Zahnstellungs-und Kieferanomalien des Hundes mit Dehungsplatten und durch kierferchirurgische Mafnahmen, *Kleintierpraxis* 21:79, 1976.

Calabrese CT et al: Altering the dimensions of the canine face by the induction of new bone formation, *Plast Reconstr Surg* 54:467, 1974.

Cechner PE: Malocclusion in the dog caused by intramedullary pin fixation of mandibular fractures: two case reports, *JAAHA* 16:79, 1980.

Colyer F: *Variations and diseases of the teeth in animals,* London, 1936, John Bale.

Dinc C, Triadan H: Tierzahnheilkunde, Kiefer orthopadie, *Kleintierpraxis* 34:11, 1989.

Eisenmenger E, Zetner K: *Veterinary dentistry,* Philadelphia, 1985, WB Saunders.

Eisner ER: Malocclusions in dogs and cats, *Vet Med* 83:1006, 1988.

Elzay R, Hughes RD: Anodontia in a cat, *JAVMA* 154:667, 1969.

Field EA et al: The removal of an impacted maxillary canine and associated dentigerous cyst in a chow, *J Small Anim Pract* 23:159, 1982.

Follin ME, Ericsson I, Thilander B: Occurrence and distribution of root resorption in orthodontically moved premolars in dog, *Angle Orthod* 56:164, 1986.

Gruneberg H, Lea AJ: An inherited jaw anomaly in long-haired dachshunds, *J Genet* 30:285, 1940.

Leighton RL: Surgical correction of prognathous inferior in a dog, *Vet Med Small Anim Clin* 72:401, 1977.

Kawase K: Orthodontic techniques for malocclusions in the dog, *J Vet Dent* 7:9, 1990.

Kind RE, Mays RA: Use of an inclined plane for correction of ectopic mandibular canine tooth in a dog, *Vet Med Small Anim Pract* 71:52, 1976.

Kratochvil Z: Oligodonty and polydonty in the domestic and wild cat, *Acta Vet Brno* 40:33, 1971.

McKeown M: Dental arch shape—genetics or environment? *J Irish Dent Assoc* 19:99, 1973.

Michieli S et al: Surgical lengthening of the mandible: a laboratory model, *Oral Surg* 50:207, 1980.

Pearce RG: Anomalies of the English bulldog, *Southwest Vet J* 22:218, 1969.

Phillips JM: "Pig jaw" in cocker spaniels. Retrognathia of the mandible in the cocker spaniel and its relationship to other deformities of the jaw, *J Hered* 36:177, 1945.

Proell F, Wyrwoll R: Experimentelle Untersuchungen uber das Wachstum des Unterkiefers und der Zahne, *Deutsche Zahn Mund- und Kieferheilkunde* 1:81, 1934.

Proffit WR: *Contemporary orthodontics,* ed 2, St Louis, 1992, Mosby–Year Book.

Ritter R: Konnen Anomalien des Gebisses gezuchtet werden? *Deutsche Zahn-, Mund- und Kieferheilkunde* Bd.4 H.4 p 235, 1937.

Ross DL: Orthodontics for the dog. I. Bite evaluation, basic concepts and equipment, *Vet Clin North Am* 16:955, 1986.

Ross DL: Orthodontics for the dog. II. Treatment methods, *Vet Clin North Am* 16:939, 1986.

Scott EJ: An experimental study in growth of the mandible, *Am J Orthod* 24:925, 1938.

Selhorst F: Orthodontische und kieferorthopadische Behandkunger und Versuche an Hunden, master's thesis, Munich, 1964, University of Munich.

Skrentny TT: Preliminary study of the inheritance of missing teeth in the dog, *Wien Tierarzt Monaschr* 51:231, 1964.

Stockard CR, Johnson AL: *Genetic and endocrinic basis for differences in form and behavior,* Am Anat Memoir 19, Philadelphia, 1941, Wistar Inststitute.

Whitney GD: Removal of retained deciduous teeth in dogs, *Mod Vet Pract* 54:46, 1973.

Windle BCA, Humphreys J: On some cranial and dental characteristics of the domestic dog. Proceedings of the Zoological Society, 1889.

Wisdorf H, Hermanns W: Persistent milk teeth (canines) in the upper jaw of a cat, *Kleintierpraxis* 19:14, 1974.

Yamagata J: Dental malocclusion and odontorthosis in dogs, *Jpn Vet Med Assoc* 32:194, 1979.

9

Oral Neoplasms

The oropharynx is the fourth most common site of malignant neoplasia in dogs and cats. Many tumor types, both benign and malignant, occur in the oral tissues of dogs and cats (Tables 9-1 and 9-2). In dogs, on the basis of specimens submitted for biopsy, the four most common tumor types (epulis, fibrosarcoma, malignant melanoma, and squamous cell carcinoma) account for more than 80% of all oral neoplasms. In cats, squamous cell carcinoma alone accounts for 70% of all neoplasms, whether benign or malignant.

Most oral masses seen on physical examination in dogs are benign; the most common are generalized gingival hyperplasia and epulis (osseous or fibromatous) lesions. Many firm smooth gingival masses are permitted to remain untreated in old dogs; thus fibrous/osseous epulides and gingival hyperplasia are underreported in lists of surgical biopsy specimens. A standard nomenclature for the canine epulides has been suggested, and three types are recognized. They are fibromatous epulis, ossifying epulis, and the locally aggressive acanthomatous epulis. Another benign neoplasm is infectious papilloma, a viral disease that is seen occasionally in young dogs (see Figs. A-31, p. 57; and A-56, p.63). Transmissible veneral tumors occasionally occur in the canine oropharynx. Tumors of the dental laminar epithelium are rare in both dogs and cats; ameloblastoma is the most frequently diagnosed tumor of this sort; ameloblastic fibroodontoma and complex and compound odontoma are rare.

Feline dental tumors include inductive fibroameloblastoma and ameloblastoma. Benign oropharyngeal tumors are rare in cats, although fibroma and papilloma have been noted.

Nonneoplastic diseases that may appear as single oral masses are common (see Atlas for examples). They include infectious, inflammatory lesions (see Chapters 3 and 5), endodontic lesions (see Chapter 6), and traumatic lesions (see Chapters 3 and 10).

▶ HISTORY AND CLINICAL SIGNS

Animals with oral neoplasms are brought in for examination because the owner notices an oral mass or because of excessive salivation, bleeding from the mouth, difficulty in mastication, dysphagia, or halitosis. Metastases from the primary tumor may result in mandibular, retropharyngeal, or cervical lymph node enlargement, occasional anorexia because of mechanical interference with mastication or deglutition, or respiratory disease because of lung metastasis.

Oral tumors are most prevalent in older animals. Exceptions include oral papillomatosis in young dogs (mean age of 1 year), papillary squamous cell carcinoma (sometimes found in dogs younger than 6 months of age), inductive fibroameloblastoma in cats (younger than 18 months of age), fibrosarcoma in large-breed dogs (mean age of about 5 years), and occasional acanthomatous epulides in dogs (see Fig. 9-5).

TABLE 9-1		Oral tumors: canine
No. of cases	Percentage of cases	Tumor type
657	22.8	Epulis: fibrous/fibromatous/fibrodentitious
170	5.9	Epulis: osseodentitious
241	8.4	Epulis: acanthomatous
22	0.8	Ameloblastoma
17	0.6	Fibroma/neurofibroma
3	0.1	Round cell tumor
28	1.0	Papilloma/papillomatosis
111	3.9	Plasmacytoma
16	0.6	Mast cell tumor
56	1.9	Lymphosarcoma/malignant histiocytosis/lymphohistiocytic sarcoma
5	0.2	Hemangioma
16	0.6	Hemangiosarcoma
2	0.05	Lymphangioma
7	0.2	Lipoma
199	6.9	Fibrosarcoma
6	0.2	Neurofibrosarcoma
10	0.3	Spindle cell sarcoma
8	0.3	Myxosarcoma
2	0.05	Odontogenic sarcoma/odontogenic fibrosarcoma
1	0.03	Osteoma
50	1.7	Osteosarcoma
2	0.05	Chondroma
3	0.1	Chondrosarcoma
55	1.9	Sarcoma, type not stated
707	24.6	Malignant melanoma
361	12.6	Squamous cell carcinoma
119	4.1	Carcinoma (anaplastic, papillary, ductal, or type not stated)
1	0.03	Malignant lymphoepithelial neoplasm
TOTAL: 2875		

Data from Surgical Biopsy Service, Department of Pathology, School of Veterinary Medicine, University of Pennsylvania; courtesy M. Goldschmidt and F. Shofer.

Male dogs are at greater risk for development of malignant oral tumors than are females. This sex distribution is most pronounced with malignant melanoma (four times as frequently in males as in females). Fibrosarcoma occurs twice as commonly in males. There is no sex predilection for gingival, lingual, or lip squamous cell carcinoma.

Breeds that are at a significantly higher risk for oral cancer include the golden retriever, German short-haired pointer, weimaraner, Saint Bernard, boxer, and cocker spaniel. Melanomas develop more frequently in breeds with heavily pigmented oral mucosae. Beagles and dachshunds have a lower risk than all breeds combined.

In dogs the gingivae are the most frequent sites of involvement for fibrosarcoma (87%), squamous cell carcinoma (81%), and malignant melanoma (55%). Most tumors of buccal or labial mucosa are melanomas (76%), and 66% of hard palate tumors are melanomas.

TABLE 9-2		Oral tumors: feline
No. of cases	Percentages of cases	Tumor type
27	3.1	Epulis: fibrous
4	0.6	Epulis: osseodentitious
3	0.5	Epulis: acanthomatous
12	1.6	Ameloblastoma
3	0.5	Fibroma
1	0.2	Round cell tumor
5	0.7	Plasmacytoma
1	0.2	Mast cell tumor
1	0.2	Giant cell tumor
2	0.3	Hemangioma
2	0.3	Hemangiosarcoma
22	3.4	Lymphosarcoma
3	0.5	Lymphohistiocytic sarcoma
46	6.3	Fibrosarcoma
2	0.3	Neurofibrosarcoma
1	0.2	Myxosarcoma
3	0.5	Osteosarcoma
8	1.3	Sarcoma, type not stated
10	1.6	Malignant melanoma
444	69.5	Squamous cell carcinoma
61	9.4	Carcinoma (type not stated)

TOTAL 639

Data from Surgical Biopsy Service, Department of Pathology, School of Veterinary Medicine, University of Pennsylvania; courtesy M. Goldschmidt and F. Shofer.
During the time period covered above, 22 oral eosinophilic granuloma complex lesions also were reported by the Surgical Biopsy Service.

Tumors that are primarily nasal may invade through the palate and manifest as ulcerative or protuberant palatal masses; the history of nasal discharge is important in differentiating the tumor's origin.

▶ DIAGNOSTIC TECHNIQUES

The advanced age of most animals with oral neoplasms makes essential a thorough evaluation of systemic health. In addition to a thorough history and physical examination, a minimum data base is a complete blood cell count and serum chemistry screen.

Radical surgery or radiotherapy that requires numerous anesthetic episodes may not be advisable if significant cardiac, kidney, liver, neuromuscular, or hematopoietic dysfunction is evident. The clinician, in planning chemotherapy, should reject drugs that are activated by the liver, such as cyclophosphamide, if hepatic disease is present.

To determine the presence and extent of bone invasion, skull or jaw radiographs should be taken in all animals with gingival or palatine tumors or when any tumor is fixed to underlying bone. Lateral, oblique, and intraoral projections may be needed. Radiographic evidence of an osteolytic or osteoblastic reaction is present in most dogs with squamous cell carcinoma, malignant melanoma, and acanthomatous epulis (Fig. 9-1). Fibrosarcoma can be osteolytic, or it can appear radiographically as a soft tissue mass arising from otherwise normal bone. The actual incidence of bone invasion probably is higher than reported inasmuch as 40% of existing bone must be destroyed before lesions are seen radiographically.

Thoracic radiographs should be obtained for all animals with suspected oral malignancy. On the basis of the interpretation of thoracic radiographs, one study revealed lung metastases in 14% of dogs with malignant melanoma, 10% of dogs with fibrosarcoma, and 3% of dogs with oral squamous cell carcinoma. Despite negative thoracic radiographic findings, the incidence of false-negative thoracic radiographs is high; at least 13% of dogs with malignant melanoma had lung metastases at autopsy in one study.

The most critical procedure in the evaluation of a patient with oral neoplasia is obtaining and examining a biopsy specimen. It allows the clinician to establish the diagnosis, formulate a treatment regimen, and give the owner an accurate prognosis. The biopsy must avoid areas of superficial necrosis and must sample the deeper, viable tissue. Excisional biopsy, a wedge biopsy, or a needle punch technique can be used (see also Chapter 2). Electrosurgery should not be used on small samples because the entire biopsy specimen will be coagulated. If the results of the biopsy do not correlate with the gross appearance of the oral mass, a second, deeper, and larger biopsy specimen should be obtained.

On the basis of a study of necropsy findings in 91

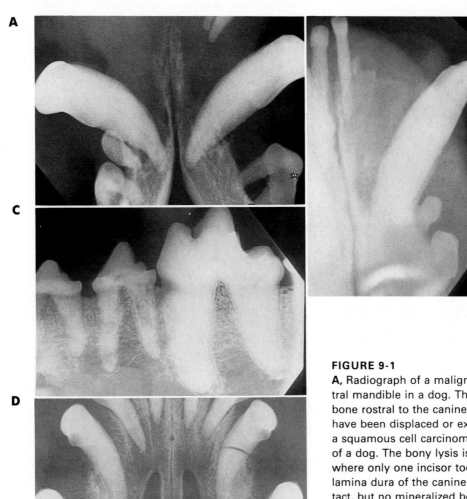

FIGURE 9-1
A, Radiograph of a malignant melanoma of the rostral mandible in a dog. There is lysis of most of the bone rostral to the canine teeth, and incisor teeth have been displaced or exfoliated. **B,** Radiograph of a squamous cell carcinoma of the rostral mandible of a dog. The bony lysis is confined to one side, where only one incisor tooth remains. The distal lamina dura of the canine tooth on that side is intact, but no mineralized bone is visible on the mesial side of that tooth. **C,** Radiograph of the mandible of a dog reveals an early malignant melanoma. There is lysis of bone and tooth root centered over the distal root of the fourth premolar tooth. **D,** Radiograph of a dog with bilateral fibrosarcomas affecting the bone mesial and medial to the canine teeth. The lamina dura has disappeared and is replaced by a widened space filled with neoplastic tissue that has fine lines of calcification arranged perpendicular to the long axis of the tooth.

dogs with malignant oral neoplasms, surgical removal or biopsy of regional lymph nodes is recommended for purposes of staging the disease. Necropsy results may represent a biased sample because they reflect animals with advanced disease or recurrence of disease; however, at autopsy, metastases to regional lymph nodes had occurred in 73% of dogs with squamous cell carcinoma, 60% of dogs with melanoma, and 19% of dogs with fibrosarcoma. Cytologic examination of lymph node aspirates, which may be adequate for diagnosing metastatic melanoma and squamous cell carcinoma, is less satisfactory for other oral neoplasms. Nodes with a positive test result for tumor can be treated with radiotherapy or radiotherapy and adjuvant chemotherapy; if radiotherapy is used, it may be possible to include the node in the primary treatment field and thus include lymphatics between the primary and the lymph node lesions.

▶ STAGING

The World Health Organization has formulated a tumor staging classification—primary tumor, regional nodes, metastasis (TNM)—for canine and feline tumors of the lips and oral cavity; stage grouping has been suggested for oral cavity tumors (see box on p. 302). In general, the prognosis after any type of treatment worsens significantly as the stage of the tumor increases from I to IV.

▶ TREATMENT PRINCIPLES

The management of oropharyngeal neoplasms depends on accurate diagnosis and staging of the disease and knowledge of (1) the biologic behavior of individual tumor types and (2) the advantages and limitations of available treatment modalities. There is no protocol available that is adequate for all tumors; therapy must be individualized. For oral malignancies, early treatment by the most radical treatment available is the key to the limited current success in the management of some oral tumors.

Surgery

Techniques for resection of oral tissues are described in detail in Chapter 10. Recommendations for surgical treatment of specific tumors are described in

the section on treatment of major tumor types.

If radical surgery has been used to treat an oral malignancy, the en-bloc surgical specimen is submitted for study with a request that the margins are to be examined for microscopic evidence of adequacy of resection.

Cryosurgery

After an initial burst of enthusiasm for cryosurgery in the 1970s, it now is clear that there is no particular advantage, and considerable disadvantage, to the use of cryosurgery for treatment of major oral tumors. The major disadvantages are as follows:

- The inability to control the extent of tissue destroyed
- The inability to reconstruct the oral tissues at the time of the initial procedure because of the need for the cryogen-destroyed tissue to necrose and separate
- The unpredictable complications, including secondary bleeding (bleeding after separation of the necrotic segment)

Cryosurgery may be of occasional minor value in painlessly destroying superficial pedunculated masses.

Electrosurgery

Use of the electroscalpel or electrocoagulation may reduce blood loss during major oral surgical procedures (see Chapter 10). Small pedunculated masses are readily resected with a needle or loop-tipped electroscalpel. Use of an electrosurgical instrument to destroy large oral tumors is inappropriate; the bony structure interferes with separation of the tissue at the time of electrodesiccation or fulguration, and the surrounding vascular structures are likely to be severely affected by extension of tissue heating. This can result in severe postoperative edema for several days, possibly with life-threatening airway obstruction after procedures in the caudal oral cavity.

Radiation Therapy and Hyperthermia

Treatment with orthovoltage or higher-energy radiation of oral tumors has been used for many years. In theory this should be an excellent way to treat rapidly growing oral malignancies; the treatment site is readily accessible, and rapidly growing cells with

World Health Organization Staging System for Tumors of the Oral Cavity

Feline or Canine Tumors of the Oral Cavity

The following classification applies to the rostral two thirds of the tongue, the floor of the mouth, the buccal mucosa, the gingival and alveolar bone, and the hard palate.

T—Primary tumor

Tis   Preinvasive carcinoma (carcinoma in situ)
T0   No visible primary tumor
T1   Tumor 2 cm or less maximum diameter
    a. without bone involvement
    b. with bone involvement
T2   Tumor 2-4 cm maximum diameter
    a. without bone involvement
    b. with bone involvement
T3   Tumor more than 4 cm maximum diameter
    a. without bone involvement
    b. with bone involvement

N—Regional lymph nodes

N0   Regional lymph nodes not palpable
N1   Movable ipsilateral nodes
    N1 (a) Nodes not considered to contain growth
    N1 (b) Nodes considered to contain growth
N2   Movable contralateral or bilateral nodes
    N2 (a) Nodes not considered to contain growth
    N2 (b) Nodes considered to contain growth
N3   Fixed nodes

M—Distant metastasis

M0   No evidence of distant metastases
M1   Distant metastases present—specify sites:

Stage grouping

I	T1	N0, N1 (a), or N2 (a)	M0
II	T2	N0, N1 (a), or N2 (a)	M0
III	T3	N0, N1 (a), or N2 (a)	
IV	Any T	N1 (b)	M0
	Any T	N2 (b) or N3	M0
	Any T	Any N	M1

From Owen LN: *TNM classification of tumors in domestic animals*, Geneva, 1980, World Health Organization.

a high metabolic activity should be maximally sensitive to the effects of the radiation. In fact, historical overall success in treating malignant lesions has been poor for most tumor types because of the following reasons:

- Rapidly growing tumors, such as malignant melanoma or squamous cell carcinoma, may outgrow their blood supply; thus areas of tumor with hypoxic cells may be immune to the effects of the radiation.
- The bones of the jaws and face are of varying thickness and cortical density; thus some areas of tumor are likely to be more protected than other areas because of their location within or behind bone. This factor may be of less concern if a high-energy radiation source (cobalt radiotherapy or linear accelerator unit) is available.
- Effects on adjacent tissues are significant. The skin within an orthovoltage radiation portal typically will lose hair, which will not regrow, and the lens of the eye will become opaque if it is not shielded. Thus the animal will look different and may be blind in one eye. Other effects seen after extensive radiation therapy in humans, such as keratoconjunctivitis sicca, xerostomia after scarring of salivary gland tissue, mucositis, or extensive periodontal disease and endodontic abscessing after osteoradionecrosis of alveolar bone may become important as survival times increase with improved techniques.
- Radiation therapy of benign lesions (such as acanthomatous epulis or eosinophilic granuloma) is successful in curing the initial lesion; however, there is an approximately one in five likelihood of development of a malignancy at the site of radiation months or years later.
- Limitations of anesthesia and equipment affect outcome. Better results may be obtainable with some tumor types by use of higher total dose or lower but more frequent per treatment dose.

Thus radiotherapy as the only treatment of oral malignancy is of moderate value at best. The beneficial effects of radiotherapy can be extended if it is combined with radiosensitizing drugs or hyperthermia as a way of increasing the susceptibility of the tumor cells to the radiation. The long-term value of combinations of drugs such as etanidazole or mitoxantrone

and radiation, particularly for squamous cell carcinoma in cats, is currently under active investigation.

An initial series of cases in dogs has shown that hyperthermia combined with radiation can produce long-term results similar to those after radical surgery but without the tissue loss that results from surgery. In this technique the tissue-heating mechanism must be carefully controlled. Hyperthermia can be used as the only means of tissue destruction; however, the extent and effects of treatment cannot be easily controlled, making it an impractical means of therapy in a practice situation.

Radiation therapy should be planned and conducted by a veterinary radiation oncologist or under the direct supervision of one.

Chemotherapy and Immunotherapy

Although chemotherapy or immunotherapy eventually may be a treatment of choice for certain tumors, no firm recommendation can be made regarding the use of these treatments at present because available data are insufficient or suggest inadequate results. The exception to this general statement is the use of radiation-sensitizing agents in combination with radiotherapy.

▶ PROGNOSIS

The prognosis for any malignant tumor in the oral cavity is poor. Nontonsillar squamous cell carcinomas have the best prognosis because they remain localized, with metastases developing late in the course of the disease. They are amenable to both surgery and radiation. Fibrosarcoma, although a localized disease, has a poorer prognosis. This reflects the local aggressiveness, radioresistance, and palatine location typical of this tumor, making surgical resection more difficult. Melanomas have the poorest prognosis, with less than 20% of patients surviving 1 year after surgical resection. Metastases from the primary tumor site and local recurrence are responsible for treatment failures.

More aggressive surgical procedures, in conjunction with aggressive radiotherapy, allow a better prognosis for animals with nontonsillar squamous cell carcinoma and fibrosarcoma. Chemotherapy, immunotherapy, and hyperthermia are areas that require further investigation through prospective studies.

Benign oropharyngeal tumors have a good prognosis. The prognosis for papillomatosis is excellent inasmuch as this tumor undergoes spontaneous remission or responds to simple surgical excision or cryosurgery. Epulides often are surgically controllable or curable with conservative surgical techniques. The exception is acanthomatous epulis, which typically requires radical surgery or radiotherapy. The prognosis for dental tumors is very good when aggressive surgery or irradiation, or both, are used. Failures result because of inadequate surgical resection.

► APPEARANCE, BIOLOGIC BEHAVIOR, AND TREATMENT OF MAJOR TUMOR TYPES

Malignant Melanoma in Dogs and Cats

Typically occurring in older dogs that have some oral pigmentation, malignant melanoma is the most common and most difficult oral malignancy to treat.

The lesion may be pigmented (see Figs. A-4, p. 50; and A-104, p. 77) or nonpigmented (amelanotic) although there is often a gray cast to amelanotic melanomas (see Fig. A-50, p. 61). These lesions grow very rapidly. The surface usually is ulcerated and protuberant, and often an overwhelming odor accompanies the lesion because of necrosis caused by the lesion outgrowing its blood supply. Typical locations are the gingivae (see Fig. A-50), palate (see Fig. A-104), dorsal surface of the tongue (see Fig. A-4), and mucosal surface of the lips. The mandibular lymph nodes often are involved, and lung metastasis is common at the time of diagnosis. The diagnostic microscopic feature is the presence of melanocytes. The only morphologic criterion that is useful for prognosis is the mitotic index; survival time after treatment is shorter if the mitotic index is more than 2.

Cure of this lesion by any treatment method is uncommon. Radical surgical treatment of small lesions (for example, en-bloc resection with 2 cm or greater margins) occasionally is successful. At best, surgery for larger lesions is palliative; it may eliminate or control the local disease but does not prevent growth of metastatic lesions (Table 9-3).

TABLE 9-3	Results after radical surgery alone for oral neoplasms in dogs and cats			
Tumor type	Mandible	Maxilla	Maxilla or mandible	Combined
Acanthomatous epulis (n = 131)	OYS = 100% (121) (two recurrences)	OYS = 100% (10)		OYS = 100% (131)
Squamous cell carcinoma (n = 84) (nontonsillar)	OYS = 91% (24) MST = 14 mo (30)	MST = 11 mo (11)	OYS = 84% (19)	OYS = 88% (43) MST = 13 mo (41)
Fibrosarcoma (n = 63)	OYS = 50% (19) MST = 14 mo (14)	MST = 9 mo (18)	OYS = 42% (12)	OYS = 47% (31) MST = 11 mo (32)
Malignant melanoma (n = 72)	OYS = 21% (37) MST = 9 mo (20)	MST = 9 mo (5)	OYS = 0% (10)	OYS = 17% (47) MST = 9 mo (25)
Osteosarcoma (n = 48)	OYS = 35% (20) MST = 10 mo (11)	MST = 13 mo (5)	OYS = 42% (12)	OYS = 38% (32) MST = 11 mo (16)

TOTAL NO. OF CASES = 398

Data from references at end of chapter.

OYS, one year survival; *MST,* mean survival time.

Data are shown as either OYS (%) or MST (in months) because data are not reported consistently; the figure shown in parentheses to the right of each entry is number of cases, with total number of cases for each tumor type shown as n = ___.

Radiation therapy and chemotherapy (for example, with cisplatin) have been used to attempt to control local or metastatic disease, with little documented beneficial effect to date. It is likely that improved results will be available for local control if a practical method can be found to give an increased tissue dose (about 800 Gy) per treatment episode because of the dose fractionation response of malignant melanoma.

Malignant melanoma is uncommon in cats.

Nontonsillar Squamous Cell Carcinoma in Dogs

Although nontonsillar squamous cell carcinoma typically is a disease of older animals, the age range is much wider than malignant melanoma, with occasional cases occurring in younger animals.

Bleeding from the mouth is a common clinical sign. The lesions most often are found on the gingivae (see Fig. A-49, p. 61) and less often on the mucosa of the lips and tongue (see Figs. A-3, p. 50; A-18, p. 54; A-33 and A-34, p. 57). (The tongue is a common site in cats; see p. 306). The lesion may be protuberant or ulcerated. The surface usually is regularly rough (like a cauliflower) and an even pink-red color. Bone invasion is common with gingival lesions. Lymph node metastasis is common later in the disease, and lung metastasis occurs but is less frequent and occurs later than with malignant melanoma. The aforementioned biologic behavior relates to gingival, buccal, and lingual squamous cell carcinomas. Tonsillar squamous cell carcinomas in dogs, which are much more frequently metastatic, are not considered further here because this discussion is limited to oral cavity lesions.

Microscopic features are ridges and nests of polyhedral squamous epithelial cells, with varying extents of invasion of connective tissue and bone. In dogs younger than 6 months of age at the time of diagnosis the histologic appearance is of papillary projections of squamous epithelium. A tumor of similar microscopic appearance in humans is caused by a papillomavirus; however, no evidence of canine oral papillomavirus infection could be found in affected tissues from three young dogs with papillary squamous cell carcinoma of the gingiva.

Treatment must be aggressive to have any likelihood of curing the animal. Radical surgery (minimally 1 cm margins in en-bloc resections) is the simplest alternative (see Figs. 10-59 and 10-67), providing 1-year survival of 80% or more in reported series (Table 9-3), usually because of metastatic disease. If an adequate margin cannot be planned because of the size or the location of the tumor, or both, the only other treatment likely to produce a satisfactory long-term result is enhanced radiation (radiation combined with hyperthermia).

In many cases squamous cell carcinoma that has invaded bone does not respond well to orthovoltage radiation therapy alone, probably a result of dose-distribution difficulties when a deep, wide area requires treatment rather than a shielding effect of the bone itself. Dogs with tumors located on the maxilla had a longer tumor-free interval (mean 12 months) compared with mandibular tumors (3 months); ros-

A 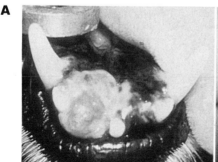 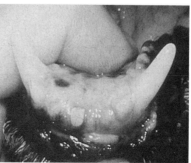 **B**

FIGURE 9-2
Squamous cell carcinoma of the rostral mandible of a dog. **A,** Before radiation treatment. **B,** At 4 months after treatment. *(Courtesy of Dr. S. Evans.)*

trally located tumors (Fig. 9-2) had a longer survival time (28 months) than dogs with caudally located tumors (10 months). Dogs younger than 6 years of age had a longer mean survival (39 months) than dogs older than 6 years (10 months).

Squamous Cell Carcinoma in Cats

Squamous cell carcinomas in cats occur in several sites: the lower premolar-molar gingiva, the upper premolar gingiva (see Figs. A-83 and A-84, p. 71), the tongue, and occasionally the lip (see Fig. A-35, p. 58). The tongue lesions occur most often in the ventral mass of the tongue caudal to the frenulum (see Figs. A-21 and A-22, p. 55); these lesions may not be visible externally but are readily palpable as firm masses.

Treatment of mandibular squamous cell carcinoma by hemimandibulectomy can be curative if the lesion is small (see Figs. 10-69 and 10-70) (Table 9-3). Maxillary and tongue lesions rarely respond well to treatment of any kind. Drug-enhanced radiation causes regression of some lingual squamous cell carcinomas (Fig. 9-3). In one study of 52 cats with oral squamous cell carcinoma treated by various combinations of surgery, radiation, chemotherapy, and hyperthermia, median survival was 2 months, and only two cats were alive longer than 1 year. Use of mitoxantrone and scattered-field radiation resulted in a median survival period of 180 days (1 year survival, 30%). In another study of six cats treated by surgery and radiation, the median survival period was 14 months (1 year survival, 66%).

Fibrosarcoma in Dogs and Cats

There are two age peaks for oral and maxillary fibrosarcoma in dogs. In smaller dogs they typically occur in older animals (8 + years), whereas in larger dogs (≥25 kg) the peak age is 4 to 5 years.

Fibrosarcoma may affect the dental margins and palate (see Figs. A-85, p. 71; and A-105, p. 77), appearing as protuberant, ulcerated lesions of variable surface coloration (although not gray or black except if a section of pigmented epithelium is distorted by an underlying tumor). It also may arise from the nasal cartilages, lateral surface of the maxilla, or palate and appear as a very slowly enlarging smooth mass cov-

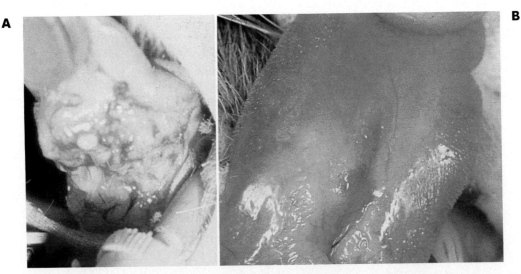

FIGURE 9-3
Squamous cell carcinoma of the ventral tongue of a cat. **A,** Before radiation and etanidazole treatment. (The rostral end of the tongue is retracted dorsally by a tongue forceps.) **B,** At 4 months after treatment. *(Courtesy of Dr. S. Evans.)*

ered by normal epithelium (see Figs. 10-61, 10-64, A-51, and A-52, p. 62).

Animals with ulcerated fibrosarcomas may be seen because of bleeding from the mouth or halitosis; however, many nonulcerated fibrosarcomas are seen because the owner felt a mass or noticed facial asymmetry. The characteristic microscopic pattern is of stubby, spindle-shaped cells, often arranged in sheets; edema or inflammatory reaction, particularly superficially, often occurs.

Of the three most common oral malignancies, fibrosarcomas are the least likely to metastasize. They are thus appropriate tumors to consider for aggressive local treatment. However, because the tumor typically infiltrates into adjacent tissue without a clearly demarcated boundary, it is very easy to undertreat. Radical surgery or hyperthermia-enhanced radiation therapy is the treatment of choice. The widest margins available (2 cm if practical) in that location is taken for surgical treatment (see Figs. 10-61 and 10-64); 1-year survival is reported in 40% to 50% (Table 9-3). In a group of 17 dogs with fibrosarcoma treated with orthovoltage radiation alone, 13 survived for 6 months or less, 2 for 9 months, and 2 for more than 1 year; long-term effects of the radiation were present in all of the dogs that survived the radiation treatment period. In five dogs treated by radiotherapy and hyperthermia, median survival time was 21 months.

Acanthomatous Epulis

Acanthomatous epulis is not a malignancy (epulis lesions as a group are benign); however, it behaves locally as a bone-invasive malignancy. Pathologists still debate the correct name for this lesion. The suggestion was made recently that it should be termed *basal cell carcinoma,* which is incorrect because it does not arise from skin. It also has been described as a peripheral ameloblastoma and some years ago was referred to as adamantinoma.

The clinical appearance is similar to a protuberant gingival squamous cell carcinoma: a rough surface of an even yellow-pink color (see Figs. 10-60, 10-65, and A-48, p. 61). The lesions arise from the periodontal tissue subgingivally, with branching sheets of epithelial cells that are large and polyhedral, with prominent intercellular bridges. There may be pe-

ripheral palisading similar to that of ameloblasts. The cells are not keratinized, and the basement membrane is smooth and intact. The most typical locations are the upper and lower incisive and canine teeth and the upper carnassial teeth.

It is an ideal tumor to treat because it does not metastasize and the borders are more clearly demarcated than those of fibrosarcoma. Treatment is surgery or radiation therapy. The latter is effective in preventing recurrence of the lesion and permits retention of bone and teeth in that location (Figs. 9-4, 9-5); however, a likelihood of about 1 in 5 exists for development of a malignancy (of several possible types) at the irradiated site months or years later. Radical surgery (see Figs. 10-60 and 10-65) is almost always curative (Table 9-3).

Fibrous-Osseous Epulides

Fibrous-osseous epulides manifest as firm, nonpainful masses covered by intact epithelium of normal color. They are most common on the rostral gingivae in medium- or large-size dogs (see Fig. A-54, p. 62). They may be pigmented if arising from pigmented epithelium (see Fig. A-55, p. 62). The major microscopic feature is the presence of subgingival stroma. The fibrous and osseous types are differentiated by the extent of osteoid matrix present. The differentiation between generalized gingival hyperplasia and fibrous epulis is not microscopically clear; clinical extent (localized mass or generalized periodontal tissue response) is the major differentiating feature. Gingival hyperplasia, which can be familial, is described in Chapter 4.

Treatment most often is not necessary. If these firm, nonulcerated masses interfere with function of the teeth or are abraded and bleed, they can be removed surgically. Electrosurgery is very useful. The lesion is removed down to the underlying bone, which is left bare of epithelium. If the adjacent tooth is left in place, there must be a collar of intact gingiva surrounding it (see Gingivoplasty, Chapter 4).

Osteosarcoma

Osteosarcoma affects the bone of the mandible (see Fig. A-53, p. 62) and, less often, the maxilla. It may manifest as a palpable mass or as an ulcerated lesion.

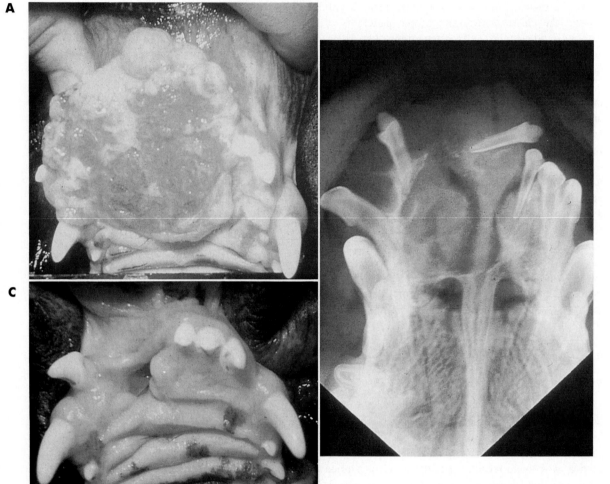

FIGURE 9-4
Large acanthomatous epulis of the premaxilla and palate of a dog. **A,** Before radiation treatment. **B,** Pretreatment radiograph demonstrates significant bone lysis and displacement of teeth. **C,** At 5 months after radiation treatment. A small oronasal fistula is present next to the incisive papilla. *(Courtesy of Dr. S. Evans.)*

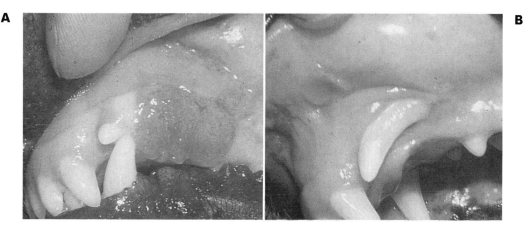

FIGURE 9-5
Acanthomatous epulis in an 8-month-old sheltie. **A,** Before radiation treatment. **B,** At 1
month after treatment. The dog has a rostrally displaced upper canine tooth, which is
common in this breed (see Chapter 8). *(Courtesy of Dr. S. Evans.)*

Often extensive radiographic evidence of bone invasion is apparent. Local lymph node and lung metastases are common, although less likely than for limb
osteosarcoma. Surgical treatment, performed early
and radically, can be curative in some cases (1-year
survival 30% to 40%; Table 9-3).

Lymphoid and Plasma Cell Tumors in the Oral Cavity

Microscopic accumulations of lymphoid or plasma
cells are common in oral tissues and usually are a
response to stimulation by oral flora. Larger, tumor-
like masses of lymphoid or plasma cells are less common but can occur anywhere in the mouth, typically
on the gingivae, buccal mucosa, soft palate, and pharynx. The external appearance is a flat or protuberant
pink mass with an even but roughened surface. Oral
lymphosarcoma most often is part of disseminated
lymphosarcoma; typically the skin lesions are the reason for veterinary examination, and the oral lesions
are a minor part of the clinical syndrome. The plasma
cell tumors generally are benign and nonfunctional;
surgical resection, including a margin of clinically
normal tissue, is curative (see Fig. 10-66). If the mass
is extensive or recurs after resection, radiation therapy
or chemotherapy by means of one of the systemic

lymphosarcoma or plasma cell tumor protocols is indicated. Metabolic abnormalities such as hypercal-
cemia, seen in association with lymphosarcoma or
plasmacytoma in other locations, are rare with oral
masses.

Tumors of the Tongue in Dogs

The tongue is a less common site for oral tumors
in dogs than in cats, although squamous cell carcinoma
also is the most common type. Of 57 canine lingual
cases in a multisite study, 21 were squamous cell
carcinoma (see Fig. A-3, p. 50), 7 were granular cell
myoblastoma, 7 malignant melanoma (see Fig. A-4,
p. 50), 5 mast cell tumor, and 17 were of 11 other
tumor types; 51% occurred on the dorsal surface. Four
of 16 (25%) dogs with squamous cell carcinoma were
alive at 12 months after treatment (surgery in two
cases, surgery and radiation in two other cases). Six
of seven granular cell myoblastoma cases showed local cure and no distant spread of the lesion after surgical treatment (median period 31 months). Surprisingly perhaps, all four dogs with malignant melanoma
treated surgically in this series were free of local disease (median period 22 months); however, only one
dog with mast cell tumor was free of local disease
after surgical treatment.

▶ **SUGGESTED READINGS**

Beck ER et al: Canine tongue tumors: a retrospective review of 57 cases, *JAAHA* 22:525, 1986.

Bostock DE, Curtis R: Comparison of canine oropharyngeal malignancy in various geographical locations, *Vet Rec* 114:341, 1984.

Bostock DE, White RAS: Classification and behavior after surgery of canine epulides, *J Comp Pathol* 97:197, 1987.

Bradley RL et al: Mandibular resection for removal of oral tumors in 30 dogs and 6 cats, *JAVMA* 184:460, 1984.

Bradley RL et al: Oral neoplasia in 15 dogs and four cats, *Vet Med Surg (Small Anim)* 1(1):33, 1986.

Brewer WG, Turrel JM: Radiotherapy and hyperthermia in the treatment of fibrosarcomas in dogs, *JAVMA* 181:146, 1982.

Brodey RS: A clinical and pathologic study of 130 neoplasms of the mouth and pharynx in the dog, *Am J Vet Res* 21:787, 1960.

Brodey RS: Alimentary tract neoplasms in the cat: a clinicopathologic survey of 46 cases, *Am J Vet Res* 27(116):74, 1966.

Brodey RS: The biological behaviour of canine oral and pharyngeal neoplasms, *J Small Anim Pract* 11:45, 1970.

Burstone MS et al: Familial gingival hypertrophy in the dog (boxer breed), *Arch Pathol* 54:208, 1952.

Clavieras J: A propos de deux cas de rage bovine, *Rev Med Vet* 111:800, 1960.

Cohen D et al: Epidemiologic aspects of oral and pharyngeal neoplasms of the dog, *Am J Vet Res* 25:1176, 1964.

Cotter S: Oral pharyngeal neoplasms in the cat, *JAAHA* 17:917, 1981.

DeMonbreun WA, Goodpasture W: Infectious oral papillomatosis of dogs, *Am J Pathol* 8:43, 1932.

Diamond SS et al: Multilobular osteosarcoma in the dog, *Vet Pathol* 17:759, 1980.

Dorn CR, Priester WA: Epidemiologic analysis of oral and pharyngeal cancer in dogs, cats, horses and cattle, *JAVMA* 169:1202, 1976.

Dubielzig RR: Proliferative dental and gingival diseases of dogs and cats, *JAAHA* 18:577, 1982.

Dubielzig RR et al: Inductive fibroameloblastoma, an unusual dental tumor in young cats, *JAVMA* 174:720, 1979.

Dubielzig RR et al: The nomenclature of periodontal epulides in dogs, *Vet Pathol* 16:209, 1979.

Emms S, Harvey CE: Preliminary results of maxillectomy in the dog and cat, *J Small Anim Pract* 27:291, 1986.

Evans SM, Shofer F: Canine oral nontonsillar squamous cell carcinoma: prognostic factors for recurrence and survival following orthovoltage radiation therapy, *Vet Radiol* 29(3):133, 1988.

Evans SM et al: Technique, pharmacokinetics, toxicity, and efficacy of intratumoral etanidazole and radiotherapy for treatment of spontaneous feline oral squamous cell carcinoma, *Int J Radiat Oncol Biol Phys* 20:703, 1991.

Gorlin RJ, Peterson WC: Oral disease in man and animals, *Arch Dermatol* 96:390, 1967.

Gorman NT et al: Chemotherapy of a recurrent acanthomatous epulis in a dog, *JAVMA* 184:1158, 1984.

Harvey HJ: Cryosurgery of oral tumors in dogs and cats, *Vet Clin North Am [Small Anim Pract]* 10:821, 1980.

Harvey HJ et al: Prognostic criteria for dogs with oral melanoma, *JAVMA* 178:580, 1981.

Harvey CE: Oral surgery: radical resection of maxillary and mandibular lesions, *Vet Clin North Am* 16:983, 1985.

Head KW: Tumours of the upper alimentary tract, *Bull WHO* 53:145, 1976.

Hoyt MRF, Withrow SJ: Oral malignancy in the dog, *JAAHA* 20:83, 1984.

Hutson C et al: Treatment of mandibular squamous cell carcinoma in 6 cats with surgical excision and radiation therapy, manuscript submitted for publication, 1990.

Kosovsky JK et al: Results of partial mandibulectomy for the treatment of oral tumors in 142 dogs, *Vet Surg* 20:397, 1991.

Langham RF et al: Oral adamantinomas in the dog, *JAVMA* 146:474, 1965.

Langham RF et al: X-ray therapy of selected odontogenic neoplasms in the dog, *JAVMA* 170:820, 1977.

LaRue SM et al: Shrinking-field therapy plus mitoxantrone for the treatment of oral squamous cell carcinoma in the cat, Proceedings of the ACVS, San Francisco, Oct 1991.

Lombard C: Contribution a létude des tumeurs des joues, des levres, de la langue et du maxillaire inferieur, chez les mammiferes domestiques, *Rev Med Vet* 111:783, 1960.

Ogilvie GK et al: Papillary squamous cell carcinoma in three young dogs, *JAVMA* 192:933, 1988.

Page R: Cisplatin, a new antineoplastic drug in veterinary medicine, *JAVMA* 186:288, 1985.

Penwick RC, Nunamaker DM: Rostral mandibulectomy: a treatment for oral neoplasia in the dog and cat, *JAAHA* 23:19, 1987.

Postorino NC et al: Feline oral squamous cell carcinoma: a retrospective study of 52 cats, *Vet Cancer Soc Newsletter* 12:6, 1988.

Preister WD, McKay FA: The occurrence of tumors in domestic animals, *Nat Cancer Inst Monogr* No. 54, 1980.

Salisbury KS, Lantz GC: Long-term results of partial mandibulectomy for treatment of oral tumors in the dog, *JAAHA* 24:2285, 1988.

Salisbury KS et al: Partial maxillectomy in the dog: comparison of suture materials and closure techniques, *Vet Surg* 14:265, 1985.

Salisbury KS et al: Partial maxillectomy and premaxillectomy in the treatment of oral neoplasia in the dog and cat, *Vet Surg* 15:16, 1986.

Shapiro W et al: Cisplatin for treatment of transitional and squamous cell carcinomas in dogs, *JAVMA* 193:1530, 1988.

Stebbins KE et al: Feline oral neoplasia: a ten year survey, *Vet Pathol* 26:121, 1989.

Thompson JM: Advances in the use of hyperthermia. In *Oncology*, vol 6, *Contemporary issues in small animal practice*, New York, 1986, Churchill Livingstone.

Thompson JM et al: Hyperthermia and radiation in the management of canine tumours, *J Small Anim Pract* 28:457, 1987.

Thrall DE: Orthovoltage radiotherapy of oral fibrosarcomas in dogs, *JAVMA* 179:159, 1981.

Thrall DE et al: Malignant tumor formation at the site of previously irradiated acanthomatous epulides in four dogs, *JAVMA* 178:127, 1981.

Todoroff RJ, Brodey RS: Oral and pharyngeal neoplasia in the dog: a retrospective survey of 361 cases, *JAVMA* 175:567, 1979.

Vernon FF, Helphrey M: Rostral mandibulectomy, three case reports in dogs, *Vet Surg* 12:26, 1983.

White RAS: Wide local excision of acanthomatous epulides in the dog, *Vet Surg* 18:12, 1989.

White RAS: Mandibulectomy and maxillectomy in the dog: long-term survival in 100 cases, *J Small Anim Pract* 32:69, 1991.

White RAS et al: Clinical staging for oropharyngeal malignancies in the dog, *J Small Anim Pract* 26:581, 1985.

White RAS et al: The surgical management of bone-involved oral tumours in the dog, *J Small Anim Pract* 26:693, 1985.

White RAS et al: Sarcoma development following irradiation of acanthomatous epulis in two dogs, *Vet Rec* 118:668, 1986.

Withrow SJ, Holmberg DL: Mandibulectomy in the treatment of oral cancer, *JAAHA* 19:273, 1983.

Withrow SJ et al: Premaxillectomy in the dog, *JAAHA* 21:49, 1985.

10

Oral Surgery

Oral surgical procedures are performed very commonly: tooth extraction is probably the single most common surgical procedure in small animal practice. Some of these procedures are considered minor; however, complications do occur. By appropriate and careful use of techniques, these procedures can be performed with more control, less trauma to the patient, faster recovery and healing, and more dependable long-term results. Major procedures are practical, with excellent functional long-term results if the procedure is selected with full knowledge of the condition under treatment and the requirements and limitations of the procedure.

The oral surgeon is fortunate to work with tissues that have an abundant blood supply and an epithelial surface constantly bathed by saliva, a fluid rich in antimicrobial properties. The result is that healing of incisional wounds in oral mucosa is more rapid than for skin: phagocytic activity is greater, occurs earlier, and is due mostly to monocytes rather than polymorphonuclear leukocytes; epithelial migration occurs earlier; and epithelialization is completed earlier. The higher metabolic activity and higher mitotic rate of oral mucosa are believed to be responsible for these differences and may be due to the richer blood supply and higher temperatures of oral mucosa. Although the oral surfaces cannot be prepared before surgery with the same attention to detail available for skin preparation, and postoperative cleanliness by isolating the

affected area is impractical, infections after oral surgical procedures are rare.

In a study of sutures used in the oral tissues of normal dogs, monofilament nylon was found to cause the least reaction, polyglycolic acid and surgical gut were found to cause a mild to moderate reaction, and silk was found to cause the most severe tissue response. In another study, however, silk and Mersilene (Dacron) sutures caused a similar moderate leukocytic infiltration, and surgical gut caused a significantly greater cellular response. Most sutures with knots on the mucosal surface, whether absorbable or nonabsorbable, are sloughed within 2 to 4 weeks. Synthetic absorbable sutures appear to remain in place somewhat longer than surgical gut, they do not interfere with healing any more than do nonabsorbable sutures, and they do not require removal; they are the suture of choice for routine use during oral surgical procedures. A vertical mattress pattern ensures some contact between connective tissue surfaces as well as epithelial apposition; this technique is particularly recommended for use when the suture line will not be supported by underlying tissue, as in some palate or maxillectomy reconstruction procedures.

Wire is not recommended for use in the mouth because the small diameter of wire, compared with other suture materials, causes the sutures to saw through the tissue more readily. In addition, wire does not prevent tongue movements, and it causes lacerations in the tongue from licking. Preventing damage to oral suture lines is best achieved by attention to suture technique in providing apposition of tissues without tension or excessive tightness of sutures. In the occasional case in which glossal or pharyngeal muscle activity is particularly likely to cause breakdown of the suture line, a temporary acrylic obturator can be cemented or wired to the teeth to protect the healing tissues. Pharyngostomy or gastrostomy tubes have been recommended as a means of reducing tension on oral or pharyngeal suture lines; however, documentation of a beneficial or protective effect is not available, and esophagitis from pharyngostomy intubation may result. Unless there is some other medical reason for medium-term nutritional support (inability to swallow because of severe pharyngeal muscle trauma, for instance), tube feeding is not necessary. Gastrostomy rather than pharyngostomy intubation is preferred.

Temporary occlusion of both carotid arteries through an incision in the neck should be considered if extensive surgery is likely, particularly in an animal in poor condition or anemic because of blood loss from an oral lesion.

In this chapter, indications, techniques, complications, and prognosis are described for extractions, oral trauma, and palatal and oronasal defects. Resection of neoplasms and mass lesions is described; long-term results are described in Table 9-3. Periodontal surgery is discussed in Chapter 4, and flaps for surgical endodontic techniques in Chapter 6.

▶ TEETH EXTRACTION

Extraction, in a way, is a dentist's admission of defeat. Many owners are not willing or able to provide the frequent oral care and checkup examinations required for optimal oral health in their companion animals, and animals require anesthesia for even the most routine dental procedure. Therefore veterinary dentists must, on the one hand, carefully evaluate the balance between the need for a permanent and reliable means of treatment and, on the other, consider professional options and the owner's esthetic preferences. In some cases these considerations mandate extraction as the treatment of choice.

The most common indication for teeth extraction in dogs and cats is periodontal disease or other oral inflammatory diseases; the teeth may already be loose or their stability may be threatened by significant bone loss in animals whose follow-up oral hygiene care is likely to be ineffective (see Chapters 4 and 5). Extraction of severely crowded or rotated teeth can reduce the likelihood that periodontal disease will lead to loss of the remaining teeth. Other indications for extraction are fractured teeth that are causing the animal pain or have resulted in an apical abscess and for which endodontic treatment is inappropriate or is declined by the owner; teeth that are preventing normal occlusion (see Chapter 8 for discussion of alternatives to extraction for malocclusion); dental caries (see Chapter 7 for restorative treatment options); carnassial abscess (endodontic treatment is described in Chapter 6); and external odontoclastic resorption lesions in cats (see Chapter 7 for description and discussion of restorative options).

Techniques
Permanent teeth

No matter what specific technique is used, two principles apply. First, before any leverage is applied, the soft tissue attachment between the gingiva and the tooth is incised by running a scalpel blade or sharp-edged luxator around the inside edge of the gingival margin (Fig. 10-1). This prevents subsequent tearing of the gingiva during root elevation. Second, at all times during active instrumentation, the fingers or palm, or both, of the noninstrument hand are used to provide support to the jaw; this is particularly necessary to reduce the likelihood of fracture of the jaw (Fig. 10-2) in cats, small dogs, or any animal with extensive periodontal or endodontic bone resorption.

Generally, the tooth is loosened with a root elevator, or a wedge leverage is applied, or both. The root elevator should be narrower than the root and sharp at its tip. Root elevators are available in several sizes (see Chapter 11). Most are made of hard steel and have relatively thick blades (see p. 399). Another type of instrument, known as a *dental root luxator,* has a blade made of softer steel and is designed to be resharpened frequently (see p. 399). This instrument is designed to cut its way through the periodontal

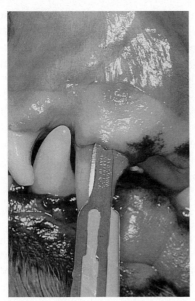

FIGURE 10-1
A scalpel blade is used to sever the soft tissue attachment around the neck of the tooth as the first step in extraction.

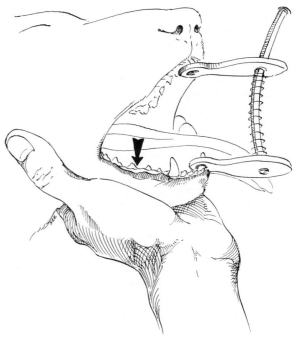

FIGURE 10-2
The palm of the noninstrument hand is used to support the jaw when force is applied to a tooth during extraction.

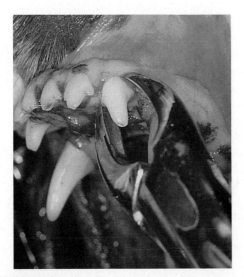

FIGURE 10-3
Dental extraction forceps applied on a tooth. The fit is poor in many cases.

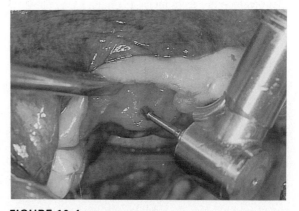

FIGURE 10-4
Alveoloplasty. Rough edges of alveolar ridge after extraction are burred smooth.

fibers but, for large teeth, is too soft to provide the wedging force used in the leverage technique without bending. Ideally both root elevators and root luxators should be available. Elevators with offset jaws (see p. 399) are useful for reaching caudal teeth, which often have serrated sides that act as saws when side-to-side motion is applied to the elevator.

Rarely does the dental extraction forceps fit the neck of a canine or feline tooth accurately (Fig. 10-3), and use of forceps alone (or prematurely) often will fracture the tooth. Thus dental extraction forceps are the final instrument used, and they are placed on the tooth only when it has already been loosened significantly. After extraction the alveolus is flushed free of debris and chips of calculus, bone, or root. Narrow ridges or prominences of alveolar bone are burred smooth (aveoloplasty; Fig. 10-4) and the alveolus is again flushed. The soft tissue is allowed to conform to the surface of the jaw. Some oral surgeons prefer to suture the soft tissues over the empty alveolus (Fig. 10-5), but generally this is not necessary unless the entire attached gingiva was deliberately or accidentally dissected free; this approach should not be taken if the tissues will be under tension after suturing.

Single root teeth

For a single root tooth, the surgeon inserts the root elevator between the gingival margin and the crown or exposed root, applying pressure while rotating the elevator through a small arc. At the end of each rotation, the instrument is held firmly against the tissues for a second or two and kept at about a 10- to 20-degree angle to the long axis of the root to avoid its slipping and injuring the gingiva or adjacent tissues (Fig. 10-6, A). A finger extended along the blade of the elevator acts as a stop should the instrument slip (Fig. 10-6, B).

The root elevator is used against all available surfaces of the root until the tooth begins to loosen. Typically the mesial and distal areas provide better "hold" for the elevator, and, in multirooted teeth the furcation area is useful also as an area where slippage is less likely to occur as force is applied.

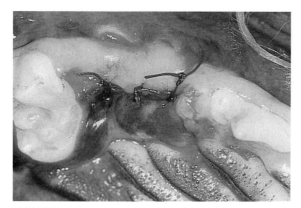

FIGURE 10-5
Gingival tissue sutured over the alveolus after extraction.

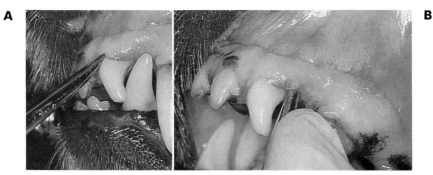

FIGURE 10-6
A, Angulation of a root elevator to maintain position between the tooth and alveolar bone. **B,** A finger is extended along the elevator to prevent trauma should the instrument slip.

Canine teeth

Canine teeth have massive roots. In large dogs it is best to incise and reflect the mucoperiosteum on the lateral surface of the tooth and then resect the alveolar bone overlying the root. The mucosal incision is best made well away from the root so that the suture line will not be directly over the resulting void (Fig.

10-7, *A*). On the upper jaw the incision is made caudally, avoiding the infraorbital/lateral nasal vessels dorsally; on the lower jaw the flap incision can be made rostrally to avoid the mental artery and attachments of the frenulum. The gingival and subgingival tissue is reflected with a sharp periosteal elevator. If a bur is used (round bur, No. 1 or No. 2, or pear-

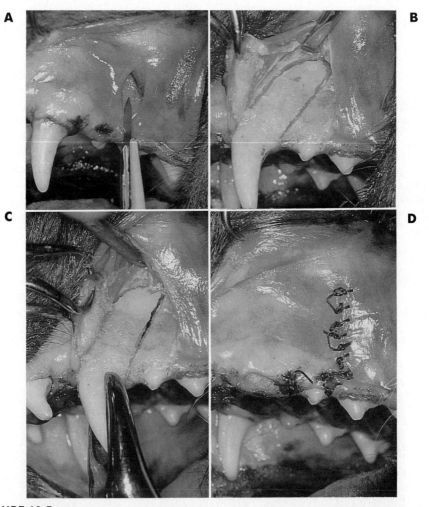

FIGURE 10-7

A, Incision for flap surgery—bone removal technique for extraction of a canine tooth; the incision is made distal to the bony juga of the root. **B,** With use of a dental bur, a channel is cut in the bone overlying the root. **C,** A dental extraction forceps is applied to the tooth and rotated. **D,** The flap incision is closed with simple interrupted sutures.

shaped bur, No. 330 or No. 331), a channel is cut full thickness through the lateral alveolar plate in a U or V along the mesial and distal margins of the root from the attachment level to the apex of the palpable juga over the root (Fig. 10-7, *B*). The tissues must be cooled with a water spray. Alternatively, a bone chisel can be used to chip away the bone overlying the root. The mesial and distal surfaces of the root are loosened with a root elevator. Once the tooth starts to move relative to the jaw, the tooth is grasped with extraction forceps and twisted until resistance is felt, then held for a few seconds (Fig. 10-7, *C*). This movement is alternated in both directions until the tooth can be lifted out. After alveoloplasty, if necessary, and flushing the alveolus, the gingival flap is sutured with simple interrupted absorbable sutures (Fig. 10-7, *D*). Digital pressure is used for several seconds to adapt the gingiva to the underlying bone, lessening the likelihood of detachment of the flap.

In narrow-nosed dogs with extensive periodontal disease, in whom the risk of creating an oronasal fistula after canine tooth extraction is greatest, damage to any remaining bone palatal to the root must be avoided. During the use of forceps, the crown of the tooth should not be levered buccally because this movement pushes the tip of the root palatally into the nasal cavity. If penetration into the nasal cavity is obvious at the time of the extraction procedure (from observing hemorrhage or emergence of flushing solution from the nostril), the alveolus and fistula are first flushed thoroughly with chlorhexidine solution. The operator then attempts to prevent formation of a permanent fistula by placing absorbable sutures through the buccal and palatal gingivae, apposing the two edges to collapse the soft tissues. The alveolus can be packed loosely with a shaped cube or granules of polylactic acid (Fig. 10-8), which will retain a blood clot within the alveolus and encourage granulation tissue formation. If the tissue edges do not meet except under tension, the edges of the alveolar bone can be crushed with the fingers or a buccal-based flap created (see p. 345) and sutured over the defect. If an oronasal fistula does form and causes nasal discharge or difficulties during eating, treatment is closure of the fistula by a single or double flap procedure (see p. 345).

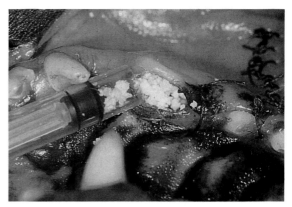

FIGURE 10-8
Granules of polylactic acid are placed in the alveolus to promote formation and retention of a blood clot and to prevent fistula formation.

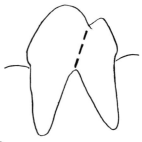

FIGURE 10-9
Separation of a multirooted tooth into single root sections to facilitate extraction.

Multirooted teeth

Multirooted teeth can be removed as one unit by loosening the roots with a root elevator before applying extraction forceps; however, this approach is hard work, and it is much easier to extract the tooth if it is first separated into single root sections (Fig. 10-9). The best implement with which to cut the tooth is a cross-cut fissure bur (Nos. 700, 701, 702, or 703, depending on size of the tooth) inasmuch as this creates a channel that is the correct width for starting the next step, the wedging process. A diamond disk or even a hacksaw blade can be used, but the risk of

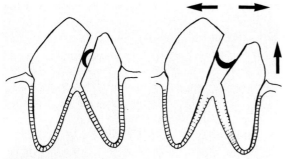

FIGURE 10-10
Rotation of a root elevator horizontally between root sections permits application of distraction and lifting force.

damaging adjacent bone and soft tissue is higher. Each single root section is levered against the other section(s) and then forcefully rotated individually. For wedge leverage to be successful, the root elevator or other wedging instrument must be applied by twisting or levering between the sections of the tooth until firm resistance to further distraction is felt. After it is held in that position for several seconds so that the periodontal fibers are stretched and torn, it is twisted the other way and again held under tension. By inserting the wedging elevator between the teeth horizontally (perpendicular to the long axis of the tooth), one root section is elevated as the elevator is rotated, greatly assisting the periodontal fiber-tearing process (Fig. 10-10). This back-and-forth twisting and holding action is continued until one of the root sections loosens. Then the surgeon applies the extraction forceps and continues the twist-and-hold sequence until that section can be lifted out.

Often the second tooth section is still rather firmly attached. The root elevator is applied between the tooth and an adjacent tooth if available and rotated outward toward the remaining section—not against the adjacent tooth unless it also is to be extracted. Then the operator applies the extraction forceps and uses the same twist-and-hold action until the remaining section can be lifted out. If little space exists between the tooth to be extracted and the adjacent tooth, the cross-cut bur can be used to cut a groove in the tooth to be extracted which will facilitate place-

ment of the elevator during the wedging process, with care taken to avoid damage to the tooth that will be retained.

Patience is the key; applying excessive torque or failing to hold the tension for a period of time and rapidly reapplying force will cause the tooth crown to crack off.

Two-rooted teeth. In the dog, these are the upper second and third premolar teeth and all of the lower premolar and molar teeth except the first premolar; in the cat, they are the upper third premolar and all of the lower premolar and molar teeth. The surgeon starts from the furcation (the area where the roots join to form the crown) and separates the tooth into mesial and distal sections. If necessary, a root elevator or periosteal elevator is used to reflect the gingiva and expose the furcation. The root elevator is inserted into the channel between the sections, and leverage force is applied as already described.

Three-rooted teeth. These are the upper fourth premolar and the first and second molars in the dog, and the upper fourth premolar in the cat. Three-rooted teeth can be removed as easily as two-rooted teeth by initial sectioning into a two-root and a one-root segment. The segment with the smallest root is separated from the main part of the tooth; then that section is levered against the rest of the tooth. Alternatively, for the carnassial tooth that has a very small palatal root, the palatal root is extracted by burring with a high-speed, water-cooled round (size 1 or 2) or pear-shaped (size 331L) bur. Once the smallest root is extracted, the two larger roots are dealt with as for a two-rooted tooth.

Deciduous teeth

When the developing bud of the permanent tooth is not in direct alignment with the root of the deciduous tooth, the deciduous root resorption process does not proceed normally as the permanent tooth develops. The permanent tooth may develop in abnormal position, and correction may require extraction of the deciduous tooth (see Chapter 8). Deciduous and permanent versions of the same tooth should not be in erupted position in the mouth at the same time. Deciduous teeth sometimes are easier to extract than permanent teeth because part of the root has been

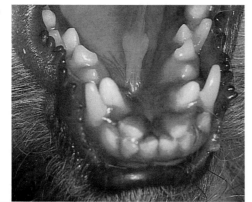

resorbed, but this is not always the case, and the unresorbed roots of the deciduous canine and incisor teeth are long (Fig. 10-11).

The danger in extracting deciduous teeth is that the developing permanent tooth may be damaged if the extraction instruments penetrate too deeply at the wrong angle. Thus extraction of deciduous teeth requires particular care and patience. Gradual work with the root elevator, with the tip constantly directed so that it is working against the root of the deciduous tooth (Fig. 10-12), is preferred to surgical extraction by exposing and removing bone, although this latter

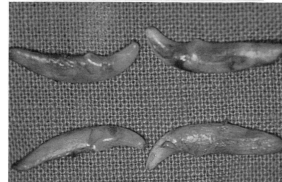

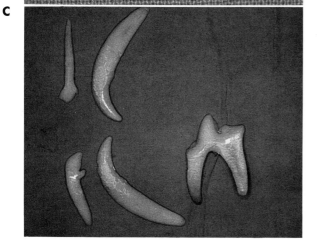

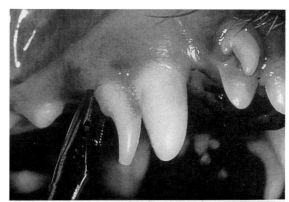

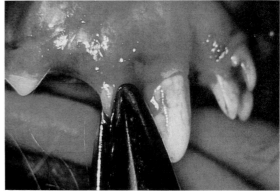

FIGURE 10-11
A, Retained deciduous incisor and canine teeth in a toy breed dog. **B,** The retained deciduous teeth following extraction. **C,** Retained deciduous teeth with very long roots from another toy breed dog.

FIGURE 10-12
Retained deciduous canine tooth extraction. **A,** The root elevator is directed against the deciduous root without levering against the permanent canine. **B,** When the tooth is loose, dental extraction forceps are applied to deliver the tooth.

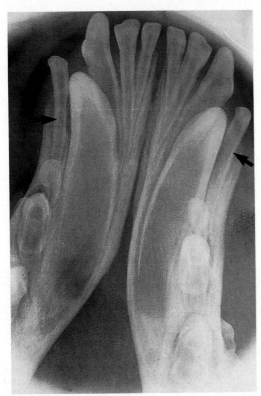

FIGURE 10-13
Radiograph of a dog with retained deciduous canine teeth *(arrows).*

technique occasionally is necessary to gain access to a fractured root segment of significant length. The temptation to lever against the canine tooth should be avoided. The crown may look very substantial, but the foundation, the root, is very vulnerable at this age. A radiograph is useful to determine the length and direction of root of the retained tooth (Fig. 10-13).

Tooth extraction in cats

Tooth extraction in cats is performed in similar fashion as for dogs, although it must be kept in mind that the skull of the cat is smaller and more fragile than that of dogs, and the teeth of cats are narrower and smaller than those of a dog of similar body weight. They tend to fracture if extraction forces are misapplied. The narrow, small mandible must be protected from fracture by gentle careful technique. The tooth sectioning and leverage technique can be used (Fig. 10-14, *A*), but the crown sections are more likely to fracture unless the force is applied very gradually. Root elevators are often too large for convenient use in cats; a No. 11 straight-edge scalpel blade mounted on a scalpel handle makes a convenient root elevator to start the process; a small root elevator (for example, No. 301) is inserted after the scalpel blade has formed an initial channel between root and bone. Thereafter, elevation and wedge pressure techniques are as for dogs.

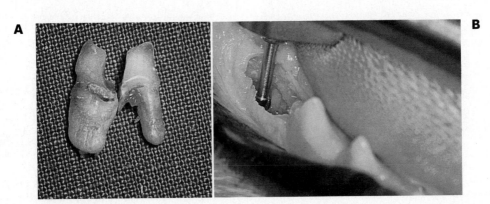

FIGURE 10-14
A, Transected and extracted lower first molar tooth in a cat. **B,** A dental bur is used to cut away root tissue—one method of extracting teeth of cats.

An alternative technique is to use a round dental bur (such as No. 331L) in a dental handpiece to cut away all of the root tissue (Fig. 10-14, *B*). With use of a high-speed handpiece the process is very quick, and the cooling water jet keeps the field clear of blood and root fragments. With this technique it is helpful if a radiograph is available to determine the length of the root to be extracted. Because of the difference in density between dentine and bone, the bur causes frequent skittering noises when root tissue is still present. A bur slightly smaller than the diameter of the root can be circled around the alveolus as it cuts away the root, or a bur slightly larger than the root is kept centered directly over the root.

After extraction, narrow ridges of alveolar bone are burred smooth, and the soft tissue is allowed to conform to the surface of the jaw. There is rarely sufficient tissue for placement of sutures after extractions in cats.

Complications
Hemorrhage

Packing the empty alveolus with gauze for a few minutes is sufficient to arrest bleeding in most cases. Some bleeding often is evident for a day or two after extraction, although this rarely is clinically significant. Packing the alveolus with polylactic acid granules or tetracycline powder will help to retain a blood clot, speed granulation, and prevent dry socket formation, although clinical evidence of poor alveolar healing after extraction rarely occurs in dogs and cats.

Fractured root

Fracture of a root with retention of the tip is common, particularly if excessive force is applied before the periodontal fibers have been loosened sufficiently (Fig. 10-15). A cracking sound may be obvious, or a sharp edge will be palpated at the end of the coronal segment. Root tips that contain necrotic pulp or are surrounded by deep periodontal pockets will cause bone lysis and subsequent fistula or abscess formation; they should be removed to prevent these unwanted sequelae. Removal of fractured root tips is achieved by one of two methods. Either a root-tip pick or narrow-bladed root elevator is inserted into the alveolus and levered between the root and alveolar bone progressively until the tip is loose and extracted, or a dental bur in a handpiece is used to cut away the remaining tooth root structure, as already described for cat tooth extractions. Occasionally, a root tip will be dislodged into the mandibular canal or into the nasal cavity (Fig. 10-15, *B* and *C*); removal may require burring away interradicular or cortical bone to enlarge the working space.

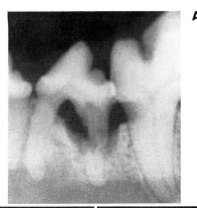

A

B

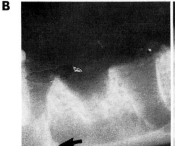

C

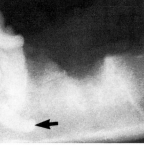

FIGURE 10-15
A, Oblique bone loss and fracture of the distal root of the lower fourth premolar is treated by extraction. **B** and **C,** Fractured mesial root tip *(arrow)* has been pushed into the medullary canal of the mandible.

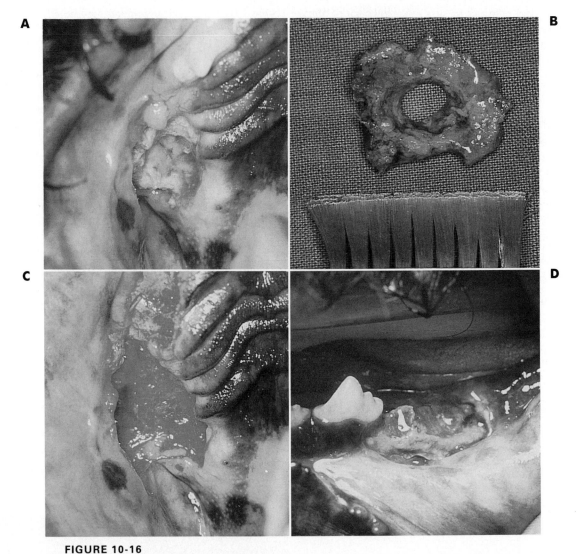

FIGURE 10-16
A, Necrotic segment of maxillary bone after tooth extraction. **B,** The necrotic segment is resected. **C,** The wound is cureted and left open to granulate. **D,** Necrotic segment of mandible following extraction.

Mandibular fracture

Fracture of the mandible is avoided by careful extraction technique. Remember that dogs with the highest risk of fracture of the jaw during tooth extraction (small dogs with extensive periodontitis) also are those with the least desirable conditions for fracture healing. Management of fractured mandible in dogs with extensive periodontal disease is described on p. 333.

Extended infection

Infections in the deeper soft tissues, such as the orbital or intermandibular areas, are seen occasionally as a result of contamination from inadvertent penetration of the elevator into these areas. Treatment is drainage of the abscess that results.

Local bone necrosis

Necrosis of bone around the extraction site occurs occasionally, particularly if the extraction procedure was excessively traumatic or caused loss of vascular supply to a segment of alveolar bone (Fig. 10-16, *A* and *D*). Conservative treatment is unlikely to be effective. Surgical treatment consists of removal of the affected bone with a curet or rongeur until healthy bleeding bone is reached (Fig. 10-16, *B*). The surgical site is left uncovered (Fig. 10-16, *C*). Management of extensive maxillary or mandibular osteomyelitis is described on p. 372.

Oronasal fistula

If the nasal cavity has been penetrated during extraction, one or two absorbable sutures are used to appose the gingival tissues to prevent formation of an oronasal fistula (see also p. 317). Management of a healed oronasal fistula is described on pp. 345-347.

▶ TRAUMA TO ORAL STRUCTURES
Jaw Fractures

Jaw fractures are common in dogs and cats. They result from external trauma (typically automobile accidents, jumping into a swung baseball bat, or, in cats, falling from a height) or from periodontitis or neoplasia predisposing the animal to pathologic fracture. Most fractures in dogs affect the mandibular body. In cats the most common site of fracture is the symphyseal area.

Animals with mandibular fractures are seen for treatment because of pain, bleeding from the mouth, unwillingness or inability to close the jaws, or obvious malocclusion. Maxillary fractures are less common; clinical signs are epistaxis, sensitivity to the side of the face, malocclusion, and bleeding from the mouth. Associated soft tissue injury may result in inability to swallow or airway obstruction.

After emergency treatment of airway obstruction and hemorrhage, the priorities for management of mandibular fractures and maxillary fractures are, first, to restore the animal's ability to use its tongue and close its jaws sufficiently for swallowing to occur; second, to restore the ability to completely close its jaws in a comfortable position; and third, to restore normal occlusion.

Diagnosis is made from physical examination by inspection of occlusion and gentle manipulation. The fracture may be sufficiently painful that a full examination requires sedation or anesthesia.

Classification and Treatment Planning

Many fractures of the mandible and maxilla do not need surgical fixation, particularly those in which the fracture lines are contained within the areas of attachment of the masticatory muscles, inasmuch as these muscles effectively splint the fracture during healing. If the fracture causes malocclusion, the aim of treatment is to restore normal or near normal occlusion during the healing process. Even for mandibular body fractures, the most common location in dogs, a tape around the muzzle for 3 to 4 weeks often is sufficient if the jaws are in normal occlusion.

Mandibular fractures are classified in several ways: open/closed (almost invariably open, because there is so little soft tissue coverage of attached gingiva over the dorsal part of the mandible); simple/fragmented but without loss of mandibular length/comminuted, with collapse and loss of mandibular length; anatomic location (symphysis, body, ramus); direction of fracture line relative to muscular pull; occlusion; and quality and vascularity of bone present. Additional considerations regard the presence of teeth in the fracture line, as well as the anatomy of the mandible relative to use of specific fixation devices. Attention to each of these factors influences the decision concerning which treatment technique is most appropriate.

Mandibular Fractures
Traumatic symphyseal separation

Symphyseal separations that result in instability of the two sides of the mandible relative to each other—but without malocclusion and with healthy mandibular bone—heal readily after placement of an encircling wire if there is not other orthopedic injury (Fig. 10-17). This is the most common oral injury in cats. Sufficient fixation can be obtained by wiring the two sides together caudal to the canine teeth with use of a hypodermic needle or suture passer to feed the wire subcutaneously. The fixation device usually can be removed in 2 to 3 weeks.

If the fracture is comminuted, symphyseal collapse and distortion of the angle of the canine teeth may occur; a single wire may cause the canine teeth to collapse medially, resulting in malocclusion. Normal occlusion can be obtained by a combination of circummandibular and figure-of-8 wiring around the canine teeth, tightening one or other of the wires further as necessary to achieve normal canine tooth divergence, or an acrylic splint can be placed, incorporating the wire or attached to the canine teeth (Fig. 10-18) by means of the acid-etch technique (see p. 237).

If the rostral end of the mandible is severely comminuted but the canine teeth and immediately surrounding bone are intact, normal occlusion can be maintained during the 2 to 4 weeks necessary for the healing process by cementing the upper and lower canine teeth to each other with acid-etched composite resin or acrylic splints (Fig. 10-19). The cat can be fed by gastrostomy or pharyngostomy tube or by introducing fluid food into the cheek pouch while the device is in place. Once a stable fibrous union has occurred, the devices are removed and the surfaces of the teeth are restored. There is a risk of aspiration if the animal vomits while the device is in place.

Fractures of the vertical ramus

Vertical ramus (coronoid and condylar process) fractures rarely result in significant malocclusion and are best managed conservatively (tape muzzle and soft-food diet for 2 to 4 weeks). If significant malocclusion is present, a temporomandibular joint luxation or fracture-luxation is suspected (see p. 374). The muscular attachments and dental occlusion generally maintain adequate apposition of fractured fragments during healing, and the surgical approach for potential internal fixation is likely to be traumatic and fixation difficult to achieve.

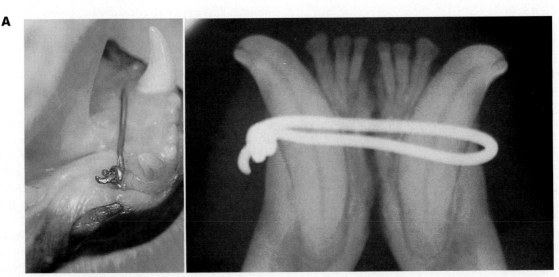

FIGURE 10-17
A and **B**, Mandibular symphyseal separation in a cat treated with an encircling wire.

Complications of fractures of the vertical ramus are temporomandibular joint disease causing continuing pain on opening and closing the mouth, which is treated by condylectomy (see p. 376), and excessive callus production (Fig. 10-20). The latter is more likely with a fragmented fracture in an animal that has yet to complete its growth (up to 18 to 24 months of age for the mandible in some giant-breed dogs) because limitations of space between the temporal bone and zygomatic arch may prevent the animal from opening its mouth. This complication is treated by resection of the coronoid process and callus (see p. 366).

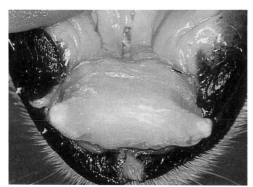

FIGURE 10-18
Management of a comminuted rostral mandibular fracture with circummandibular wire and acrylic splint to maintain correct separation and angulation of the canine teeth.

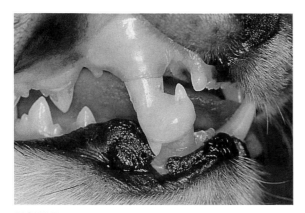

FIGURE 10-19
Management of a severely comminuted rostral mandibular fracture with a composite splint between the upper and lower canine teeth.

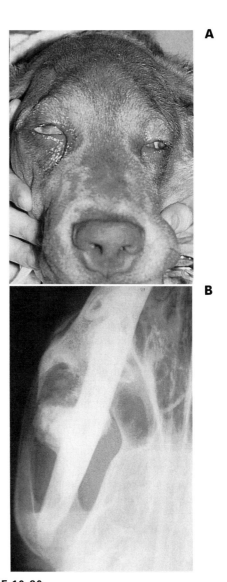

FIGURE 10-20
A and **B**, Fracture of the coronoid process of the mandible in a young dog that has resulted in a large callus, causing exophthalmos and preventing normal opening of the mouth.

Fractures of the body of the mandible

Fractures of the midpart of the mandibular body can be managed by applying a loose muzzle for 2 to 3 weeks if the canine teeth are able to occlude normally when the animal's mouth is gently closed.

Even in cats and small dogs the mandible is thick enough to accommodate simple osseous wires, cross pins and wires, plates and screws, and intramedullary pins; their placement, however, depends on the viability of the bone, as well as stability of the fracture. These orthopedic techniques are more involved and perhaps more time-consuming than use of a simple muzzle or alternative techniques in which the teeth are used as fixation points, such as with dental wire and acrylic splint. The upper and lower teeth can be wired together on one or both sides to retain normal occlusion in animals with combined mandibular-maxillary fractures; however, feeding into the cheek pouch or through a gastrostomy or pharyngostomy tube will be necessary for the 3- to 4-week period during which the device is in place.

Dental or surgical fixation generally is indicated if the fractured ends are distracted by muscular pull or if fracture fragmentation or tissue loss has occurred. In dogs, dental fixation generally is recommended for fractures rostral to the third premolar tooth and surgical fixation for fractures caudal to the third premolar tooth. In cats, fractures of the body of the mandible caudal to the canine teeth are not appropriate for dental fixation; however, such fractures are uncommon in cats. Each of these above techniques is described later in this chapter.

Effect of muscular pull

The mandibular insertions of the masticatory muscles are located at the caudal end of the body of the mandible. The effect of temporal/pterygoid/masseter contraction is to swing the mandible dorsally. The dorsal surface of the mandible can be considered the "tension" side and the ventral surface the "compression" side.

A complete mandibular body fracture that is oblique ventrorostrally will tend to remain apposed as a result of muscular pull ("favorable fracture," Fig. 10-21, *A*) and usually will heal well with minimal fixation (such as tape muzzle). A complete mandibular

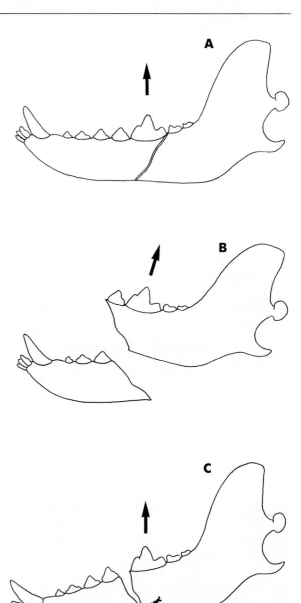

FIGURE 10-21
Mechanical effects of muscular pull on mandibular body fractures. **A,** Ventrorostral fracture line. Masticatory muscle pull will tend to keep the fracture ends apposed ("favorable" fracture). **B,** Transverse, or ventrocaudal, fracture line. Masticatory muscle pull will result in fracture line distraction ("unfavorable" fracture). **C,** Unfavorable fracture with ventral fixation only will distract dorsally with muscular pull.

body fracture that is transverse or oblique ventrocaudally (Fig. 10-21, *B*) is likely to result in dorsal distraction of the caudal fragment. The rostral fragment will tend to hang ventrally because there is no muscular pull to counteract the weight of the fragment and the tongue lying on top of it ("unfavorable" fracture). For unilateral fractures, this distraction may be minimal, and an "unfavorable" fracture may still be successfully managed conservatively if the fragments meet in correct position when the jaws are kept closed with a muzzle, although dental or surgical fixation is preferred. For bilateral mandibular body fractures that are transverse or oblique ventrocaudally, the rostral mandible hangs directly ventrally as a dead weight and must be held in normal occlusion by surgical or dental fixation for functional healing to occur. Fixation that is applied ventrally only may "gap" dorsally as a result of masticatory muscular pull (Fig. 10-21, *C*).

Teeth in the fracture line

In a normal dog or cat most of the dorsal half of the body of the mandible is occupied by teeth. Thus mandibular body fractures very often involve teeth or, more commonly, the alveolus surrounding the roots of teeth. Management of fractures of teeth is described in Chapters 6 and 7.

Otherwise intact teeth are at risk as a result of mandibular fracture in three ways: the fracture results in exposure of large areas of the periodontal attachment of the tooth, risking periodontal disruption and avulsion (see discussion of tooth avulsion-luxation in Chapter 6); the blood supply to the endodontic system that enters at the apex of the root is torn, causing endodontic disease; and the fixation system causes further endodontic or periodontal disruption or physical damage to the tooth itself.

Even when it is obvious that a tooth in a fracture line is severely compromised (Fig 10-22), extraction is not always indicated. Teeth often are useful as "spacers" across a fracture site to maintain normal bone length and rotational alignment, even if the tooth is extracted after satisfactory bone healing. This approach is not suitable if the tooth provides the only continuity across a fracture site. If the ventral cortex is not fragmented and a tooth is involved but still solidly embedded in bone, it is generally best to leave

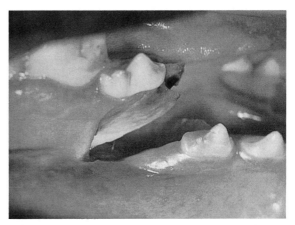

FIGURE 10-22
Oblique mandibular fracture with exposure of the roots of the fourth premolar tooth.

the tooth in place during fracture healing to provide a more rigid and anatomically correct fixation. The tooth can be extracted after fracture healing, or an alternative procedure such as hemisection and root canal therapy (see Chapter 6) can be performed to permit long-term retention of part of the tooth in the mouth.

When a tooth is in an unstable fracture site and is itself unstable, it should be extracted. This leaves a gap in the dorsal cortex, which may require more radical management (see later discussion).

Fixation techniques for mandibular body fractures

Muzzle. A cloth, leather, or plastic muzzle can be placed around the nose and mandible. This permits the fracture to be held in fixation because the canine teeth interdigitate. To be most effective, this technique should be limited to animals with intact canine teeth and unilateral fractures with little or no comminution or loss of contact of the fractured ends on that side. A simple test is to close the animal's jaws gently; if the canine teeth are in normal occlusion or slide easily into normal occlusion as the upper and lower teeth interdigitate, a muzzle should be adequate.

A muzzle can be custom-made for a dog with adhesive surgical tape. First a layer with the adhesive

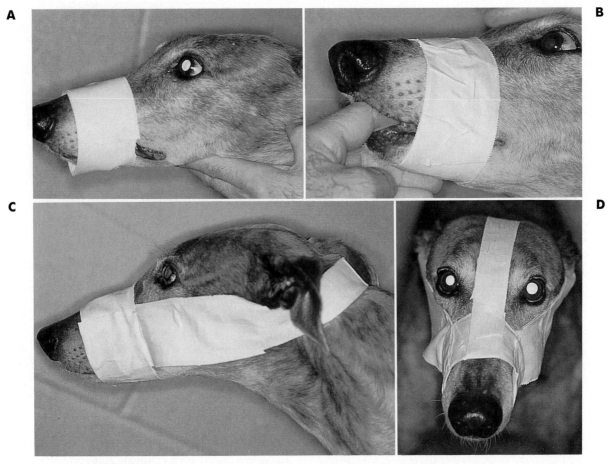

FIGURE 10-23
Tape muzzle. **A,** The first layer is placed with the adhesive side of the tape facing outward. **B,** The muzzle is fitted so that the mouth can be opened moderately. **C,** The neck loop is added. **D,** A dorsal piece is added in cats and short-muzzle dogs.

side outward is formed into a loop, encircling the muzzle and mandible (Fig. 10-23, *A*). It is made loose enough so that the incisor teeth do not meet, but the tips of the canine teeth overlap (Fig. 10-23, *B*), which keeps the jaw in correct alignment but allows the dog to suck in food of a fluid consistency. A second layer is then added, with the adhesive side facing inward, directly on top of the first layer. The retaining loop around the neck is added—also adhesive side out for the first layer, then adhesive side in (Fig. 10-23, *C*). For cats and short-muzzled dogs, an additional piece

is placed from the muzzle, looped over the top of the head (avoiding the eyes) to the neck loop (Fig. 10-23, *D*).

Dental wiring and splints. Teeth that are solidly implanted in bone can be used as points for attachment of a fixation device.

The classic technique used in human oral surgery is interdental wiring. However, this procedure is now rarely used in canine and feline oral surgery because the dental anatomy does not lend itself to this technique; the large interdental spaces and short or absent supragingival "neck" of the teeth mean that seating the wires and obtaining firm fixation of a mandibular segment with wires alone is awkward at best. Dental wires are still used, although mainly to reinforce an acrylic splint. If interdental wires are to be used alone, it is often necessary to undercut the crown of one or more teeth with a dental bur to permit retention of the wires when tightened. Techniques that require wires to be tightened around the necks of teeth, or undercutting of tooth substance, will cause periodontal disease.

The technique that has come into general use for dental fixation of jaw fractures in dogs is splinting with acrylic or composite material. This technique is useful for dogs with stable teeth that have fractures from the incisor areas as far caudal as the third premolar teeth. It requires at least one, and preferably two, firmly seated teeth on either side of the fracture that are large enough for attachment of the splint. Sufficient tooth structure rarely exists in cats to place a unilateral mandibular splint. The occlusal pattern of the dog permits a splint to be placed on the buccal surface of the mandibular premolar teeth, but not on the molar teeth because the upper fourth premolar and molar teeth overlap the lower molar teeth buccally. It is possible to place a splint on the lingual side of the lower molar teeth; however, care must be taken to minimize its size and to avoid formation of any rough edges that will irritate or lacerate the tongue.

The surfaces of the teeth to be used for attachment of the splint are thoroughly polished with flour pumice, rinsed, and dried and then acid-etched, rinsed, and dried as described for the composite bonding restorative technique (see Chapter 7). If there is sufficient space, a dam of wax or plastic modeling material is placed around the teeth. One method of making the splint is to pour acrylic powder onto the area to be splinted and then add the liquid; this powder-liquid sequence is continued until the splint has reached the desired thickness. An alternative method is to mix the powder and liquid in a small paper cup until it is a thick puttylike consistency. A layer of liquid is painted onto the prepared tooth surfaces and then the acrylic putty is pushed onto the surface of the teeth and molded into place.

With either technique the splint must be kept still

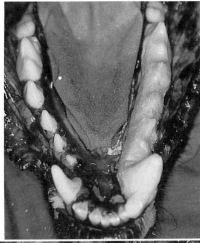

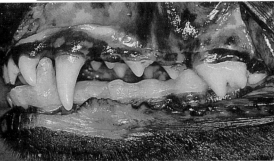

FIGURE 10-24
Mandibular acrylic splint stabilizing a fracture of the mandibular body at the level of the first premolar tooth. **A,** The splint includes the third incisor, canine, and premolar teeth and lingual surface of the first molar tooth. **B,** The occlusion is checked to ensure that the splint does not prevent closure of the mouth.

with the fracture in correct occlusion for the next several minutes until the acrylic has set (Fig. 10-24, A and B). Wires can be incorporated into the acrylic before setting. These can be circumdental (to improve retention) or simply placed on the surface of the tooth and between teeth to strenghten the splint, particularly for a long splint in the premolar area. Care must be taken to ensure that the upper canine teeth can close with the lower canine teeth in normal occlusion (Fig. 10-24, B), usually accomplished by oversizing the splint and then reducing it with an acrylic bur. The owner should be instructed to irrigate the area daily or twice daily while the splint is in place. The splint is removed 2 to 6 weeks later, depending on the age of the dog and severity of the fracture. The splint is removed by scoring with a dental bur and snapping sections free. The teeth are polished. After splint removal, the gingival tissue often is acutely inflamed or ulcerated (see Fig. 10-33, *C*); irrigation with chlorhexidine solution should be continued for several more days.

An interdental bridge also can be made with composite material, which is more rigid than acrylic. This technique is particularly useful for splinting together the upper and lower canine teeth of cats to ensure fixation of a comminuted symphyseal fragment in normal occlusion (Fig. 10-19). The basic acid-etch/composite technique is described in Chapter 6. Dentinal pins can be used to reinforce the attachment of the composite splint; technique for placement of these pins is described in Chapter 7. One pin is placed in each tooth. The pins can be bent towards each other. Where possible, the operator should angle the drill obliquely into the tooth to prevent the pins from penetrating into the pulp chamber.

It is possible to hold a severely fractured mandible in correct occlusion by wiring the upper and lower teeth together on one or both sides. The wires can be placed circumdentally or through the furcation area of multirooted teeth and then twisted together. The fixation of canine or incisor teeth can be secured by circumdental wires held in place in notches, or dentinal pins can be incorporated in a composite splint, as already described. With the jaw held rigidly closed, the animal must be fed through a gastrostomy tube, which creates a risk of fatal aspiration if the animal vomits. However, this technique rarely is necessary. An alternative, which permits rapid opening of the mouth in an emergency, is to loop orthodontic elastics or Masel chain over hooks bonded to the surface of the upper and lower teeth.

Osseous wiring. If significant comminution and collapse of the fracture site are not present, osseous wiring of fractured ends is an excellent technique. This is particularly applicable for fractures caudal to the lower third premolar tooth because adequate bone is available but space is insufficient for placement of

an acrylic dental splint. The following principles and techniques apply to using osseous mandibular wires.

1. Be aware of the anatomy of the roots (Fig. 10-25). A radiograph will clarify root length and direction for the individual animal and will help prevent penetration of the root or area adjacent to the root apex that would damage the endodontic blood supply.
2. The approach for wire placement can be made either through the mucosa of the cheek or through the skin over the lower jaw. Avoid making the incision directly over the likely position of the wire. Make the holes for the wire with a round bur in a water-cooled dental handpiece or with a Kirschner wire in a Jacob's chuck.
3. Place two wires, one dorsally and one ventrally, so that both compression and tension sides are stabilized (Fig. 10-26, *A*). If there is a dorsal gap but no ventral bone loss, an osseous wire can be used ventrally and an interdental splint dorsally. The dorsal wire should be below the mucogingival junction, or an interdental wire or splint should be used. If the fracture is oblique, a triangulated wire can be used (Fig. 10-26, *B*).
4. After snugging the wires into place, turn in the cut ends.
5. Close the mucosal or skin incisions over the wires.

Plates and screws. Rigid internal fixation of many mandibular fractures can be achieved with a plate placed on the buccal surface of the mandible, which is large and flat in many dogs. The problem is that the screws that hold the plate in position very likely will damage roots or the blood supply to the roots. The position of the plate should be planned; carefully laying it on a parallel-position intraoral radiograph (Fig. 10-27) of the mandible will make it obvious whether any damage will result. In large and giant breed dogs, which may exert considerable occlusal force on the mandible during fracture healing, a plate placed on the ventral third of the lateral surface of the mandible will provide excellent fixation and can span a defect in the bone (Fig. 10-28). This should be combined with dorsal fixation by intradental fixation (see p. 329), or the animal should be prevented from

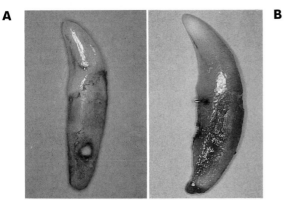

FIGURE 10-25
A and **B**, Wires used to maintain fixation of mandibular fractures that were placed through canine or incisor teeth.

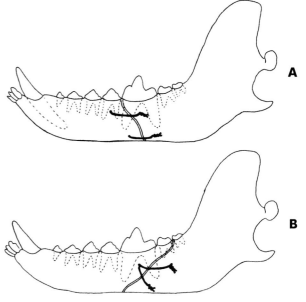

FIGURE 10-26
A, Dorsal and ventral osseous wiring of a mandibular body fracture. The wires penetrate between the roots of the teeth. **B**, Triangulated osseous wiring for fixation of an oblique mandibular body fracture.

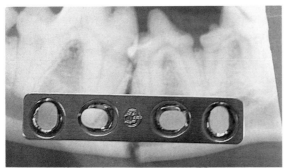

FIGURE 10-27
Trial placement of a plate on the radiograph of the mandibular body to ensure that two screws are on each side of the fracture line and that no screw penetrates a root. **A**, This four-hole plate will inevitably cause penetration of a root by a screw. **B**, Careful placement of this five-hole plate will allow four screws to avoid roots.

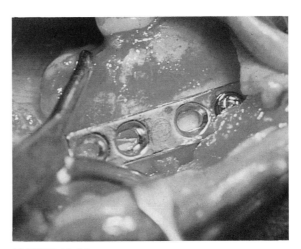

FIGURE 10-28
Plate fixation of a mandibular fracture in process.

using its jaws by placing a tape-muzzle for 3 to 4 weeks. The plate is placed through an incision through the ventral skin of the mandible or by extending an intraoral laceration. Plates that can bend to conform to the shape of the mandibular body should be used.

Half-pins and external splints. Practical pin and bolt systems have been developed for use with an external splint in humans; however, many dogs, and all cats, are too small for routine use of such appliances. These systems occasionally may be indicated—as a way of maintaining occlusion while the defect heals in—for management of fractures with extensive bone loss. The device is lighter and more adaptable if an acrylic side bar is used. Either bolts with heads or pins with 1-cm length turned perpendicular to the long axis of the pin are used so that the bold head or turned end of the pin is encased in the acrylic bar.

Intramedullary pins. Pins placed into the mandibular canal severely traumatize the mandibular alveolar artery, depriving the lower canine, incisior, and premolar teeth of their endodontic blood supply or causing direct damage to the tooth roots (Fig. 10-29; see also Chapter 6). The mandibular canal is curved; a pin driven to the full length of the canal will cause the fracture line to gape dorsally. Given these complications and the fact that practical alternatives are readily available, the use of mandibular intramedullary pins cannot be recommended.

Ventral longitudinal pin. A large Kirshner wire or small Steinmann pin can be shaped to the external ventral cortex of the mandible. It can be held in place with partial cerclage wires, and longitudal fixation can be strengthened by turning the ends of the pin dorsally for 3 to 5 mm and seating the turned ends in holes drilled in the ventral cortex.

Combination techniques. Dorsal fixation with an interdental splint or wire can be combined with a ventral osseous wire or plate to achieve optimal fixation with minimal fixation metal in bone.

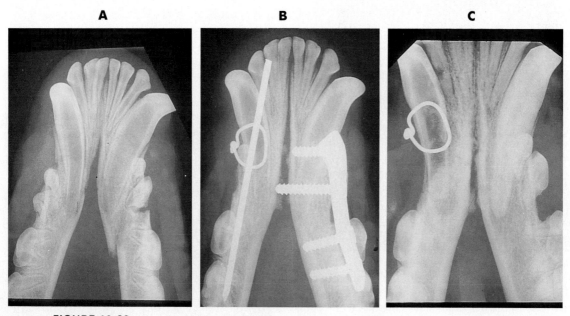

FIGURE 10-29
Bilateral fracture of the rostral end of the mandible. **A,** Treated on one side by intramedullary pin and hemicerclage wire. **B,** Immediate postoperative radiograph. **C,** One canine tooth (left side) has failed to develop normally 5 months postoperatively.

Management of bony defects

If comminution or necrosis secondary to extensive and prolonged bone exposure has resulted in a defect that will cause severe malocclusion, alternative techniques are indicated. If fixation at both ends of the defect is adequate, the defect eventually will fill in; for defects of more than 4 to 6 mm, this may take several months. To speed up the filling-in process, the fractured ends can be held in occlusally correct fixation (by an interdental splint, osseous wire, half pins, or plate and screws) and the defect filled with cancellous bone chips and covered with healthy oral epithelium. The fracture site is radiographed every 4 to 6 weeks, and the fixation system is removed only when there is radiographic evidence of healthy bone bridging the defect. An alternative technique is to use an autogenous cortical bone graft by harvesting a rib. The rib is opened along its long axis to expose the medullary canal and cancellous bone, then placed so that it rests in a ventral channel in the mandibular segments at either end of the defect, spanning the defect. It is held in place with cerclage wires (Fig. 10-30).

Management of pathologic fractures and mandibular nonunion

Mandibular nonunions result from inadequate fixation. For a unilateral fracture that is stabilized to some extent by the contralateral intact mandible, fibrous healing may be adequate for comfortable function in many dogs and cats. If both right and left mandibles are fractured, satisfactory healing is much less likely without excellent fixation. For young dogs with traumatic fractures, excellent fixation generally can be obtained for both mandibles by use of the techniques already described. For aging, small-breed dogs with severe periodontal disease, bilateral pathologic mandibular fractures often are orthopedic disasters (see Fig. A-74, p. 68. All periodontally involved teeth in the area of the fractures are extracted, and the soft tissues are allowed to heal while the mandibles are supported in a muzzle; a stable mandible may result. Fixation may be possible with a single pin shaped and laid on the ventral cortexes of both mandibles and held in place with partial cerclarge wires. Often these cases are hopeless; permanent placement of a loose

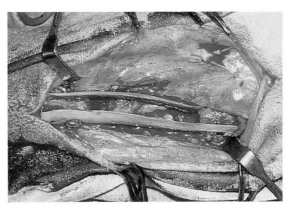

FIGURE 10-30
Autogenous rib graft used to span a defect in a mandible. *(Courtesy of Dr. R.J. Orsher.)*

muzzle may be the only practical way to manage the functional and esthetic problems (Fig. 10-31). Pathologic fractures also can result from neoplastic invasion. In these cases, management of the neoplasm is of far greater importance than fracture fixation.

Salvage treatment of mandibular fracture

One practical option for treatment of a unilateral, severely infected, comminuted fracture or nonunion with extensive bone loss is hemimandibulectomy (see p. 364).

Maxillary Fractures

Maxillary fractures often are less evident clinically than are mandibular fractures because the lower jaw does not hang. Muzzle trauma may be evident externally.

Minor malocclusion in an area that has adequate attached soft tissues can be set and held in normal occlusion by suturing the soft tissues only (Fig. 10-32).

Fixation of teeth that are held in an unstable section of maxilla is best achieved with an acrylic splint applied by means of the acid-etch technique (see Chapter 6). This provides stabilization of the fractured palate or maxilla and permits rearrangement of the unstable teeth to a normal occlusal position that is retained

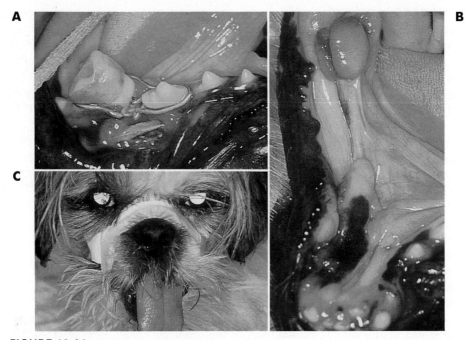

FIGURE 10-31
A, Unstable fracture with wire fixation in a dog with severe periodontal disease. **B,** Following removal of metal and involved teeth, the soft tissues have healed as a nonunion. **C,** The dog manages comfortably with a tape muzzle.

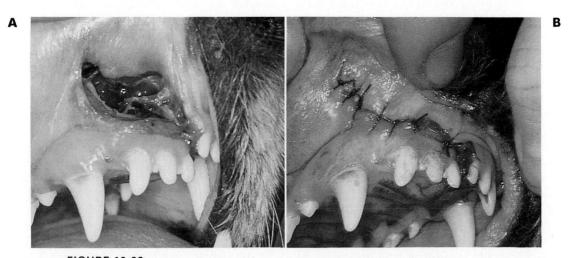

FIGURE 10-32
Premaxillary trauma with incisor malocclusion (**A**) in a dog stabilized by suturing the avulsed soft tissues (**B**).

while the device is in place (Fig. 10-33). The lower teeth should not hit against the device; the splint should be trimmed as necessary to ensure adequate occlusion. The owner is instructed to irrigate the gingiva-splint interface daily with cholorhexidine solution. The splint is removed 3 to 4 weeks later; the gingival tissues beneath the splint often are acutely inflamed at this time (Fig. 10-33, C) but respond rapidly to simple irrigation with chlorhexidine.

If the teeth are severely fractured and unsalvageable and therefore unavailable for fixation of an acrylic splint, small-diameter cross pins can be placed to stabilize large maxillary or palatal fragments. An alternative technique is to embed several wires in bone and encase them in an acrylic splint, which may permit more control in location of the wires, thus avoiding roots of healthy teeth. If a maxillary fracture has healed with teeth in a maloccluded position, the teeth may be movable by orthodontic techniques (see Chapter 8); extraction or crown shortening and pulpotomy (see Chapter 6) also are used to permit the animal to close its mouth comfortably.

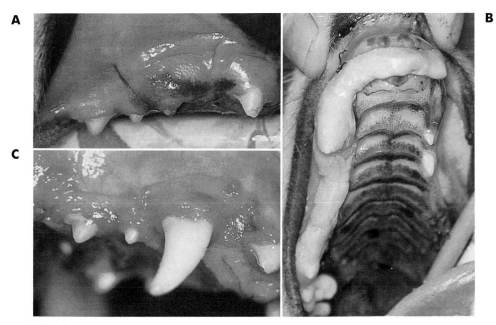

FIGURE 10-33
Acrylic splint used to stabilize a maxillary fracture and luxated canine tooth in a dog. **A,** Only the tip of the canine tooth is visible. (The most obvious tooth is the third incisor.) **B,** The splint in place. **C,** Following removal of the splint, several weeks later, the maxillary fracture and canine tooth are stable. There is gingival inflammation and ulceration.

Oral Soft Tissue Trauma
Gingival trauma

Occasionally the entire incisor gingiva is avulsed by an automobile injury (Fig. 10-34); clean edges are sutured with absorbable material, and sutures are placed around or between teeth if necessary. Flaps from tears in the attached gingiva are best trimmed off if they are too small to be sutured back into place. If the entire attached gingiva around a tooth has been lost, a gingival flap or graft procedure is indicated (see Chapter 4).

Palatal trauma

Injuries of the palate are described later under Palatal Defects.

Tongue trauma

To treat trauma to the tongue, surgical incisions or clean lacerations are sutured with absorbable material, both to control hemorrhage and to appose the epithelial edges (see Fig. A-17, p. 53). Jagged lacerations require careful conservative débridement before suturing. Treatment of irregular lacerations or avulsions is irrigation of the affected areas with dilute chlorhexidine, as well as nursing care to assist with feeding until the areas heal. Tongue injury from electric cords rarely requires much by way of definitive management; the injured tissues are best left to necrose so that the maximum amount of tongue tissue is retained (see Fig. A-16, p. 53). Use of a pharyngostomy or gastrostomy tube for several days may be necessary for feeding. Once the necrotic portion of the tongue has sloughed, the remaining stump is rapidly covered by epithelium (see Fig. A-16). To save as much tongue as possible, débridement of the lesion should be avoided until the margin of the necrotic section is obvious. Because soft tissue lesions heal rapidly, débridement often is not necessary. Barbed objects such as fish hooks or bone spicula may require incision along the object during removal to prevent further damage. Dogs and cats that have lost the entire free portion and some of the root of the tongue often manage well by sucking in food and water or by tossing chunks of food to the back of the tongue. Sloughing of part of the tongue as a result of chewing on electrtic cords is more likely to be troublesome in cats; even

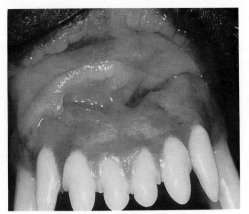

FIGURE 10-34
Avulsion injury of the incisor gingiva.

though they can eat and drink, they may be unable to groom effectively. One solution to this problem is to acquire an additional cat, which may socialize by grooming the disabled cat.

Foreign bodies caught around the tongue can saw their way into the frenulum, causing a granulating mass similar in appearance to a squamous cell carcinoma seen in this location in cats (see Fig. A-23, p. 55). Treatment is transection of the linear foreign body.

Lip trauma

Simple lacerations are sutured with separate layers on the mucosal and skin surfaces. Abscesses are lanced and drained, with care taken to avoid the parotid duct as it courses over the side of the face.

Necrosis of part of the lip can be caused by electric cord injury or bite wound abscesses and may result in stricture of the oral commissure and inability to open the mouth. This can be corrected by incising the scar at the commissure and closing the mucosa and skin as two layers to lengthen the commissure (Fig. 10-35).

Avulsion injuries may cause severe skin loss. Because the mandible is an exposed prominence, insufficient skin may be available to cover bare areas. Every effort should be made to retain skin at the rostral end. This can be done by reattaching the avulsed skin to the gingival attachment if the skin is healthy (Fig.

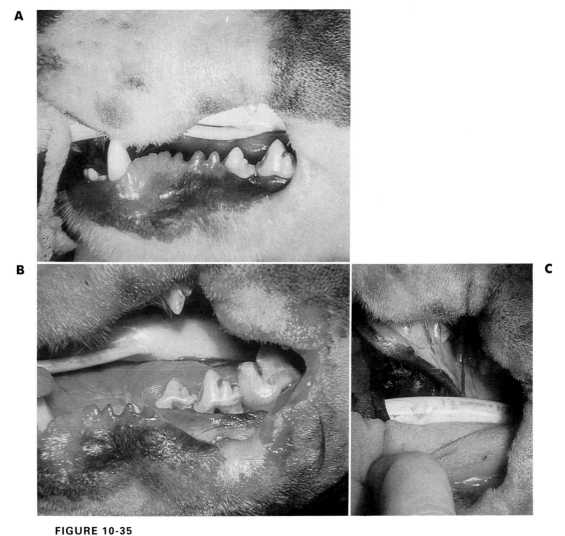

FIGURE 10-35
A, Injury resulting from chewing electric cord, causing extensive scarring of the lip and necrosis of part of the mandible. **B,** The commissure is enlarged by incising skin and mucosa. A necrotic section of the mandible is also visible. **C,** Following commissuroplasty, the dog can open its mouth wide.

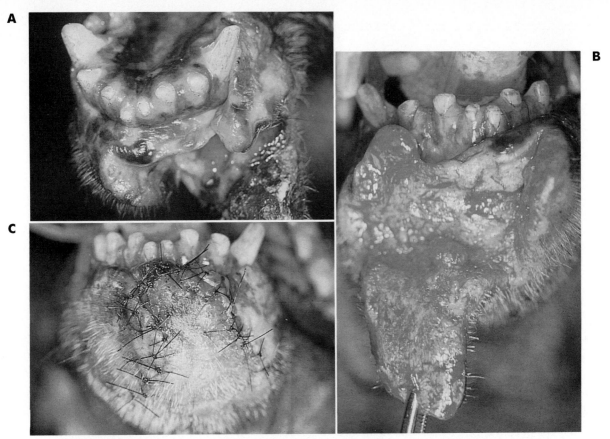

FIGURE 10-36
Injury of skin of the rostral end of the mandible. **A,** At the time of presentation, several days after the injury. **B,** Following conservative debridement. **C,** Following closure of skin and mucosal edges.

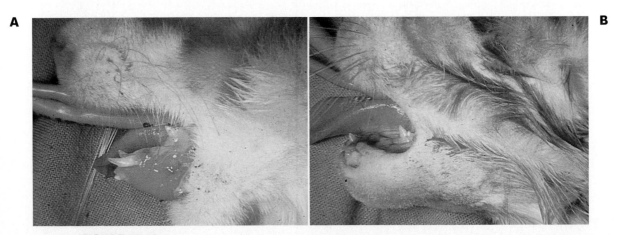

FIGURE 10-37
Avulsion of the lower lip in a cat. Before (**A**) and after (**B**) suturing the lip in place with sutures placed around teeth.

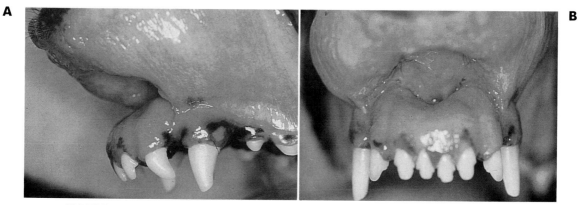

FIGURE 10-38
Midline avulsion of the nasal cartilages and upper lip from the maxilla, with formation of an oronasal fistula.

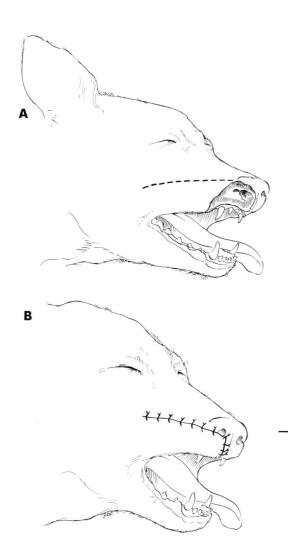

10-36) or by rotating a flap of skin from the intermandibular area; the donor area can be repaired easily by use of the loose skin of the neck. Lip skin can be held in place at its rostral end by placing sutures through the skin and around adjacent teeth (Fig. 10-37); a soft rubber drain or plastic tubing can be used to form tension-relieving sutures.

Avulsion of the upper lip is less common but more spectacular if the nasal cavity is exposed (Fig. 10-38). Disrupted tissues are débrided and kept in normal apposition by sutures that are placed through the avulsed lip; they can be anchored to one or more incisor or canine teeth. A full-thickness upper lip skin pedicle flap can be formed and sutured in place to cover avulsion defects of the area around the philtrum (Fig. 10-39); the buccinator muscle may have to be severed to obtain sufficient freedom of movement for the flap. The effect is to bring the lip commissure forward on that side, which does not interfere with the animal's ability to fully open the mouth.

FIGURE 10-39
A, Avulsion injury of the upper lip. **B,** Closure with a rostrally rotated flap.

▶ PALATAL DEFECTS

Defects of formation of the palatal structures may be inherited, or they may result from an insult during the critical stage of fetal development when the two palatine shelves fuse to separate the oral and nasal cavities. A wide variety of dog and cat breeds have been affected. The sporadic nature of these conditions and the wide range of breeds that are affected suggest that in most cases the cause is an intrauterine insult. Breeding studies have shown evidence of an inherited pattern, with incomplete penetrance in the Shih Tzu breed and possibly in pointers, bulldogs, and Swiss sheep dogs. Additional congenital defects, such as meningocele, may also be present occasionally.

Primary palate (incisive bone) congenital abnormalities appear as harelip. They may be associated with abnormalities of the secondary palate (hard and soft palate). Except for being externally visible, harelip rarely results in clinical signs. Repair, which is performed for esthetic reasons, is described on p. 369.

Clefts of the secondary palate or acquired defects of the palate or maxilla are more serious, although they are rarely visible externally. Affected animals usually are seen by the veterinarian because of nasal discharge. They also may have a history of cough, respiratory distress, poor weight gain, and general unthriftiness. The prognosis without surgical repair is guarded because of the risk of lower airway aspiration. Surgical correction of congenital cleft palate in dogs usually is possible if the animal can survive and grow to a suitable size for anesthesia and surgery. Milk substitute or puppy food fed by tube several times daily is necessary in most dogs and cats to avoid recurrent, and eventually fatal, aspiration pneumonia. The larger the animal at the time of surgery, the more tissue is available for repair; most procedures for corrections of congenital defects are performed on animals of 2 to 4 months of age.

Congenital cleft hard palate is almost always in the midline and usually is associated with a midline soft palate abnormality (Fig. 10-40). Soft palate defects without hard palate defects may occur in the midline or may be unilateral. The prognosis for successful repair of congenital absence of the soft palate (Fig. 10-41), as opposed to cleft soft palate, is poor; there is no useful purpose served by extending the life of animals with this abnormality.

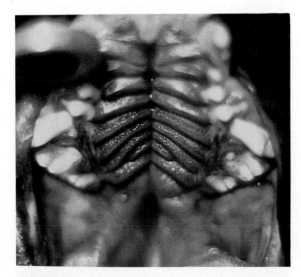

FIGURE 10-40
Midline congenital cleft of the hard and soft palates of a bulldog puppy.

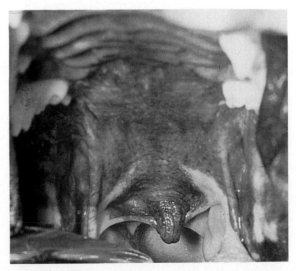

FIGURE 10-41
Absence bilaterally of the soft palate in a puppy. A midline rump of muscular tissue is covered by epithelium.

Palatal Reconstruction
Principles of palatal surgery

By careful planning and meticulous technique, it is possible to restore normal swallowing function to dogs and cats with cleft palate. The best chance of success is with the first procedure. Because the vascular supply will be distorted by unsuccessful procedures, it is better to refer the case initially rather than try the repair once or twice.

The following guidelines are recommended.

1. Treat only animals showing clinical signs; some small rostral defects will not cause nasal regurgitation.
2. Choose the procedure to be used with care, taking into account the length and breadth of the defect and the length and breadth of tissues available. Consider more radical alternatives if they are more likely to achieve first-time functional success (for example, premolar/molar teeth extraction and creation of a buccal flap).
3. Make flaps as large as possible to reduce tension and to provide overlap between the flap and the adjacent healthy tissue.
4. Suture connective tissue surfaces or cut edges together; intact epithelium will not heal to any other surface. This requires that clean, healthy, sharply incised, cut-tissue edges be made available on both apposed edges of sutured tissue.
5. Provide two-layer closure if practical, usually possible with soft palate closure and sometimes possible for hard palate closure.
6. Do not locate a suture incision over a defect if possible; use asymmetric flaps if necessary. Location of the incision over a defect will cause the tissue to become dry compared with closure that lies over an adjacent tissue surface.
7. Retain blood supply to the flap. For palatal flaps, always use full-thickness mucoperiosteum, locate the incisions away from the palatine artery (which exits from the palatine bone 0.5 to 1 cm medial to the upper carnassial tooth), and then identify and preserve the artery by blunt dissection. For buccal flaps, find a tissue plane that will leave much of the connective tissue attached to the mucosal flap.
8. Hemorrhage often is severe; use firm pressure frequently, and do not hesitate to ligate one or both carotid arteries. Incised edges that will be closed over defects should not be made with an electroscalpel nor should bleeding vessels on the cut edges undergo electrocoagulation, which increases the likelihood of wound breakdown. Electrocoagulation can be used safely for control of bleeding vessels away from incised edges, provided that the current settings are the minimum for the specific purpose.
9. At all costs, avoid creating tissue closure that is under tension, inasmuch as dehiscence is inevitable with tension.

Congenital midline defects of the hard palate

Two procedures are in general use. These are the overlapping (rotating) flap technique and the medially repositioned double flap technique.

Overlapping flap technique. This is commenced by making incisions in the muco-periosteum at the defect on one side and 2 to 3 mm from the dental margin on the other side (Fig. 10-42, *A*). The flaps are raised with a periosteal elevator (Fig. 10-42, *B*). When raising the flaps, the operator dissects carefully around the palatine artery (Fig. 10-43); when the artery is identified, further careful dissection close to it will release it from fibrous tissue. It can be stretched to accommodate the rotation of the flap (Fig. 10-43, *B*). The flaps are sutured so that one flap is turned and lies under the other (Fig. 10-42, *C*), with the connective tissue surfaces in contact. The sutures are placed in a horizontal mattress pattern; they are preplaced, then tied so that the tissues are apposed snugly (Figs. 10-42, *C*, and 10-43, *B*).

Medially repositioned double flap technique. Two symmetric flaps are formed by making incisions at the edges of the defect, undermining the mucoperiosteum laterally, and then suturing the flaps over the defect. It is often necessary to make relieving incisions on one or both sides so that the mucoperiosteal flaps can be moved medially to appose each other (see Fig. 10-53). Unless the relieving incisions are long, risking damage to the palatine vessels, this technique usually results in tension at the suture line,

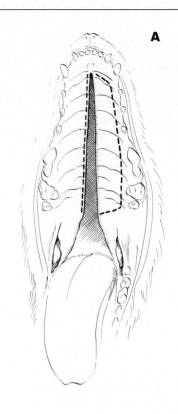

FIGURE 10-42

Overlapping flap technique for closure of midline hard palate defects. **A,** Incisions to create the flaps. **B,** Dissection with a periosteal elevator. **C,** The rotated and sutured flaps (*inset,* horizontal mattress pattern used to appose the flaps).

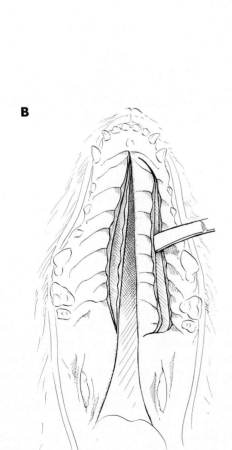

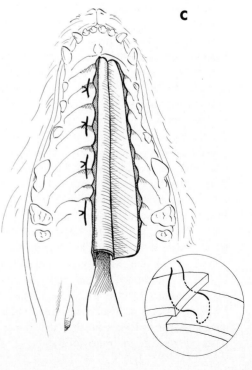

A

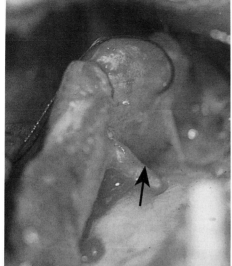

B

which is located directly over the defect. This will be followed by partial breakdown of the repair (Fig. 10-44). The relieving incision gapes, and a lateral oronasal defect may result, particularly in narrow-nosed dogs (Fig. 10-45). For these reasons the overlapping flap technique previously described is preferred for midline hard palate defects (Fig. 10-46). For any major palatine surgery, soft food is recommended for about 2 to 3 weeks, particularly if the bone of the palate or the palatine artery is left exposed. Granulation and epithelization generally are completed in 3 to 4 weeks (Fig. 10-46).

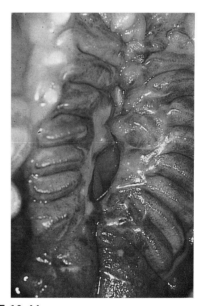

FIGURE 10-43
A, Identification of the palatine artery. The flap has been raised, and the artery is dissected free *(arrow).* **B,** The dissected artery *(arrow)* can stretch to accommodate the rotation of the flap.

FIGURE 10-44
Medially repositioned double flap technique was used in two attempts to close a midline hard palate defect in a bulldog, with partial dehiscence and reformation of a palate defect.

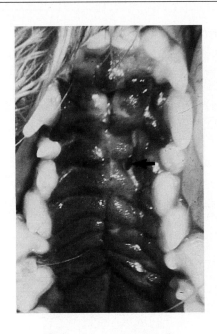

FIGURE 10-45
Lateral palate defect *(arrow)* formed through a relieving incision made when performing the double flap technique.

A **B**

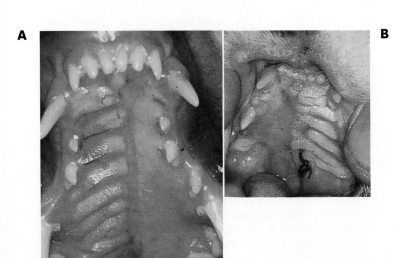

FIGURE 10-46
Successful repair several weeks following the overlapping flap technique in a dog (**A**) and in a kitten (**B**). The palate surface has epithelialized.

Midline soft palate congenital defects

If fusion of the palatal shelves was unsuccessful but the soft palate mucosa and muscle are present and deflected to the pharyngeal walls, functional results are excellent with use of a double flap technique. Incisions are made along the medial margin of the palate on each side, and blunt-ended scissors are used to separate the palate tissue to form dorsal and ventral flaps on each side (Fig. 10-47). The two dorsal flaps are sutured in a simple interrupted pattern to form a complete nasal epithelium, and the two ventral flaps are sutured to form a complete oral epithelium (Fig. 10-47, *B*). The palate is closed to the midpoint or caudal end of the tonsils (Fig. 10-48).

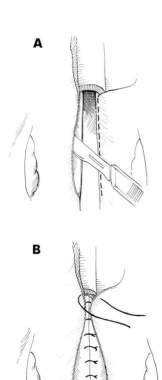

FIGURE 10-47
Double flap technique for closure of a midline defect of the soft palate. **A,** Incision to create the dorsal and ventral flaps. **B,** The nasal flaps have been sutured, and closure of the oral flaps is commencing.

Acquired Palatal Defects

The most common cause of acquired defects between the nasal and oral cavities is the loss of maxillary bone associated with severe periodontal disease or tooth extraction; this defect usually is referred to as an *oronasal fistula*. Trauma (dog bites, electric cord injury), severe chronic infections, surgery, and radiation therapy of palatal tumors are other causes.

Oronasal fistula

Oronasal fistula most commonly occurs after loss of the canine tooth (Fig. 10-49). If an abnormality is obvious at the time of tooth extraction (as evidenced by bleeding from the nose during the procedure or the appearance of fluid from the external nares when the socket is gently flushed), absorbable sutures can be placed in an attempt to collapse the sides of the alveolus and prevent formation of a fistula.

Two methods are in common use to close an established fistula.

Single buccal-based flap procedure. The defect is repaired by creating a buccal flap (Figs. 10-49 and 10-50), advancing it over the defect and suturing it to cleanly incised epithelium on the palatal margin (Figs. 10-49, *C,* and 10-50, *C*) with absorbable simple interrupted sutures. The incisions must extend dorsal to

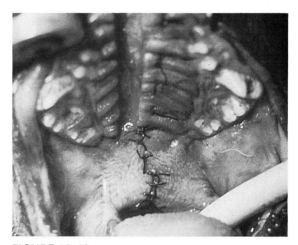

FIGURE 10-48
Completed repair of soft palate midline defect in a bulldog.

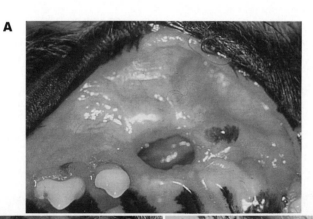

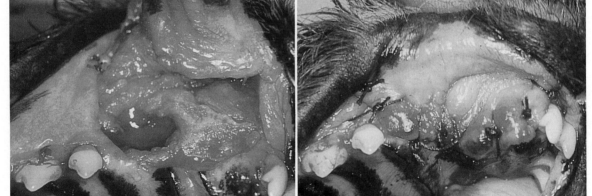

FIGURE 10-49
A, Oronasal fistula following loss of the canine tooth in a dog. The nasal cavity is visible. **B,** The buccal-based flap has been dissected. **C,** The completed flap procedure.

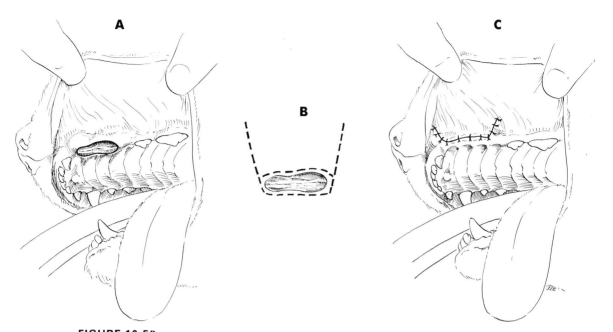

FIGURE 10-50
A, Oronasal fistula in a dog secondary to exfoliation of the upper canine tooth. **B,** Incisions for single flap repair. **C,** The flap has been dissected free, advanced to cover the defect, and sutured in place.

the mucogingival junction, and dissection to free the flap tissue must penetrate the firm connective tissue attachments of the buccal mucosa to the periosteum of the maxilla. Results are excellent with this technique if the flap is large enough and includes some connective tissue to retain vascularity.

Double flap technique. The alternative technique uses flaps in two layers; initially a flap of full-thickness mucoperiosteum palatine tissue is raised by incising with a scalpel and dissecting it from the palatine bone with a sharp periosteal elevator (Fig. 10-51, *B*). The flap remains hinged at the defect. This flap is larger than the defect. It is rotated and sutured across the defect, apposing it to a scarified surface on the lateral edge of the defect (Fig. 10-51, *C*). Then a buccal-based flap is raised and rotated to cover the first flap (Fig. 10-51, *D* and *E*). The buccal flap can be based

labially (apically), as in the aforementioned single flap technique (Fig. 10-50), or caudally (Fig. 10-51, *D*). No matter where the flap is based, it consists of full-thickness buccal mucosa and enough supporting connective tissue to ensure viability of blood supply. The buccal flap is made long enough to cover the defect and the donor site for the palate-based flap. It is sutured with single interrupted absorbable sutures that join freshly incised epithelial edges all the way round the edges of the flap (Fig. 10-51, *G*). Depending on the site and direction of origin of the buccal flap, there may be need to appose the edges of the donor area together.

With either technique a successful result depends on creation of flaps that are sufficiently large, that are not under tension when sutured, and that have an adequate blood supply.

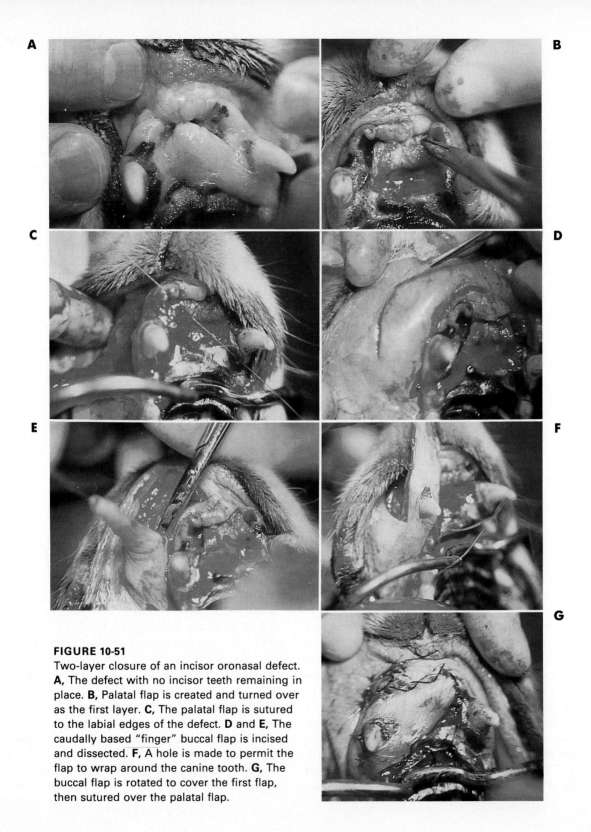

FIGURE 10-51

Two-layer closure of an incisor oronasal defect. **A,** The defect with no incisor teeth remaining in place. **B,** Palatal flap is created and turned over as the first layer. **C,** The palatal flap is sutured to the labial edges of the defect. **D** and **E,** The caudally based "finger" buccal flap is incised and dissected. **F,** A hole is made to permit the flap to wrap around the canine tooth. **G,** The buccal flap is rotated to cover the first flap, then sutured over the palatal flap.

Acquired hard palate defects

Most defects in the hard palate can be closed by some form of mucoperiosteal flap. Because the mucoperiosteum has so little elasticity, it cannot be stretched to cover a large area. Therefore it is essential to plan the position of the flap or flaps in advance so that a large enough area of tissue can be obtained to prevent tension and to ensure healing. Rotation and advancement flaps can be created. In general, one should use the technique that will provide the largest flap. For small, circular defects, rotation flaps usually are best (Fig. 10-52). For long midline or paramidline defects (such as those resulting from midline palatal separation in cats who have fallen from a height or who have been hit by a car), the overlapping technique described previously for congenital defects can be used if the epithelium at the defect has matured. Alternatively, relieving incisions can be made to allow two lateral flaps to be apposed (Fig. 10-53).

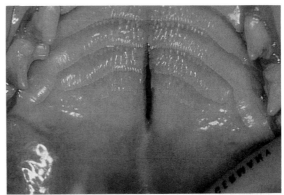
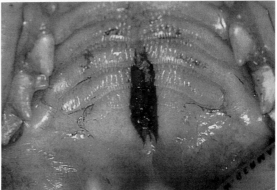
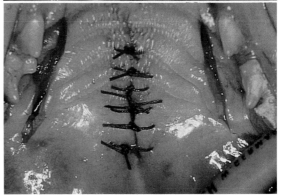

FIGURE 10-53
A, Midline defect of the palate in a cat. **B,** Incisions made at the edges of the flap and dissected to form two dorsal flaps that are sutured first. **C,** Relieving incisions are made laterally to permit the palatal mucoperiosteum to be slid medially for closure as a second layer.

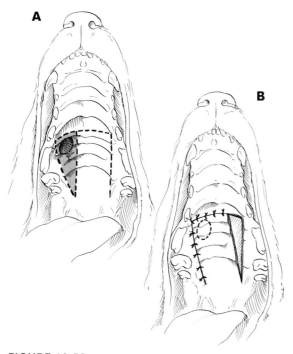

FIGURE 10-52
A and **B,** Rotation flap technique for closure of a hard palate defect.

Fresh midline lacerations in palates of cats (Fig. 10-54) may not need surgical repair if there is no bubbling through the defect from the nose, because the stump of the vomer bone or nasal septum plugs the defect until a blood clot forms and healing commences. Fresh defects with obvious communication into the nasal cavity can be closed successfully by simply placing sutures to join the tissue edges, as for a clean skin wound.

Large defects that cross the midline require the use of an advancement flap, which necessitates the elevation of the mucoperiosteum caudally to include part of the soft palate so that sufficient tissue can be pulled forward to prevent tension on the suture line (Fig. 10-55). With flaps of any shape, it is essential that the epithelium around the defect be removed to provide a surface for healing (Fig. 10-56). For very large defects (covering more than half the width of the palate), a buccal-based flap can be formed and sutured across the defect, although the teeth and remaining palatal mucosa adjacent to the defect must first be removed (Fig. 10-56).

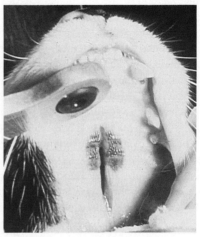

FIGURE 10-54
Fresh traumatic midline palate laceration in a cat.

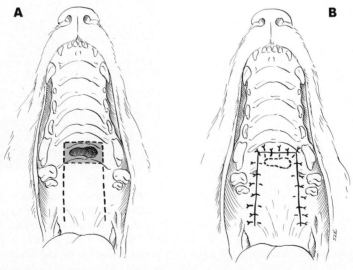

FIGURE 10-55
Advancement flap technique for closure of wide defects of the caudal hard palate.

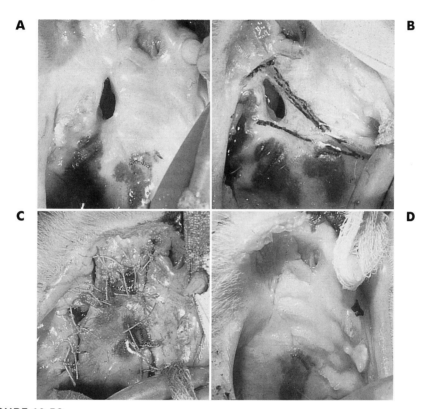

FIGURE 10-56
A, Traumatic palatal defect in a cat following several previous attempts at surgical closure. **B,** Incisions for an advancement flap and creation of an edge to which the flap can be sutured. The premolar teeth have been extracted to permit use of a buccal-based flap should the advancement flap fail. **C,** Advancement flap sutured across the defect. **D,** Successful healing several weeks later.

An alternative method is to create a permanent or removable acrylic/Silastic or metal obturator (Fig. 10-57). This technique requires a minimum of two anesthesia episodes, first to prepare the impressions (Fig. 10-57, *B*) from which a stone cast will be made (see Chapter 8). From this cast the dental laboratory creates the prosthesis (Fig. 10-57, *C*), which is then trial fitted and adjusted (Fig. 10-57, *D*) at the second anesthesia episode. Techniques and materials for making dental impressions and acrylic devices are described in Chapters 7, 8, and 11.

Another alternative for large hard palate defects, particularly in cats or small dogs with very limited tissue available, is to use the tongue. An incision, which is made in the dorsum of the free edge of the tongue, is deepened to form two flaps. The edges of the palate defect are incised and undermined. The edges of the tongue flaps and palate defect are apposed with absorbable sutures (Fig. 10-58). The animal is fed with a syringe through the cheek pouch. Three to four weeks later, the tongue is separated from the palate tissue, leaving enough tongue tissue attached to the palate to close as a bilateral flap over the defect.

► RESECTION OF ORAL MASSES

The occurrence, diagnosis, biologic behavior, treatment, and results of treatment of oral tumors are described in Chapter 9. This section describes the specific surgical techniques used in managing oral tumors.

Conservative resection of oral masses is indicated occasionally. Viral papillomatosis lesions are easily resected by transecting the stalk of the lesion with an electroscalpel. Benign gingival lesions, such as gingival hyperplasia or fibrous/osseous epulis lesions, are likely to regrow after resection at a tissue level that does not include the bone from which they arise. Their slow growth and nonulcerative nature, however, make regrowth nonproblematic. If gingival tissue is resected, a collar of gingiva should be retained around the tooth (gingivoplasty is described in Chapter 4).

Other neoplastic masses should not be treated by conservative surgery. If the diagnosis is doubtful, a biopsy specimen should be obtained (see Chapter 9).

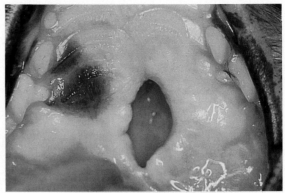

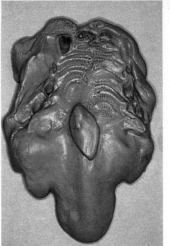

FIGURE 10-57
A, Large midline palate defect in a cat. **B,** Rubber impression of the palate and defect. **C,** Acrylic obturator made of softer acrylic on the part to fit into the defect (original height). **D,** Height following reduction to permit space for nasal airflow but retaining the rounded overhang that will keep the obturator in place. **E,** The obturator in place. **F,** The cat tolerated the device well.

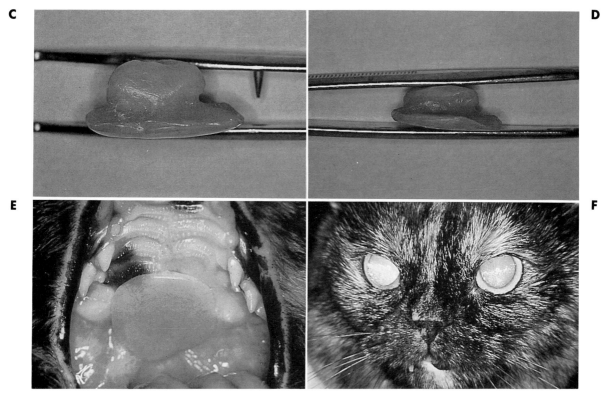

FIGURE 10-57, cont'd
For legend see opposite page.

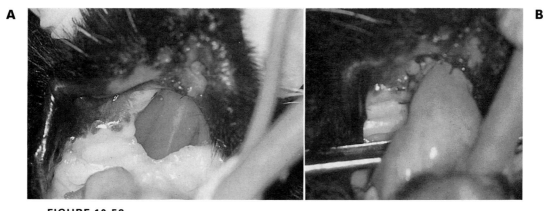

FIGURE 10-58
Use of the rostral end of the tongue to provide tissue for closure of a palate defect in a cat. **A,** Large irregular palate defect. **B,** Tip of the tongue incised and sutured to the incised edge of the defect.

Radical surgery (partial or hemimandibulectomy, premaxillectomy, or partial maxillectomy) may provide a cure in some cases of oral malignancy and is tolerated surprisingly well by dogs and cats. Small malignant lesions should be treated radically. Heroic treatment of large lesions is a wasted effort unless designed solely as palliation.

Esthetically, maxillectomy in most circumstances causes minor facial abnormality; a concavity on the side of the face can be felt and, less often, seen. After mandibulectomy the tongue often hangs out on one side, although this can be partially corrected by narrowing the commissure of the lips on that side to form a fold to contain the tongue. The quality of life provided by these procedures is excellent; the multiple anesthesia episodes required for radiotherapy and the systemic sickness and multiple office visits required for chemotherapy are avoided. Combined therapy may be indicated, particularly for lesions with local or distant metastasis (see Chapter 9).

Maxillectomy and Premaxillectomy

Maxillectomy and premaxillectomy are procedures in which segments of the maxilla or premaxilla are removed, including teeth. The tissue is removed en bloc, meaning that surgically significant vessels cannot be located and ligated before transection of the tissue containing the vessel. Hemorrhage therefore can be brisk and must be planned for. Unilateral carotid artery ligation is recommended, particularly for the first several such procedures performed by a surgeon.

Maxillectomy

The operator first decides on the extent and location of the palatal, gingival, and buccal mucosa incisions, planning to stay at least 1 cm (or more if available, particularly for fibrosarcoma and malignant melanoma) away from gross or radiographically visible margins of the lesion (Fig. 10-59). A rectangular excision should be avoided because the corners are areas most susceptible to dehiscence. It is better to extract an additional tooth or two on either side of the desired area of excision so that the resected area can be "tapered" at each end, particularly if the planned en bloc resection runs to the level of the third premolar tooth.

Because of the outward turn of the dental arch at the level of the carnassial tooth, it is best to resect all premolar and molar teeth for lesions extending to this level (Fig. 10-60).

The epithelium of the maxilla and palate is incised with a cold scalpel and is reflected with a periosteal elevator to expose the underlying bone. Hemorrhage often is profuse, particularly when the palate is incised. This usually can be controlled by pressure until the resected tissue is lifted out, when the vessels themselves can be located and ligated or electrocoagulated (the use of electrocoagulation along incised epithelial edges that will be sutured should be avoided). The maxilla and palate are fractured along the incision lines with a dental bur or diamond wheel, osteotome, or oscillating bone saw. The line of incision may include the infraorbital canal. If so, the infraorbital artery must be identified and ligated as the tissue to be resected is levered up. Remaining attachments are separated, and the section is removed en bloc. The nasal passage will be exposed at this point if the resection is adequate (Fig. 10-59, *B*). Resection that does not expose the nasal cavity is unlikely to be adequate as primary treatment of a maxillary oral malignancy.

Hemorrhage is controlled, blood clots are removed, and the remaining tissues are examined. If areas of turbinate were partially severed or traumatized during the resection, they are cut with scissors to leave a clean edge. Hemorrhage that cannot be controlled by ligation or pressure may respond to surface application of a mixture of several drops of a phenylephrine (0.05 mg/ml) and lidocaine (20 mg/ml) given at a maximum dose of 0.1 to 0.2 ml/kg body weight in dogs or 0.05 to 0.1 ml/kg body weight in cats. The use of dilute epinephrine is to be avoided, particularly when the anesthetic agent used is halothane.

The defect between the nose and mouth is covered with a buccal flap that is created by incising the buccal mucosa and gently undermining it until sufficient tissue is formed to cover the defect without tension (Fig. 10-59, *C*). Much of the connective tissue layer is left attached to the buccal mucosa to ensure viability of the flap in its new position. The tissues are apposed with interrupted synthetic absorbable sutures. A vertical mattress pattern (or interspersed simple inter-

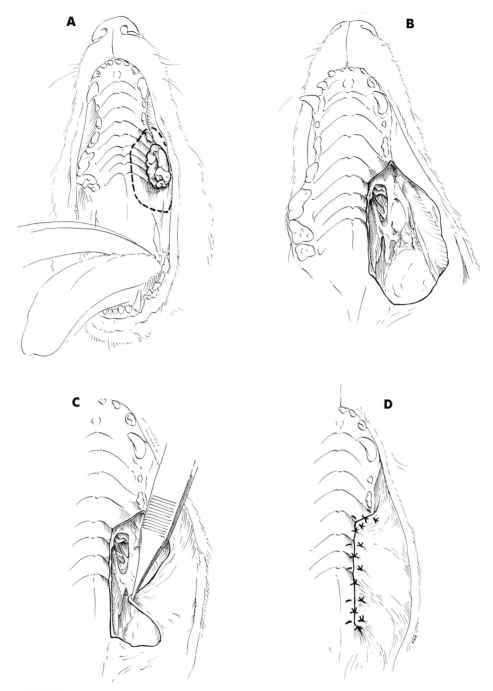

FIGURE 10-59
A, Proposed incisions for partial maxillectomy as treatment of an oral malignancy in a dog. **B,** Following en-bloc resection. **C,** Creation of the buccal-based flap. **D,** Closure of the oronasal defect.

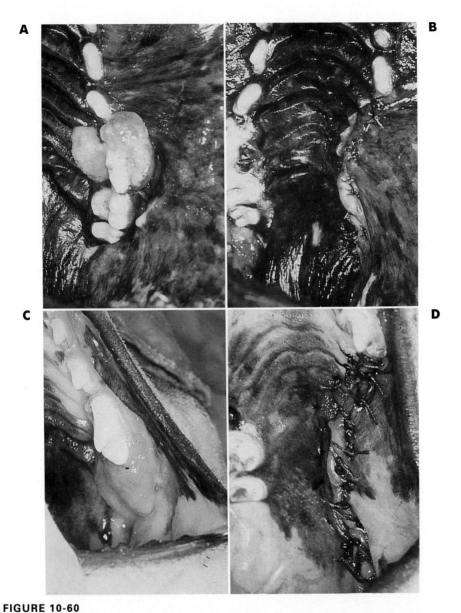

FIGURE 10-60
A, Acanthomatous epulis lesion treated by partial maxillectomy. **B,** There is a sharp corner to the flap at the rostral end. This flap dehisced a few days after surgery. **C** and **D,** Squamous cell carcinoma treated by partial maxillectomy with tapered ends to the flap; this flap did not dehisce.

rupted and vertical mattress sutures) ensures that connective tissue surfaces are in contact while apposing the epithelial cut edges (Fig. 10-59, *D*). Drains are not necessary. The connective tissue surface of the flap that faces the nasal cavity heals by granulation and epithelialization of the nasal mucosa. There is some nasal discharge for 3 to 4 weeks after surgery as the nasal tissues heal.

Occasionally the extent of the tumor requires resection of a substantial portion of the buccal mucosa of the upper lip. Tissue to close the oronasal defect can be obtained by rotating upper lip buccal mucosa from more rostral or caudal uninvolved areas, or the mucocutaneous junction of the lower lip is incised. The mucosal incised edge is closed to the palatal margin, and the skin of the upper lip is sutured to the skin of the lower lip. With the latter technique the lower jaw teeth may irritate or lacerate the transposed lower lip tissue. If this seems likely, it is best to extract the lower jaw teeth (the occluding teeth in the upper jaw having been removed as part of the maxilla en bloc resection).

Premaxillectomy—rostral maxillectomy

Premaxillectomy technique is similar to that for maxillectomy. If the procedure is entirely limited to the incisor teeth for resection of an invasive benign mass, typically an acanthomatous epulis, it may be possible to resect mucosa, gingiva, and bone containing the roots of several incisor teeth without entering the nasal cavity. In this case, no closure with a flap is necessary, and the tissue will granulate and epithelialize over 2 to 3 weeks. For malignant lesions the extent of resection must be deeper.

Most rostral oral resections for malignancy include part of the premaxilla (carries the incisor teeth) and the maxilla (carries the canine and premolar/molar teeth) (Fig. 10-61). If the resection includes the canine and incisor teeth and is closed with a flap (Fig. 10-61, *D*), the lower canine tooth may push up against the flap when the mouth is closed; this tooth should be shortened (see pulpotomy, Chapter 6) or extracted. If the resection includes the entire incisor tooth arch and one or both canine teeth, the ventral support for the nasal cartilages and planum nasale is lost. The snout droops when the mouth is open (Fig. 10-61, *E*); however, there is no functional problem.

The practical limits for resection are very wide. The entire dental arcade on one side, including the palate to the midline, can be resected and the defect closed with a unilateral buccal flap (Fig. 10-62). The entire palate and both entire dental arcades can be resected as one en bloc section, with closure by bilateral buccal flaps that meet in the midline (Fig. 10-63). For more caudally located lesions that extend onto the side of the face, the caudal maxilla, malar bone, and zygomatic arch can be resected. The parotid duct is identified by inserting a length of black monofilament suture material through the duct papilla. As long as the contents of Tenon's capsule and the skin and conjunctiva of the lower eye lid are intact, the eye will remain functional and in position even if there is no bone forming the ventral or lateral limits of the orbit. In cats the relatively small size of the skull and the short, tighter upper lip compared with that of dogs make radical maxillectomy more difficult (Fig. 10-64); bilateral surgery is possible.

Radical maxillectomy or premaxillectomy may result in loss of most of the ventrolateral external skeleton of the nose. If the width of the palatal resection and height of the maxillary resection combined will result in obstruction of nasal airflow when the soft tissue flap is closed across the defect, sections of nasal conchae can be resected with scissors to create free air space in the reformed nasal cavity before the buccal flap is sutured closed.

The animal may have pain during recovery from anesthesia, but dogs usually are able to eat without difficulty the following day. Cats may take several days to adapt and require syringe feeding into the cheek pouch during this time. Breakdown of the sutures holding the flap in place may occur 2 to 3 days after surgery, although this is uncommon with the use of the vertical mattress suture technique on tissues that are not under tension. If wound disruption does occur, the animal is reanesthetized and the flap is resutured after further undermining, if necessary, to eliminate tension on the suture line. Feeding the animal through a pharyngostomy or gastrostomy tube is of doubtful value in preventing dehiscence. Antibiotics are not necessary. To protect the flap while it heals, the animal should be fed a soft diet and prevented from chewing hard objects for the next several weeks.

Text continued on p. 362.

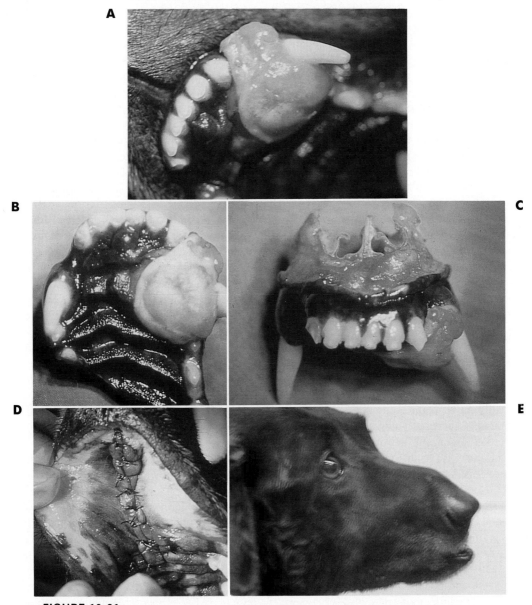

FIGURE 10-61
Premaxillectomy. **A,** Fibrosarcoma of the incisive-canine area of a dog. **B** and **C,** The surgical specimen includes the premaxilla, both canine teeth, and ventral third of the nasal septum. **D,** Surgical closure by bilateral labial flap. **E,** Drooping of the snout after surgery.

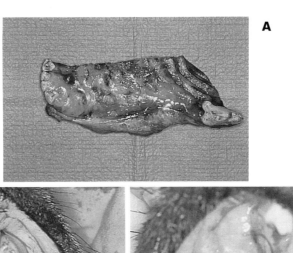

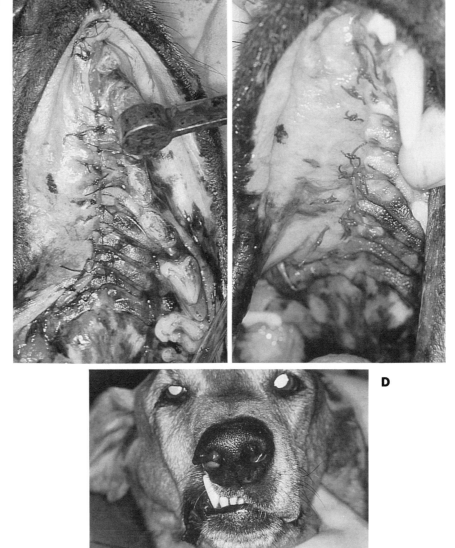

FIGURE 10-62
Fibrosarcoma of the maxilla of a dog. **A,** Surgical specimen includes the entire dental arch to beyond the midline. **B,** Surgical closure with a unilateral buccal-based flap. **C,** The flap is intact and healing 1 week later. **D,** The dog is eating and functioning well 1 week after surgery.

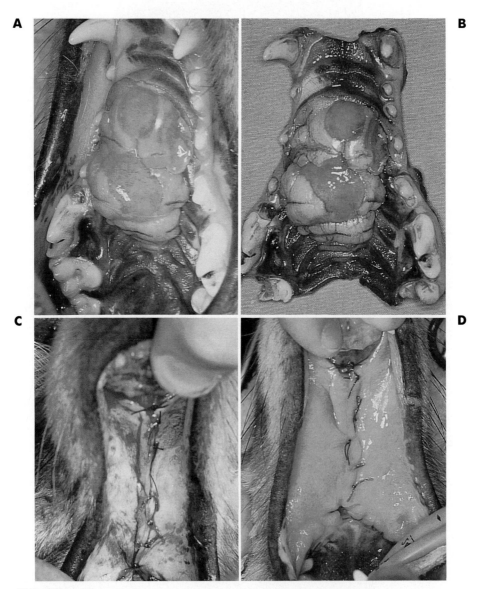

FIGURE 10-63
A, Midline fibrosarcoma on the hard palate of a dog. **B,** Surgical specimen. **C,** Double buccal flap closure. **D,** The flaps are intact and healing after 2 weeks.

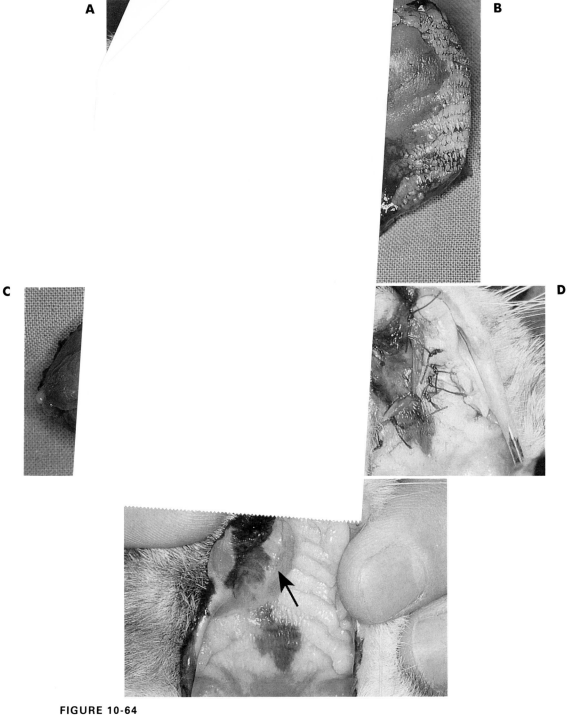

FIGURE 10-64
A, Fibrosarcoma of the palate in a cat. **B** and **C,** Surgical specimen. **D,** Closure by buccal flap. **E,** The flap healed, but recurrence of the tumor is evident *(arrow)* several months later due to inadequate surgical margins.

Dehiscence occurs most commonly when the surgical site is located caudal to the second premolar tooth. This is almost always due to tension disrupting the apposition of the two epithelial edges, most commonly as a result of poor flap design (Fig. 10-60).

The major complication is recurrence of disease. Long-term results are described in Table 9-3.

Mandibular Resection

It is possible to resect large sections of the mandible. The entire hemimandible often is resected (see discussion of hemimandibulectomy later in this section). For lesions at the rostral end of the mandible, part of the mandible can be resected bilaterally. Small lesions confined to the incisor area can be resected with a wide zone of surrounding grossly normal tissue,

A

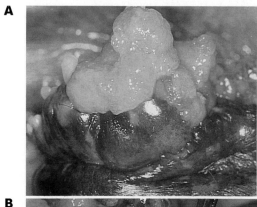

FIGURE 10-65
Rostral mandibulectomy. **A,** Acanthomatous epulis lesion. **B,** The cortex of the mandible at the resection has been burred through and the tumor section has been twisted to fracture remaining bony connections. This reveals the apex of the root of the canine tooth. **C,** Surgical specimen with intact canine tooth. **D,** Surgical site following resection. **E,** Following closure of lip to oral mucosa.

B   **C**

D   **E**

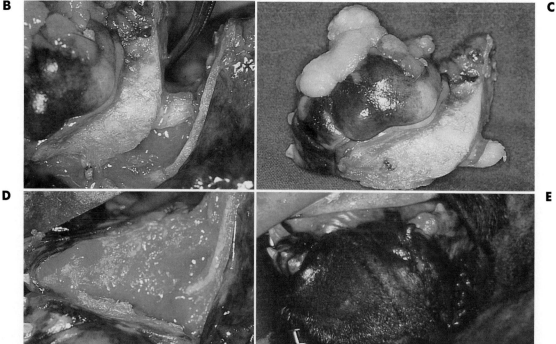

without losing the integrity of the symphysis. For lesions involving one or both canine teeth, the symphysis usually will be transected (Fig. 10-65).

Rostral mandibular resection

Unilateral rostral mandibular resection requires removal of incisor teeth and often a canine tooth. The resection should include all of the roots of any resected teeth, even if the root tip extends beyond the line of resection (Fig. 10-65). The labial mucosa is sutured to the sublingual mucosa; the awkward area during suturing is the rostral end of the incision, where the only tissue available is the incisive gingiva; the needle is pushed along the bone to obtain sufficient bite.

Resection of bilateral rostral mandibular sections to the level of the first premolar teeth provides good functional and acceptable esthetic results. Bilateral resections caudal to this level result in progressively greater problems with retention of the tongue, ability to eat, and ability to groom. The long-term results depend on the disease present (recurrence or distant metastasis of the neoplasm).

Resection of the full length of the symphysis causes the two remaining hemimandible sections to "float"; this is functionally and esthetically acceptable. It is possible to stabilize them, either by wiring the ends together in the hope of creating a "new" symphysis caudal to the original or by cross-pinning or cross-screwing the two hemimandibles. The first technique, creating a new symphysis, is not recommended because it causes the lower premolar and molar teeth to lie in a more medial position than normal, narrowing the mandibular arch and preventing the normal upper-lower arch occlusal relationship. The second technique—orthopedic stabilization with pins or screws—is not necessary and is contraindicated because of the likelihood of pin migration or development of infection around the screws as they inevitably loosen. With any procedure that requires placement of an orthopedic device in the jaws, there is a risk of impaling the roots of teeth and development of endodontic disease. It is possible to reconstruct the bony body of the mandible by means of an autogenous graft of rib that is wired to the mandibular bone at either end of the defect (see p. 333). This approach is rarely necessary.

Partial mandibular body resection

For lesions in the body of the mandible that arise from the dorsal (gingival) margin and that are not malignant but require more than simple excision level with the bone of the mandible (Fig. 10-66, *A*), resection of a dorsal segment is recommended. The lesion, including sufficient adjacent grossly normal tissue, is resected, including one or more teeth (Fig. 10-66, *B*). The gingiva, buccal, and sublingual mucosa are incised down to bone to delineate the area to be resected. The bone is then channeled along the resection lines with a dental bur in a water-cooled dental handpiece deep enough to reach close to the mandibular canal. With a rongeur or bone cutter, the segment is then levered until it cracks off the mandible. The surgeon should avoid jerking the piece away from the mandible entirely. The next step is to gently lift the segment to identify the mandibular artery as it crosses to the isolated segment. The artery is picked up with hemostats and transected. The segment is lifted out of the mouth, and the clamped ends of the artery in the remaining mandible are ligated (Fig. 10-66, *C*). Rough edges of bone are burred smooth (Fig. 10-66, *D*), and the buccal and sublingual mucosal edges are sutured across the remaining ventral strut of mandible.

Partial or segmental mandibular body resection has been described. This is generally an inadequate treatment for malignant disease and is not recommended here. Complete hemimandibulectomy (see following discussion) gives a much greater likelihood of resection of all areas of vascular invasion within bone, and it is functionally and esthetically acceptable.

Hemimandibulectomy

For lesions located anywhere in the body of the mandible, hemimandibulectomy can be performed. This procedure is well tolerated in dogs and cats, although cats usually take several days to adapt to the changed circumstances in their mouths before they are willing to eat normally. The fibrous symphysis is separated by bone cutters, scissors, or scalpel (Fig. 10-67, *A*). Incisions are made well away from the lesional tissue in the buccal and sublingual mucosa (Fig. 10-67, *B*), and the mandible is undermined by blunt dissection. The lateral attachments of the tongue (genio-

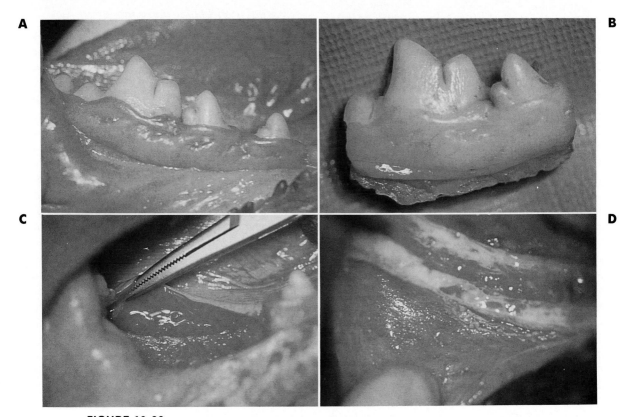

FIGURE 10-66
Resection of a dorsal section of the body of the mandible. **A,** Buccal gingival irregularity between the fourth premolar and first molar tooth is the site of a previously biopsied plasma cell tumor. **B,** Surgical specimen includes the dorsal two thirds of the mandible. **C,** The mandibular alveolar artery is clamped and ready to ligate. **D,** The mandibular canal is visible as a trough in the ventral third of the mandible.

glossus and hyoglossus muscles) are separated, leaving the mandibular and sublingual gland ducts intact if they can be identified. This frees the mandible so that it can be swung independently, which facilitates dissection of the masseter and pterygoid muscles from their attachments (Fig. 10-67, *C*). These muscles are reflected laterally and medially, exposing the vertical ramus of the mandible.

Exposed or incised vessels are ligated. The mandibular artery branches from the maxillary artery and enters the medullary canal of the mandible through a foramen located on the medial surface of the mandible

on an oblique line connecting the last molar tooth and the muscular process. The vessel is hidden beneath the rostral attachments of the pterygoid muscle, which must be dissected carefully to avoid transecting the vessel (Fig. 10-68). If the vessel is torn and bleeds, dissection into the pharyngeal tissues should be avoided because this approach may damage the hypoglossal nerve. First, the operator places a sponge firmly in the area of bleeding, then rotates the mandible medially to increase pressure on the area of the vessel while lateral attachments are dissected. After a few minutes the pharyngeal tissue is reexamined. If

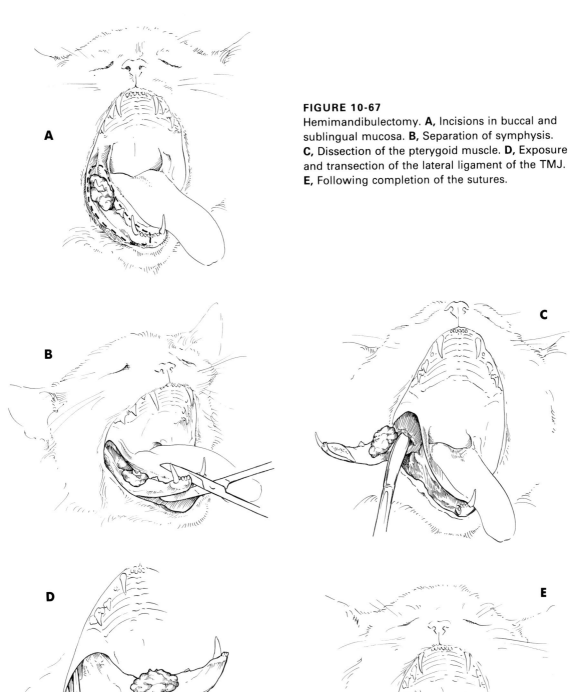

FIGURE 10-67

Hemimandibulectomy. **A,** Incisions in buccal and sublingual mucosa. **B,** Separation of symphysis. **C,** Dissection of the pterygoid muscle. **D,** Exposure and transection of the lateral ligament of the TMJ. **E,** Following completion of the sutures.

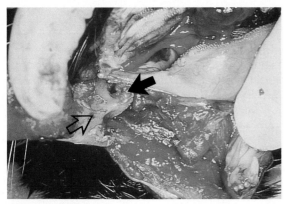

FIGURE 10-68
Hemimandibulectomy. The mandible is retracted laterally. The attachments of the pterygoid muscle have been dissected. The mandibular artery has been ligated and transected; the foramen housing the artery is shown *(open arrow)*. The medial end of the condylar process has been dissected *(closed arrow)*.

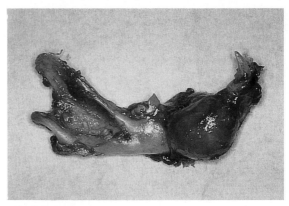

FIGURE 10-69
Hemimandibulectomy. Surgical specimen from a cat with squamous cell carcinoma.

there is still significant bleeding, the carotid artery is ligated on that side through an incision in the neck.

After the temporomandibular ligaments, particularly the thick lateral ligament, are exposed by rotating the mandible, they are incised (Figs. 10-67, *D*, and 10-68). The temporal muscle attachments on the rostral and dorsal edges of the coronoid process are dissected free with scissors that nibble against the bone, and the mandible is lifted out (Fig. 10-69). A drain can be placed in the cavity beneath the suture line, exiting through the skin. The incision is closed by absorbable sutures apposing the incised oral mucosal edges (Figs. 10-67, *E*, and 10-70). The opposite mandible will swing over toward the midline, which may result in the remaining mandibular canine tooth impinging on the palate when the mouth is closed; to prevent this, the tooth is extracted, or 2 to 3 mm of the crown is burred away without exposing the pulp cavity.

Commissuroplasty. The lip commissure on the involved side can be shortened to prevent constant lateral extrusion of the tongue in dogs. Commissu-

roplasty is performed by resecting the mucocutaneous junction tissue of the upper and lower lips to the level of the first premolar or canine teeth (Fig. 10-71). Then the mucosal incised edges of the upper and lower lips are sutured, followed by the incised edges of the skin of the upper and lower lips (Fig. 10-71, *B*, and *C*). Because the commissuroplasty may dehisce if the dog is allowed to open its mouth fully during the first 2 weeks of the healing period, a loose muzzle (Fig. 10-23) should be kept in place for 1 week after suture removal. Tension-relieving button sutures have been recommended; they are not necessary if a muzzle is used.

Coronoid process resection

Lesions of the coronoid process of the ramus of the mandible can be resected by an approach through the zygomatic arch and the masseter muscle. The periosteum of the zygoma is incised and reflected (Fig. 10-72, *A*, and *B*); full-thickness resection of the zygoma is performed with a dental bur, osteotome, or rongeur (Fig. 10-72, *C*). The temporal, masseter, and pterygoid muscles are reflected from the coronoid process (Fig. 10-72, *D*), which can then be partially or completely removed with a dental bur, rongeur, or osteotome (Fig. 10-72, *E*). The incision is closed by apposing the periosteum of the zygomatic arch and

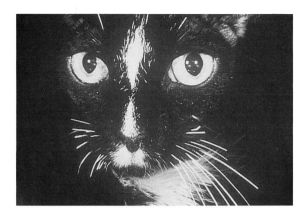

FIGURE 10-70
Head of a cat several weeks after hemimandibulectomy for squamous cell carcinoma. This cat lived for
3 more years, eating and grooming well, before
dying of renal failure.

A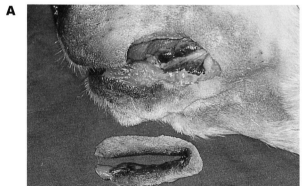

FIGURE 10-71
Commissuroplasty. **A,** Resection of the mucocutaneous junction to the level of the first premolar
tooth. **B,** Completion of closure of the mucosal layer.
C, Completion of skin closure.

B 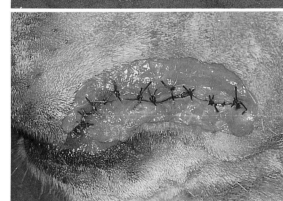   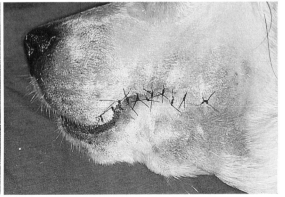 **C**

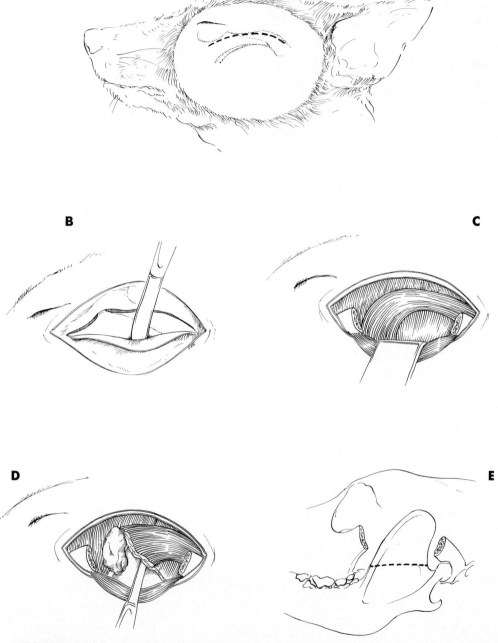

FIGURE 10-72
Zygomatic arch and coronoid process surgery. **A,** Incision over the zygomatic arch. **B,** Reflection of the zygomatic periosteum. **C,** After resection of the zygoma, the temporal muscles cover the coronoid process. **D,** Dissection of the temporal muscles to reveal the coronoid process. **E,** Extent of resection of the coronoid process.

the orbital fascia. Even with very extensive dissection and resection, surgical drainage and antibiotic therapy usually are not necessary.

Results of mandibular resection procedures

Table 9-3 summarizes the results of mandibulectomies in several large series of cases in dogs and cats. Almost all these animals were able to eat and drink satisfactorily. Dehiscence of the lip commissuroplasty incision occurred in one dog. Drooling and grooming abnormalities were present in some animals but were not severe enough to result in euthanasia.

▶ MISCELLANEOUS ORAL SURGICAL PROCEDURES

Tongue

Management of traumatic tongue injuries is described on p. 336.

Congenital anomalies

Macroglossia (grossly enlarged tongue) has been treated by resection of the rostral section of the tongue, with good clinical results. Many brachycephalic dogs have tongues that seem grossly long compared with their jaw length, although they have good control of function and the tongue does not become traumatized from exposure. A short frenulum in a dog, which caused difficulty in eating and drinking, was treated successfully by incising the frenulum for 2 cm.

Mass lesions

Tongue masses can be resected with good results if the resection can be confined to the free rostral portion or the dorsocaudal portion. Protuberant, ulcerated lesions on the tongue should be examined by biopsy before resection (or before euthanasia if the lesion appears to be too extensive for surgery or radiation therapy). Eosinophilic granuloma of the tongue, which can be treated medically with good results (see Chapter 5), appears similar to an invading neoplasm in some cats and dogs. Surgical resection of part of the tongue is likely to result in significant hemorrhaging; thus electrosurgery is useful. Ideally, tongue tissue is removed as a wedge so that the mucosa

can be apposed with synthetic absorbable sutures. The wedge technique can be used to remove lesions from the dorsal part of the root of the tongue. Neoplastic lesions such as squamous cell carcinoma in cats that are deep in the root of the tongue or that cause the tongue to be tied down to the adjacent soft tissues are not amenable to resection in veterinary patients. Tongue neoplasms are described further in Chapter 9.

Lips and Cheeks

Management of injuries of the lips and cheeks is described on p. 336.

Congenital abnormalities

Harelip. The most obvious congenital abnormality that affects the lips is harelip, in which the two sides of the primary palate fail to fuse normally. This condition is sporadically seen in a wide variety of breeds and probably is caused by intrauterine trauma or stress rather than by a genetic defect, although affected puppies have been born to affected parents. When the harelip is unilateral in dogs, it is almost always on the left side, as is also the case in affected children.

Treatment is by reconstruction of the lip (Fig. 10-73). Attempts to close the defect by simple sliding skin procedures rarely are successful because there is no connective tissue bed to support the flap. The floor of the nasal vestibule must be reformed by creating flaps of oral and nasal tissue that are sutured with synthetic absorbable sutures. It is often necessary to remove one or more incisor teeth that would otherwise erupt into or through the repair (Fig. 10-73, *B*, and *C*). The skin is closed over the defect by forming overlapping flaps on either side; absorbable subcutaneous sutures are then placed. The philtrum (the midline crease between the lips) should be preserved or reformed as symmetrically as possible (Fig. 10-73, *D*).

Results depend on the care that is taken to form the flaps with minimal tension and accurate apposition of epithelial edges, resulting in minimal distortion of the lip edge. Surgery of this type can be performed at any age, although the anesthesia risk suggests delaying the procedure until the animal is several months old; delayed surgery for harelip without secondary

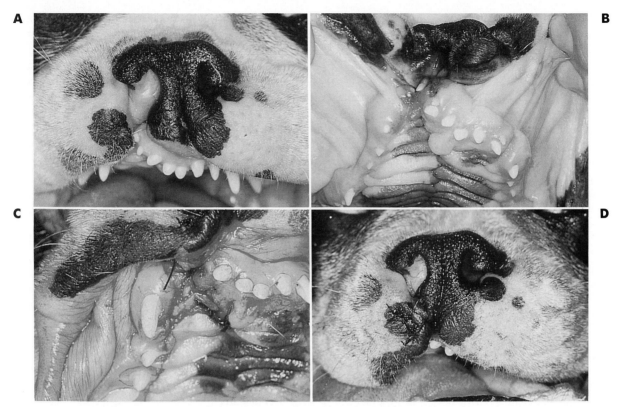

FIGURE 10-73
Harelip in a dog. **A,** Before surgery, facial view. **B,** Oral view, showing incisor teeth facing into the defect. **C,** Following surgical closure of the oral defect. **D,** Following reformation of the philtrum.

cleft palate is not a problem because airway aspiration is not a complication. If a cleft of the secondary palate is also present, additional surgery is indicated (see p. 340).

Lip-fold dermatitis. The most frequent congenital abnormality that affects the lips and cheeks is the abnormal lip-fold conformation seen in some dogs, particularly spaniels. The indentation of the lips forms a channel that causes saliva to flow onto the skin of the lip. The result is a foul-smelling chronic, moist dermatitis. Diagnosis is by inspection of the lips (see Fig. A-47, p. 60). The major differential diagnosis is halitosis caused by periodontal disease or uremia, or

both, which may coexist. Conservative treatment (frequently washing the lip-fold area with chlorhexidine solution, followed by application of a corticosteroid ointment) may be helpful; however for severe cases, surgery is much more successful. Treatment is by resection of the folds, making a V-shaped incision through the skin and mucosa (Fig. 10-74, *C*). The two layers (mucosa and skin) are sutured separately (Fig. 10-74, *D*). Results usually are excellent. Most affected dogs require treatment of both sides.

Drooping lip in giant-breed dogs. Giant-breed dogs with heavy pendulous lower lips that predispose the animal to drooling can be treated by bilateral man-

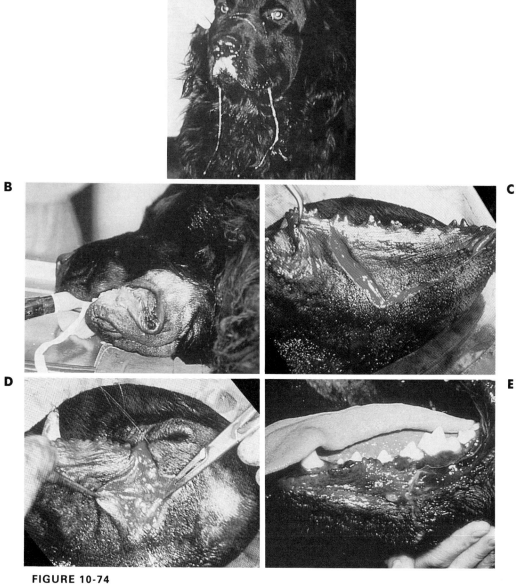

FIGURE 10-74
A, Giant-breed dog with ropes of saliva hanging from the mouth. **B,** The lip fold before surgery. **C,** Skin and mucosal incisions. **D,** Closure. **E,** Healing of the mucosal incision at the time of suture removal.

dibulosublingual duct ligation through a small incision in the sublingual mucosa, combined with resection of part of the lower lips (as already described for lip-fold dermatitis; Fig. 10-74).

A more involved form of cheiloplasty has been described for this condition; a flap of the lower lip is isolated and is sutured to a defect created in the upper lip, forming a sling that channels the saliva back into the oral cavity. Both techniques result in significant reduction in the esthetic problem created by this condition (Fig. 10-74, E).

Tight lip in Shar-pei dogs. Shar-pei dogs often have very tight lower lips, referred to by breeders as "meat mouth." They have little or no depth to the lower rostral mucolabial fold (vestibule). This results in the lower lip extending up over the incisal edge of the lower incisor teeth, causing malocclusion and difficulty in mastication.

Many surgical methods of tight lip correction have been employed, such as removal of a wedge of lower lip or removal of lip and a portion of the mandible. The most successful to date is vestibuloplasty, which is designed to increase the depth of the vestibule, allowing the lower lip to swing free of the incisor teeth.

Vestibuloplasty. General anesthesia is administered, and the dog's head is suspended by a rope loop located caudal to the upper canines. This allows the mandible to be available at unobstructed eye level for the operator.

The incision is begun caudal to the frenulum that is present just caudal to the lower canine teeth (Fig. 10-75, A). A complete deep frenectomy is performed, avoiding the mental artery that exits from the mental foramen deep to the frenulum. The incision is carried around to the opposing frenulum where the same procedure is performed (Fig. 10-75, B). The ventral extent of the labial incision is almost to the ventral border of the mandible, with careful dissection of the underlying mucosa (Fig. 10-75, B).

Once the lip has been fully dissected, a sharp No. 15 or No. 11 scalpel blade is used to fenestrate or scarify the periosteum at the ventral border of the releasing flap by firmly directing the blade at right angles to the mandible in multiple cuts. This fenestration will prevent subsequent creeping of the at-

tachment beyond the fenestration to its original position.

The lateral ventral border of the mucosal flap is sutured down and back on itself to the underlying tissues at four to six sites. The frenulum incisions are sutured in like manner down and back (Fig. 10-75, C).

On completion the lip will appear to dip ventrally at an alarming angle (Fig. 10-75, D), which is the desired result. To avoid alarm the client should be told before surgery what to expect. The dog is fed soft food for 1 week. Suture removal is not necessary for this procedure.

Neoplastic and hyperplastic lesions of the lips

The principles of surgical management for lip and cheek lesions include (1) biopsy of all lesions suspected of being malignant, (2) wide excision of known malignant lesions (Fig. 10-76), (3) maintenance of a functional commissure so that the mouth can open (which may require lengthening of the commissure or use of rotation flaps), (4) separate closure of the incisions in the mucosa and the skin when the resection is full thickness, and (5) avoidance of the parotid salivary duct when possible or ligation or transposition when avoidance is not possible. By rotating tissue from the side of the face or lower lip, it is possible to close successfully very large lip defects.

Severe Chronic Maxillary or Mandibular Osteomyelitis

Fortunately, generalized maxillary or mandibular osteomyelitis is uncommon. This condition usually results from chronic periodontitis. Large areas of necrotic bone, with reactive new bone surrounding it, are seen on examination of the mouth. The maxilla or mandible may be grossly swollen. Nasal discharge is not common. Medical treatment of osteomyelitis in this location is often unavailing, although drugs that are particularly effective against the spectrum of bacteria associated with severe periodontitis, such as amoxicillin–clavulanate, clindamycin, tetracycline, or metronidazole, should be tried before resorting to radical surgery. Conservative surgical treatment, such as limited curettage of obviously necrotic bone, fol-

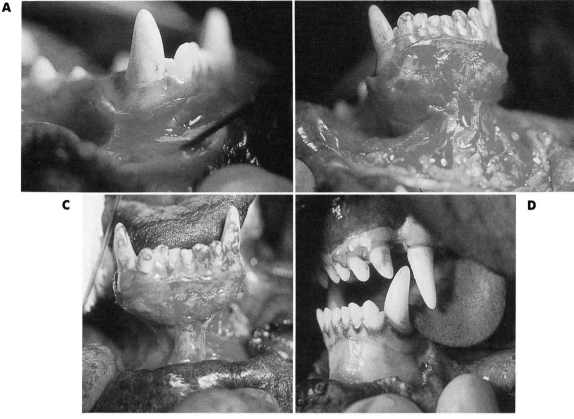

FIGURE 10-75
Vestibuloplasty in a Shar-pei dog with meat mouth. **A,** Initial incision in the lower lip. **B,** Vestibuloplasty incision is continued around to the opposite side and to the ventral aspect of the mandible. **C,** The mucosa is sutured laterally in a more ventral location. **D,** Appearance 2 months after surgery.

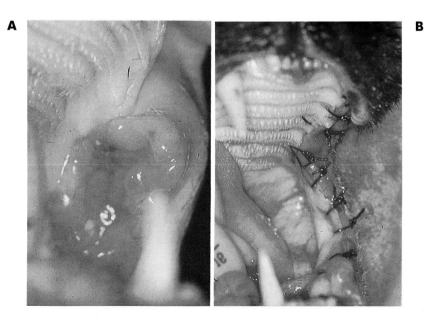

FIGURE 10-76
Resection of a lip mass.
A, Fibrosarcoma of the upper lip of a cat. **B,** Following lip resection and partial maxillectomy, the lip commissure has been extended caudally.

lowed by a prolonged course of antibiotics, usually is successful only temporarily. Radical resection of affected tissue back to normal bone is much more likely to cure the condition.

Temporomandibular Joint
Conditions and Surgery

Temporomandibular joint (TMJ) abnormalities occur in cats and less often in dogs, usually as a result of trauma. Fractures of this area can be very difficult to define clearly on radiographs. Fractures that affect the articular condyle may not heal in an acceptable position and may cause long-term dysphagia; treatment is condylectomy (see p. 376). Although theoretically it is possible to reconstruct the TMJ by osteoplasty or by insertion of a biocompatible cushion between the condyloid process of the mandible and the mandibular fossa of the temporal bone, such procedures rarely are performed in dogs and cats. One reason is that the TMJ is in a difficult-to-reach location, protected by the caudal end of the zygomatic arch; it is impossible to reach the medial end of the condyloid process or joint space without sacrificing or damaging the lateral end (Fig. 10-77). The second reason is that condylectomy is a practical procedure, with excellent long-term cosmetic and functional results in dogs and cats.

Joint luxation

Traumatic luxation occurs in cats and occasionally in dogs. Luxation usually is in a rostrodorsal direction, causing rostromedial displacement of the mandible on that side and preventing full closure of the mouth because the canine teeth on the opposite side hit against each other (Fig. 10-78, *A* and *B*). Luxation is treated by closing the animal's jaws together while a wood or plastic rod separates the upper and lower carnassial teeth on the side involved (Fig. 10-78, *C*), then pushing the involved mandible caudally until the condylar process slips back into place (Fig. 10-78, *D*). For the less common caudal luxation, reduction is obtained by forcing the mandible rostrally while the carnassial teeth are held separated, then releasing the mandible.

Dysplasia

Clinical signs and diagnosis of TMJ dysplasia are described in Chapter 3.

Treatment of recurrent jaw-locking episodes (Fig. 10-79) is by surgical resection of a section of the zygomatic arch (see p. 366), by resection of a dorsal section of the coronoid process (see p. 366), or by condylectomy. These techniques all provide good long-term results. The simplest and quickest to per-

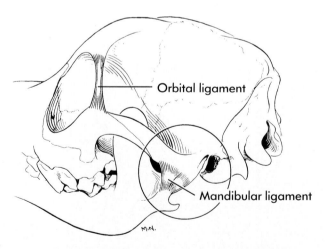

FIGURE 10-77
Location of the mandibular ligament and condylar process of the TMJ beneath the zygomatic arch. *(From Evans HE: Miller's anatomy of the dog, ed 3, Philadelphia, 1993, WB Saunders.)*

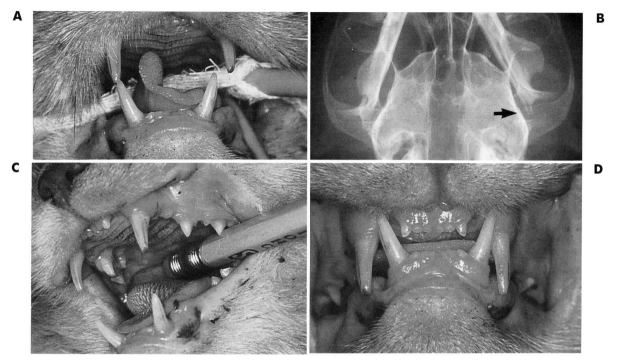

FIGURE 10-78
Temporomandibular joint luxation in a cat. **A,** Malocclusion of the canine teeth resulting from the luxation. **B,** Ventrodorsal radiograph shows increased TMJ space on the luxated side *(arrow).* **C,** Use of a pencil to provide a fulcrum during reduction of the luxation. **D,** Normal occlusion restored.

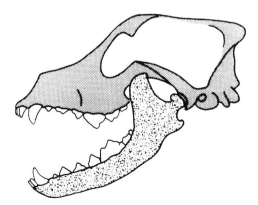

FIGURE 10-79
Diagram showing the locking of the tip of the coronoid process outside the zygoma in a dog with temporomandibular joint dysplasia.

form is resection of the zygoma, taking a section of about 2 cm on either side of the point where the coronoid process hits the zygoma.

Condylectomy

Fractures of the TMJ area and chronic luxations that have resulted in ankylosis or pain in the joint can be treated by mandibular condylectomy. The articular condyle is approached through an incision in the masseter muscle ventral to and at the caudal end of the zygomatic arch (Fig. 10-77). The parotid duct and buccal branches of the facial nerve, which run parallel to the horizontal ramus of the mandible, are identified and avoided. The strong lateral ligament of the TMJ is severed, and the articular condyle is resected with rongeurs. The articular disk can be left in place if intact and uninjured or removed with rongeurs or a curet. The masseter muscle aponeurosis and subcutaneous and skin tissues are sutured. Unilateral and bilateral condylectomy causes minor, temporary, and functionally unimportant changes in occlusion. Long-term clinical results are excellent.

Mandibular Symphysiotomy

Surgical access to the caudal oral cavity and pharynx can be enhanced by mandibular symphysiotomy.

The mandible and cranial neck area is prepared for surgery. A midventral skin incision is made from the basihyoid bone to the tip of the mandible. The mylohyoid muscle is incised, separated, and reflected. The mandible is exposed, and the symphysis is split with a scalpel. The mandibles are spread to tense the genioglossus muscle as it is incised about 1 cm from the midline. The sublingual mucosa is incised lateral to the salivary ducts. The mandibles can then be spread maximally, and the tongue is retracted caudally to expose the pharynx.

Closure is effected by suturing the oral mucosa and the genioglossus and mylohyoid muscles with absorbable suture material. The mandibular symphysis is closed with an encircling wire. There is little postoperative discomfort or interference with prehension or swallowing.

▶ SUGGESTED READINGS

References for mass resection surgery, including long-term results, are included in the list of Suggested Readings at the end of Chapter 9.

Beattie IEJ: Treatment of dislocated feline mandible, *Vet Rec* 11:493, 1982.

Bennett D, Prymak C: Excision arthroplasty as a treatment for temporomandibular dysplasia, *J Small Anim Pract* 27:361, 1986.

Blogg R: Exodontia in the dog, *Aust Vet J* 39:57, 1963.

Bone RC et al: Mandibular trauma: secondary problems in reconstruction. Paper presented at the seventy-ninth annual meeting of the American Laryngological, Rhinological and Otological Society, Inc, April 1976.

Boulton J: Dental flap operation for tooth extraction, *Can Vet J* 1:167, 1960.

Campbell JR, Nixon GS: Metal implant in the hard palate of a dog, *J Small Anim Pract* 6:255, 1965.

Counsell M et al: Mandibular osteotomy repair using high density polyethylene plates, *JAAHA* 21:685, 1985.

Currey JR: Canine exodontia. Proceedings of the Annual Meeting of the American Veterinary Medical Association, p 178, 1963.

Ellison GW et al: A double reposition flap technique for repair of recurrent oronasal fistulas in dogs, *JAAHA* 22:803, 1986.

Harvey CE: Palate defects in dogs and cats, *Compendium Small Anim* 9:403, 1987.

Harvey CE: Tooth extraction in dogs and cats, *Compendium Small Anim* 10:175, 1988.

Hoppe F, Svalastoga E: Temporomandibular dysplasia in American cocker spaniels, *J Small Anim Pract* 21:675, 1980.

Huebsch RF, Hansen LS: A histopathologic study of extraction wounds in dogs, *Oral Surg Oral Med Oral Pathol* 28:187, 1969.

Huebsch RF, Kennedy DR: Healing of dog mandibles following surgical loss of continuity, *Oral Surg Oral Med Oral Pathol* 29:178, 1970.

Johnson KA: Temporomandibular joint dysplasia in an Irish setter, *J Small Anim Pract* 20:209, 1979.

Jones RS, Thordal-Christensen A: Extraction of the upper carnassial tooth in the dog, *Mod Vet Pract* 43:68, 1962.

Kangur TT et al: The use of methylmethacrylate in the fixation of mandibular fractures in dogs: experimental results, *Oral Surg Oral Med Oral Pathol* 41:578, 1976.

Kirby BM et al: Surgical repair of a cleft lip in a dog, *JAAHA* 24:683, 1988.

Lane JG: Disorders of the canine temporomandibular joint, *Vet Ann* 22:175, 1982.

Lantz GC: Temporomandibular joint ankylosis: surgical correction of three cases, *JAAHA* 21:173, 1985.

Lantz GC et al: Unilateral mandibular condylectomy: experimental and clinical results, *JAAHA* 18:883, 1982.

McOwen JS: Intraoral dental acrylic splint for mandibular fracture: a case report, *Companion Anim Pract* 1:17, 1987.

Merkley DF, Brinker WA: Facial reconstruction following massive bilateral maxillary fracture in the dog, *JAAHA* 12:831, 1976.

Mumaw ED, Miller AS: The application of a frequency oscillation method for tooth extraction in dogs, *Lab Anim Sci* 25:228, 1975.

Nunamaker DM: Mandibular fractures. In Newton CD, Nunamaker DM, editors: *Textbook of small animal orthopedics*, Philadelphia, 1985, JB Lippincott Co.

Obialski M et al: Fallbericht: eine operative Variante zur Beseitigung einer angeborenen Gaumenspalte bei einem Rottweiler-welpen, *Kleintierpraxis* 33:43, 1988.

Peddie JF: Extraction of a dog's carnassial tooth, *Mod Vet Pract* 62:129, 1981.

Plata RL, Kelln EE: Intentional retention of vital submerged roots in dogs, *Oral Surg Oral Med Oral Pathol* 42:100, 1976.

Richman S, Schunick W: Flap operation for removal of the canine tooth. In La Croix JV, Hoskins HP, editors: *Canine surgery*, Evanston, Ill, 1939, North American Veterinarian.

Robertson JJ, Dean PW: Repair of a traumatically induced oronasal fistula in a cat with a rostral tongue flap, *Vet Surg* 16:164, 1987.

Robins G, Grandage J: Temporomandibular joint dysplasia and open-mouth jaw locking in the dog, *JAVMA* 171:1072, 1977.

Roush JK, Wilson JW: Healing of mandibular body osteotomies after plate and intramedullary pin fixation, *Vet Surg* 18:190, 1989.

Salisbury SK, Richardson DC: Partial maxillectomy for oronasal fistula repair in the dog, *JAAHA* 22:185, 1986.

Stewart WC et al: Temporomandibular subluxation in the dog. A case report, *J Small Anim Pract* 16:345, 1975.

Thomas RE: Temporo-mandibular joint dysplasia and open-mouth jaw locking in a basset hound: a case report, *J Small Anim Pract* 20:697, 1979.

Ticer JW, Spencer JW: Feline temporomandibular joint injury, *J Am Vet Radiol Soc* 19:1121, 1978.

Ticer JW, Spencer JW: Injury of the feline temporomandibular joint: radiographic signs, *Vet Radiol* 19:146, 1978.

Tomlinson J, Presnell KR: Mandibular condylectomy: effects in normal dogs, *Vet Surg* 12:148, 1983.

Verstraete FJM: Instrumentation and technique of removal of permanent teeth in the dog, *J S Afr Vet Assoc* 54:231, 1983.

Zetner K: Treatment of jaw fractures in small animals with parapulpar pin composite bridges, *Vet Clin North Am, Small Anim Pract* 22:1461, 1992.

11

Small Animal Dental Equipment and Materials

As a result of a rapidly evolving and enlarging supply of dental equipment and materials, the veterinary dentist is faced with a daunting and confusing array of choices. With time and experience, he or she will select those materials and instruments that best fit the needs. This chapter lists and briefly describes dental equipment and materials that have been found to be effective for the veterinary dental procedures described in this book. Each item is followed by a number in [brackets], which is the item number in the Henry Schein veterinary and dental supplies catalog.* These or similar items also are available from other suppliers.

A general description of the use of hand and power dental instruments is provided (see pp. 381, 382, 393, and 394). The use of specific equipment and material is described in the earlier chapters.

▶ POWER EQUIPMENT AND ACCESSORIES

Power equipment is necessary to perform many dental procedures; all dental disciplines make use of power equipment in some form.

*Available from Henry Schein, Inc., 5 Harbor Park Dr., Port Washington, NY 11050; telephone: 1-800-V-SCHEIN.

Power Units

Dental units that drive the dental burs, prophylaxis handpieces, finishing disks, and other units are driven by either electrical power or air power.

Electrically driven units

Electric engine dental units are constantly being improved in their efficiency and revolutions per minute (rpm). They employ a micromotor in the handpiece to drive the burs or disks. Although they are less expensive than air-driven units, the most common electrically driven units operate at a maximum of 30,000 rpm [100-2878] (Fig. 11-1). These units tend to vibrate to some extent, making highly accurate work more difficult; the bur tends to "walk off" the tooth surface. Irrigation must be from an external source, such as an irrigating syringe during operation on vital teeth or sectioning bone. Newer electrical units are capable of 100,000 rpm and have the added advantage that they produce substantially more torque than air units. Torque (for a dental engine, the ability to continue to rotate the bur while the working tip is pressed against a firm surface) is a mixed blessing; the work may proceed more quickly, but more heat is produced.

Some inexpensive electrical engines drive the dental handpiece through a system of pulleys and a belt rather than a power motor located in the handpiece

378

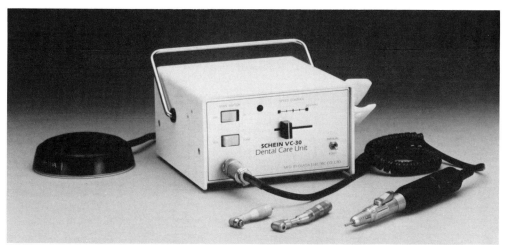

FIGURE 11-1
Electrically driven dental engine and handpiece micromotor, shown with foot pedal, prophylaxis angle, and contraangle.

(Fig. 11-2). They have substantial torque but operate at a maximum of only 10,000 to 15,000 rpm. These units are excellent if their use is limited to dental polishing and sectioning of teeth to be extracted. Care must be exercised with these belt-driven units to avoid trapping hair from the dog or cat in the moving belt.

Air-driven dental units

Air units drive a dental handpiece through high-pressure air from a compressor mounted on or distant from the unit. The compressed air is directed to an air turbine in the head of the handpiece ([100-5723 or 100-0603] (Fig. 11-3). Although the turbine can produce up to 300,000 to 400,000 rpm, this is not a true measure of tooth- or bone-cutting ability. The air units produce very little torque; consequently revolutions per minute are reduced to closer to 100,000 when the tooth surface is contacted. Air-driven units require a much lighter touch than do high-torque units. They are much easier to control, however, and the bur does not tend to walk off of the tooth surface when cutting into the tooth.

Air-driven units usually are equipped with water irrigation that is directed to the tip of the high-speed bur. They typically include a high-speed handpiece, a low-speed handpiece, and an air-water syringe (Fig.

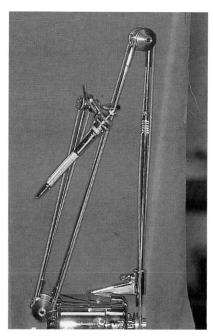

FIGURE 11-2
Electric belt-driven engine ("bench engine").

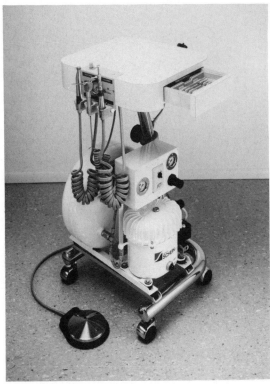

FIGURE 11-3
Air-driven dental engine and handpiece system. High-speed, low-speed handpieces and air-water syringe are attached to the base unit, which also has an instrument drawer and work surface.

11-3). Air-driven units generally are more expensive; however, they are preferred, enabling the clinician to produce the best results with minimal difficulties.

Water-cooled dental engines produce an aerosol of potentially contaminated water droplets and can result in high-speed spread of tooth or bone particles or of disintegrating metal bur or disk parts; eye and face mask protection is recommended (see Use of Power Instruments in next section).

Dental Handpieces

Dental handpieces are available in high or low speeds and are used for different functions.

High-speed handpieces

High-speed handpieces are those capable of more than 70,000 to 80,000 rpm [100-2231 or 100-1922] (Fig. 11-4). They usually are air driven, but the newer electrical handpieces are capable of high speed. The high-speed handpiece is used for tooth reduction, tooth entry, restorative procedures, and oral surgery. A fiberoptic light can be fitted in some high-speed handpieces to illuminate the cutting area [100-1922]. Miniature-head, high-speed handpieces [100-7111] are useful for limited access procedures, such as surgical endodontics.

High-speed burs are held in the handpiece by a friction-grip mechanism in the turbine head (Fig. 11-4, *A*). These burs are referred to as *friction-grip (FG) burs*. This form of bur retention provides stability, efficiency, and accuracy.

Low-speed handpieces

Low-speed handpieces are air driven through the same outlet as the high-speed handpiece, or they are electrically driven [100-6708] (Figs. 11-3 and 11-4, *B*). The principal difference is that the low-speed handpiece uses a turbine gear-reduction system to reduce the speed compared with the turbine high-speed handpiece. This makes the low-speed handpiece more expensive than the high-speed handpiece. Low-speed handpieces usually use loosely retained larger-shanked burs with a latching groove at the end of the shank; these burs are known as right angle (RA) burs. Slow-speed contraangles that use FG burs are available. Electrically driven units, which have the advantage of speed control from very low (1000 rpm) to high speed with the same handpiece, permit attachment of contraangles. Because some air-driven low-speed and most electrical units lack integral water cooling, they require an external flow of water or saline over the operating tip when operating on vital teeth or bone.

Low-speed handpieces may be used as a straight handpiece, or a contraangle or prophylaxis-angle attachment can be set into the straight handpiece. The straight handpiece accepts straight, long-shanked burs and mandrels (Fig. 11-4). These long burs are available as dental or surgical burs. The mandrel accepts

A

B

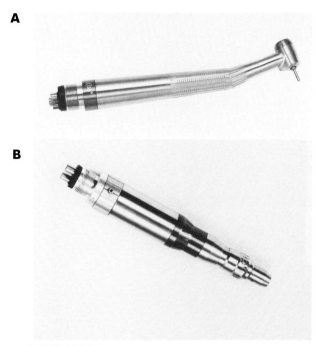

FIGURE 11-4
A, High-speed (turbine) handpiece. **B,** Low-speed dental handpiece.

A

B

C

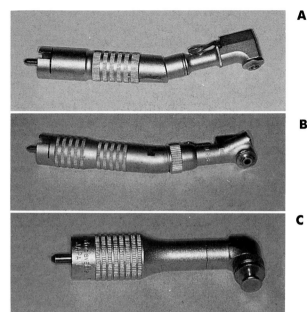

FIGURE 11-5
Low-speed dental handpiece accessories. **A,** Contraangle. **B,** Reduction gear contraangle. **C,** Prophylaxis angle.

sanding disks, mounted finishing stones, and diamond disks. The shaft of these burs and other accessories is designated HP (handpiece type).

The contraangle attachment [100-8643] (Fig. 11-5, *A*) fits onto the straight handpiece to form two angles: a 15-degree initial angle and a 90-degree angle at the working end. It redirects the working tip to 65 degrees to the horizontal, improving access to the more difficult-to-reach areas of the mouth. Latch (RA) or FG types of burs are available for use in the contraangle (although the same contraangle cannot accept both). The low speed, which is used mainly for finishing and sanding restorations, can be used for general restorative procedures. Reduction-gear (typically 10:1) contraangles (Fig. 11-5, *B*), are used with lentulo spiral root canal fillers or with drill pieces for dentinal pins.

The prophylaxis angle attaches directly onto the straight handpiece and is used with a rubber prophylaxis cup for dental polishing [100-2652] (Fig. 11-5, *C*). The prophylaxis cup is attached at a 90-degree angle to the long axis of the prophylaxis angle. Prophylaxis paste [100-7869] is placed in the prophylaxis cup [100-6461] and rotated at up to 3000 rpm (Fig. 11-6; see also p. 133). Prophylaxis angles and cups are available in two types: screw-in or snap-on button (Fig. 11-6). A to-and-fro action prophylaxis angle also is available [100-2280], which reduces the likelihood of entanglement of lip hair but is more expensive than the rotating prophylaxis angle.

Use of Power Instruments

The potential for creating trauma with power rotating instruments is very high if they are not used

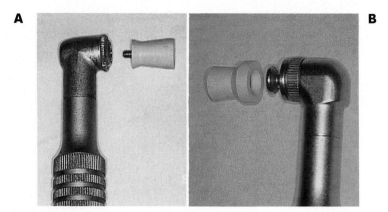

FIGURE 11-6
Working end of a prophylaxis angle and prophylaxis cup. **A,** Screw-in pattern. **B,** Snap-on button pattern.

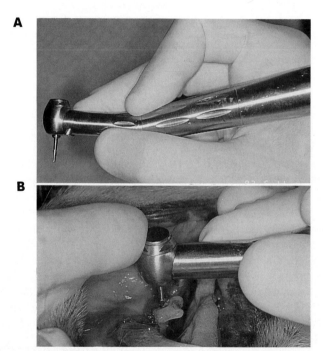

FIGURE 11-7
Using a dental handpiece. **A,** "Pen grasp" used to hold a handpiece near the working tip. **B,** Two-hand control of a dental handpiece.

correctly. The following criteria are suggested in the use of dental power instruments.

1. Select the correct bur or other tip to be used.
2. Discard cutting burs that start to lose their effectiveness.
3. Correct hand position: hold the handpiece as you would a pen, and rest the ring and little fingers against a convenient tooth or bone surface (Fig. 11-7, *A*). To provide additional control and support, rest the wrist on a convenient surface and also use the fingers of the other hand (Fig. 11-7, *B*).
4. Protect adjacent soft tissue, hair, and other areas by retracting them. A hair-dressing clip works very well for long-haired dogs to prevent entanglement of lip hair in the rotating handpiece.
5. Follow the manufacturer's recommendations for cleaning, lubrication, and care.
6. Protect the operator and other persons in the vicinity; provide eye safety glasses and face masks.

Burs

Dental burs are available in many shapes, sizes, and functions. The bur heads are mounted on three types of shank: straight handpiece (HP), latch (RA), and friction-grip (FG) (Fig. 11-8). The type of bur head chosen depends on the type of cut required. FG burs provide the greatest variety of cutting heads available (Table 11-1); however, the handpiece that is available determines what type of shank must be selected.

Long straight shank (HP) burs fit directly into the straight low-speed handpiece (Fig. 11-4, *B*), providing a straight-line cutting angle. The burs are 40 mm long, or longer, in surgical length and bur head configuration.

Latch-type (RA) burs are usually 20 mm in length and are designed to fit the RA slow-speed contraangle attachment. They are retained in the contraangle by a latch in the contraangle head that fits into a groove on the shank at the noncutting end of the bur (Fig. 11-9). This allows the bur some lateral movement, causing it to wobble slightly.

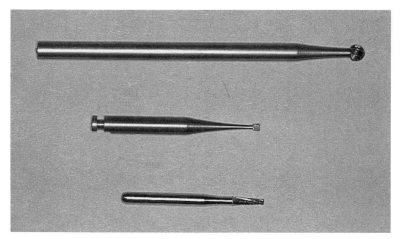

FIGURE 11-8
Dental burs, shank types. *Top,* Long HP bur for use in straight, low-speed handpiece. *Middle,* Latch (RA) bur for use in RA low-speed contraangle handpiece attachment. *Bottom,* Friction-grip (FG) bur for use in high-speed turbine handpiece (or FG contraangle attachment).

TABLE 11-1 Burs and other handpiece accessories*

Size no.	Friction grip	Right angle	Handpiece
Pear Burs			
329	100-0343		
330	100-8426		
331	100-1120		
332	100-5616		
331L	722-6892		
332L	722-6988		
333L	722-7205		
Round Burs			
¼	100-7205		
½	100-3995	100-6373	100-5860
1	100-4907	100-6319	100-7176
2	100-0288	100-6411	100-2095
4	100-4535	100-1847	100-0899
6	100-3220	100-8765	100-9086
8	100-6131	100-1401	100-6137
Inverted Cone Burs			
33½	100-0703	100-6637	
34	100-8454	100-7755	
35	100-2482	100-2431	100-8612
37	100-9299	100-2407	
Fissure Burs			
Cross-cut 669	100-9613		
Taper 700	100-7926		
700L	100-3046		
701	100-4546	100-0435	100-9229
701L	100-4546		
702	100-9464		100-9941
703	100-3108		100-6111
Cross-cut 557	100-3307	100-3795	
Straight 557L	100-9947		
558	100-3104		100-4895
558L	100-8157		
Plain 56	100-4718		
Straight 58	100-0281		

*The 7-digit numbers are Schein catalog numbers.

TABLE 11-1	Burs and other handpiece accessories—cont'd		
Size no.	Friction grip	Right angle	Handpiece
Finishing Burs			
7006	100-5193 (round)		
7606	100-4632 (cone)		
7610	100-1478 (taper)		
7612	100-6113 (taper)		
7613	100-6164 (taper)		
7408	100-3889 (egg)		
7801	100-1458 (bullet)		
Diamond Burs			
808/014	100-0928 (pear)		
863G/018	100-3922 (bullet)		
852/011	100-810 (flame)		
Acrylic Burs			
84-T			142-7975 (taper)
82-T			142-8574 (cone)
53-A			142-8842 (pear)
Diamond Wheel			
818/045	999-6151		
347/190			387-5547

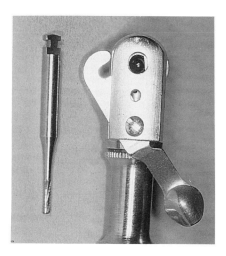

FIGURE 11-9
RA bur and contraangle showing the groove on the bur and the latch on the contraangle.

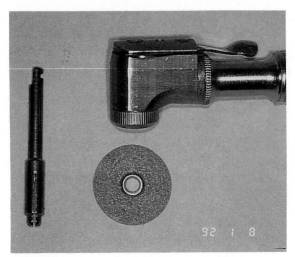

FIGURE 11-10
Mandrel with button system for attachment of finishing disks.

FG burs fit into FG handpiece heads. They are available in 20 mm lengths to be used in a high-speed turbine or low-speed FG contraangle handpiece.

Mandrels come in HP, FG, and RA shanks (Fig. 11-10). Finishing tips, diamond disks, sanding disks, polishing wheels, and cups are premounted or fitted individually onto the mandrel with screws or by a snap-on button system (Fig. 11-10).

Bur heads are made of steel, tungsten carbide, or steel coated with diamond grit of various grit sizes (from extra fine to coarse). The most durable burs are tungsten carbide and diamond-coated. Burs are made with various head shapes, depending on their function. Starter sets, containing a range of the most useful sizes and shapes, are available in FG/HP [896-0188] or HP/RA configurations.

The *pear bur* has a universally useful shape (Fig. 11-11, Table 11-1). It is available in long and short cutting head sizes. In ascending order, sizes are Nos. 329, 330, 331, and 332; longer heads are Nos. 331L, 332L, and 333L. They are used for cutting enamel, dentin, cavity or endodontic access preparation, as well as for removing caries and creating undercuts adequate for the retention of fillings.

Round burs have round cutting heads (Fig. 11-11 and Table 11-1). They are used particularly for cavity preparation, tooth entry, and creating undercutting retention in dentin. They range in size from No. 1/4 to No. 8.

Inverted cone burs are used primarily to create undercuts in dentin for the retention of restorative material (Fig. 11-11, Table 11-1).

Fissure burs, both tapered and straight fissure, available in either cross-cut or plain-cut pattern, are useful for sectioning multirooted teeth before extraction and alveoloplasty (Fig. 11-11, Table 11-1). Cross-cut burs cut faster but produce a rougher cut surface. The long-head burs (700L, 701L, 557L, 558L) are particularly useful for sectioning large teeth.

Finishing burs are constructed with 12 to 40 straight-bladed flutes on the cutting heads (Fig. 11-11, Table 11-1). They are used to shape, finish, and polish enamel, dentin, composite, and amalgam. The 12-bladed finishing burs are the most practical.

Acrylic burs are large cutting burs designed to shape and smooth acrylic devices (Fig. 11-11, Table 11-1).

Abrasives, in mounted and unmounted forms (Fig. 11-11, Table 11-1) are made of silicone carbide grit; they are used for the smooth finishing of enamel and restorative materials. Green and white finishing stones or rubber abrasive wheels also are available. The purchase of a Shofu Super Snap Kit [195-1804], with disks, minidisks, and stones, and the Moore's paper spindle set [294-8195] is an excellent way to acquire a starting range of polishing materials.

Diamond cutting disks are used to make straight, thin cuts in teeth or bone (Fig. 11-11, Table 11-1). They are available in thin (flexible) and standard types; for most purposes the standard type is adequate as well as safer.

Ultrasonic and Subsonic Dental Scalers
Ultrasonic scalers

Ultrasonic units are used for dental scaling procedures [167-5476] (Fig. 11-12, *A*). The working tip of the unit vibrates elliptically at 20 to 30 kHz. A cooling water spray directed over the tip produces an effect called *cavitation;* this energized water helps

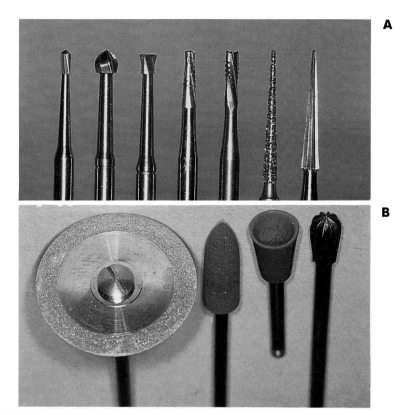

FIGURE 11-11
A, Burs for use in dental handpieces. *From left to right,* Pear shaped, round, inverted cone, tapered fissure, straight fissure, needle diamond, 12-sided finishing bur. **B,** Larger handpiece attachments. *From left to right,* Acrylic bur, rubber polishing cup for amalgam, composite finishing and polishing stone, and diamond disk.

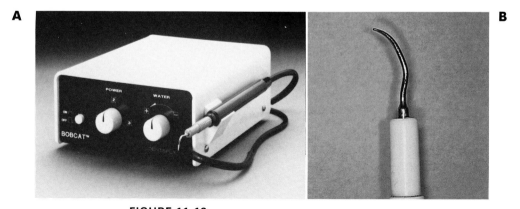

FIGURE 11-12
A, Ultrasonic dental scaler. **B,** Ultrasonic scaler tip.

dislodge the calculus deposits and stain from the tooth surface. A variety of scaling tips are available; the most serviceable for general veterinary use is a thin-curved tip that resembles a dental hand scaler [167-4055] (Fig. 11-12, *B*). Ultrasonic scalers are of two types, magnetostrictive or piezoelectric. In a magnetostrictive unit, the working tip is energized by electromagnetic energy that changes the shape of the laminated ferromagnetic rod stack in the handpiece handle, producing an elliptic oscillation pattern at the tip of the instrument. Piezoelectric units produce changes in the shape of a crystal within the handpiece, resulting in oscillating semielliptic vibrations at the working tip. The piezoelectric scalers have a smaller handpiece than do magnetostrictive scalers; however, because of the brittle nature of the crystal, they tend to be more easily damaged.

All ultrasonic units produce an aerosol that contaminates the local environment (see Chapter 4). Use of an antiseptic solution such as 0.2% chlorhexidine as the cooling fluid helps to reduce this environmental contamination. Check the manufacturer's recommendations before using anything other than water as the cooling fluid.

Subsonic scalers

Subsonic scalers are air-driven dental handpieces with a scaling tip that oscillates in a linear pattern but at less than 20 kHz [808-1753] (Fig. 11-13). The sonic scaler handpiece fits onto the high-speed outlet of an air-driven dental unit. It is cooled by water (or dilute antiseptic) that flows over the vibrating tip, forming an aerosol that has a somewhat lesser beneficial cavitation effect than a true ultrasonic unit.

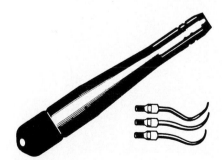

FIGURE 11-13
Subsonic dental scaler handpiece.

Roto-Pro scaler

Another form of dental scaler uses a six-sided, noncutting bur inserted in the high-speed handpiece. The Roto-Pro bur [295-8151] rotates at approximately 100,000 to 200,000 rpm, producing 10,000 to 20,000 impacts per second against the tooth (Fig. 11-14). This tends to dislodge calculus but also can scarify the surface of the tooth. These scarifications create tooth sensitivity and produce plaque-retentive areas, contributing to rapid build-up of calculus deposits. A water or antiseptic cooling spray is essential. Unless used with care and experience, these units can do more harm than good and are much less effective than the ultrasonic dental scaler.

Radiology
X-ray machines

Both human and veterinary x-ray units can be employed. Dental x-ray units are much easier to manipulate than are standard table-mounted radiology units (Fig. 11-15), but additional cost is involved. Units are available from most supply houses.

Radiographs

Intraoral radiographs commonly used in veterinary dentistry are described in Chapter 2. Equipment and procedures for developing dental radiographs also are described in Chapter 2.

Radiograph developing unit

For intraoral dental films the fastest and most convenient method of development is the use of rapid developer and fixer solutions in a "chairside" dark room (Fig. 11-16; see also Chapter 2).

▶ HAND INSTRUMENTS

Hand instrumentation is necessary for proper dental therapy. The variety of hand instruments that have been developed for the dental profession is enormous. With a comparatively small selection of dental hand instruments, the veterinarian will be able to perform almost all dental procedures.

Basic hand instruments and other materials and supplies needed for the various dental disciplines are listed in this section.

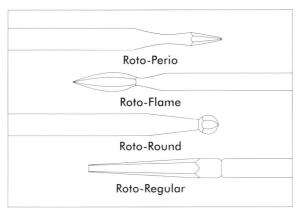

FIGURE 11-14
Roto-Pro dental scaling burs.

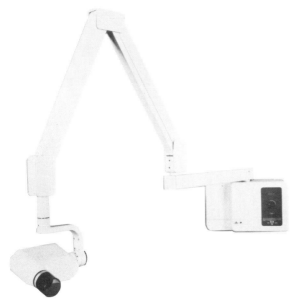

FIGURE 11-15
Wall-mounted dental radiographic unit.

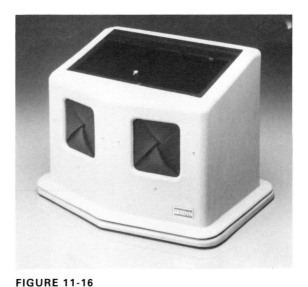

FIGURE 11-16
"Chairside darkroom," containing developer, rinse, fixer, and rinse solutions in beakers, with lightproof hand portals and a safety light lid.

Oral Examination

The following instruments are needed for all veterinary dental procedures.

Periodontal probe and dental explorer

A periodontal probe is blunt-ended and marked in graduations of 1 to 3 mm (Fig. 11-17). Some types have a color-coded tip for easy reading (for example, Hu-Friedy No. CP11 [600-3452]). Other types have indentations as depth markers. A dental explorer has a sharp point (Fig. 11-17) that is designed to identify irregularities in or on the tooth surface and to detect calculus, caries, or external resorptive lesions. A combination periodontal probe (at one end) and dental explorer (at the other end) is also in common use [100-4807] (Fig. 11-17).

Round dental mirror

A round dental mirror, with a plastic or metal handle, is used for visibility, increased reflective illumination and retraction [100-5067].

Periodontics
Periodontal curets and scalers

The parts of a curet or scaler are the handle, the shank, and the blade (Fig. 11-18). Periodontal hand instruments are generally double-ended (each end has the same shank and blade, but one end has the tip to the right and the other end has the tip to the left). The blade of a *curet* has a "face" and a single-curved back surface that forms a half-moon shape on cross section (Fig. 11-19); the two edges of a curet meet at a rounded "toe" at the tip of the instrument. The blade of a *scaler* is triangular in section and has a face and two lateral surfaces that converge toward the toe to form a sharp point (Fig. 11-19). Curets and scalers function by engaging an edge against the surface of the tooth; this edge is the junction between the face and the lateral surfaces. The working edge must be sharp for the instrument to function correctly (see discussion that follows).

Gracey curets differ from the Universal curets in that the face of the Gracey blade is at a 70-degree

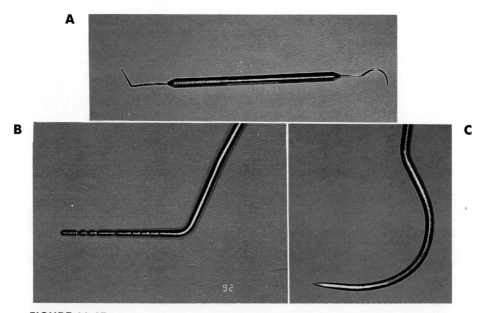

FIGURE 11-17
A, Periodontal probe–dental explorer combination. **B,** Blunt periodontal probe tip. **C,** Sharp shepherd's hook dental explorer tip.

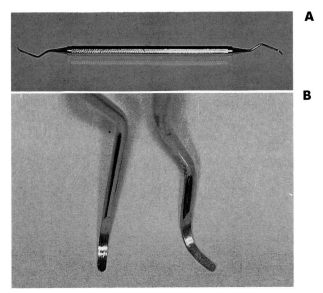

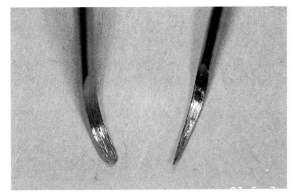

FIGURE 11-18
A, Double-ended periodontal curet. **B,** Working end (shank and blade) of a Universal curet *(left)* and Gracey curet *(right)*.

angle to the shank, whereas Universal curets have a face perpendicular to the shank (Fig. 11-18). With a Universal curet, either edge can be used, and both edges should be sharpened. With Gracey curets, only one edge is used; the correct edge is recognizable because the blade of a Gracey curet is curved in two planes (whereas a Universal curet is curved in one plane only). When a Gracey curet is examined by looking down the handle toward the blade, the blade is seen to curve away from the shank; the working edge is the long side of the blade (Fig. 11-18). Because of the offset face, it also is the edge that is farthest from the handle.

A *recommended periodontal scaler-curet set* includes the following instruments:
- McCall scaler 17S/18S [115-7959)]
- McCall scaler 13S/14S [115-7627]
- Gracey curet 1/2 [100-7016]
- Gracey curet 13/14 [100-2126]
- After-Five curet 1/2 [600-9397]
- After-Five curet 13/14 [600-1527]
- Mini-Five curet 1/2 [600-6312]
- Mini-Five curet 13/14 [600-7297]

FIGURE 11-19
Blades of a periodontal curet *(left)* and scaler *(right)*.

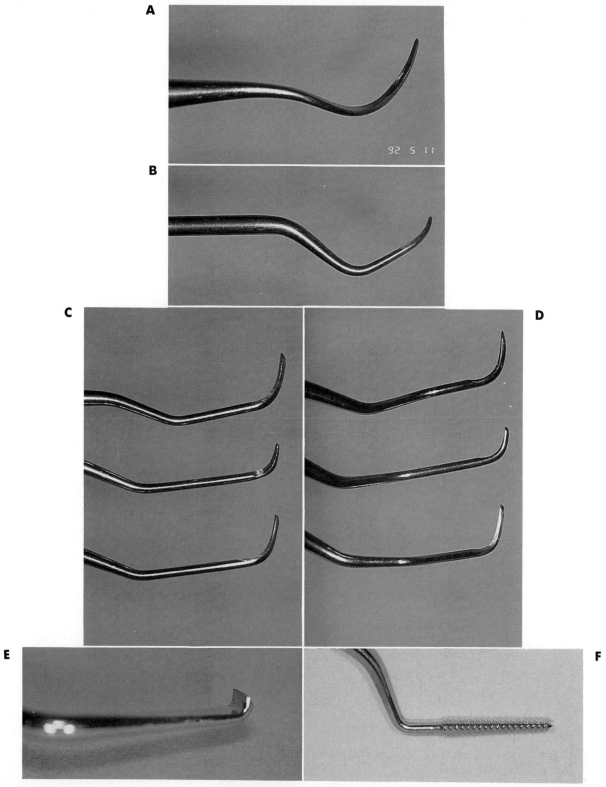

FIGURE 11-20
For legend see opposite page.

FIGURE 11-20
Periodontal scalers, curets, hoes, and files. **A,** McCall's scaler 17S/18S. **B,** McCall's scaler 13S/14S. **C,** Gracey curet 1/2 *(top),* Mini-Five curet 1/2 *(middle),* After-Five curet 1/2 *(bottom).* **D,** Gracey curet 13/14 *(top),* Mini-Five curet 13/14 *(middle),* After-Five curet 13/14 *(bottom).* **E,** Hoe (100-9588). **F,** Sugarman file (600-2081).

Miscellaneous periodontal instruments

Periodontal instruments that are used less often include hoes [100-9588] and files [600-2081] (for scaling within furcations, Fig. 11-20).

Use of hand instruments

Hand instruments, particularly periodontal curets and scalers, often need to be applied with moderate force in specific directions and with limited room for maneuver. Therefore control is very important and is best obtained by using a specific hand position known as the *modified pen grasp*.

The thumb and index finger are placed on the instrument as if writing with a pen; however, the tip of the middle finger rests against the instrument where the handle joins the shank (Fig. 11-21, *A*). These three digits form a triangle that provides support and prevents unwanted rotation of the shank as the instrument is applied. This leaves the two remaining fingers free to rest against the tooth or an adjacent tooth (Fig. 11-21, *B*). The fulcrum—the point on which the ring and little finger rest—should be close to the tooth surface being worked on. The force to remove calculus is created by rotating the wrist or rocking the wrist back and forth on the fulcrum.

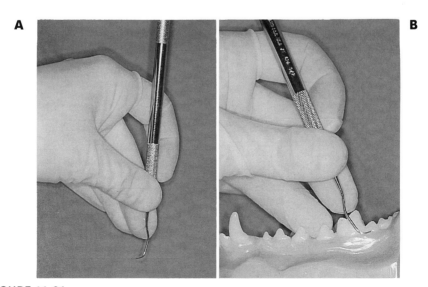

FIGURE 11-21
A, Modified pen grasp hand position for controlled use of periodontal hand instruments.
B, The remaining one or two fingers rest on an adjacent firm surface to provide a fulcrum.

Sharpening periodontal instruments

Sharpness can be easily tested. If the working edge is applied to a thumbnail or plastic rod (for example, a toothbrush handle or a ball-point pen) at the same angle and pressure as that used on a tooth and is then moved, it will glide readily if it is not sharp. However, if it is sharp, the edge will "bite" and a curl of nail or plastic material will be visible as the curet is pulled forward (Fig. 11-22).

Periodontal instruments should be sharpened immediately before use; they become dull if sharpened and then sterilized. Sharpening a curet that is sterile also avoids seeding the sharpening stone with oral organisms from the previous procedure.

To sharpen a curet or scaler, a sharpening stone and oil are needed (if Arkansas or India stones are used) [365-2875 or 600-5390]. If Carborundum stone is used, water is used to lubricate the stone. Sharpening is performed to retain the 70- to 80-degree angle between the face and the lateral surface. This is done by placing the stone and curet in position to achieve this angle and then maintaining this angle as the stone and curet are moved relative to each other. If the instrument is held so that the face of the blade is parallel to the floor, the correct angle can be easily seen from the flat surface of the stone as it is applied to the curet (Fig. 11-23). With use of a flat stone, the curet usually is held firmly and still (to maintain the face parallel to the floor) and the stone is moved with short up-and-down strokes against the lateral surface at the correct angle. The process always is finished with a down stroke to remove any irregular edges.

The blade is narrower at its tip. Thus the clinician starts with the correct angulation at the shank and gradually works toward the tip. A curet has a rounded tip ("toe") to avoid lacerating the attachment as it is placed to the bottom of the pocket; this toe is retained by continuing the sharpening movements to encircle the tip. Because a scaler is designed to have a sharp tip, the sharpening movement around the tip is not used for scalers.

Cylindric or cone-shaped stones can be used to sharpen curets and scalers by working against the face of the blade. This method is not recommended because it gradually narrows the blade (from its face to the back of the blade), making it more likely to break when in use.

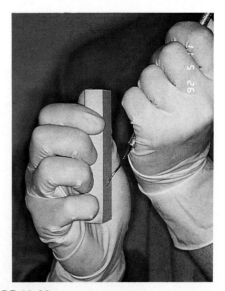

FIGURE 11-23
Sharpening a periodontal curet. The curet is held so that the face is parallel to the floor, then the flat stone is applied to the edge of the curet to form a 70- to 80-degree angle with the face.

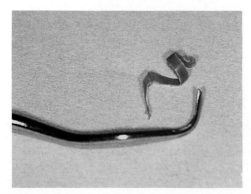

FIGURE 11-22
Curl of plastic produced by working a sharp periodontal curet against a plastic rod or pen.

Additional periodontal supplies include the following:

- Face mask, protective eye shield, prophylaxis polishing paste or pumice with fluoride (for example, Schein Zircon-F [100-7869]), disclosing solution (such as Reveal [100-2491]), fluoride gel for topical application after prophylaxis (for example, Schein Phosphated Topical Gel [100-9857])
- Subgingival irrigation solution (for example, Nolvadent chlorhexidine solution; Fort Dodge Laboratories).

▶ ENDODONTIC INSTRUMENTS AND MATERIALS

Endodontic instruments (Fig. 11-24) consist of the following:

- Root canal explorer (for example, Starlite DG16 [100-9279])
- Endodontic files and reamers (for example, Hedstrom files 60-mm length, No. 15 through 110 [100-7643, 100-8303, 100-8585]; K-files, Nos. 10 through 80, 25-mm length [100-1215, 100-5087]; reamers, Nos. 15 to 80 [100-1212, 100-3321])

- Peeso reamers [100-9385] and Gates Glidden burs [100-9919]
- Endodontic rubber file stops [100-5271]
- Endodontic spreaders (for example, single end D11 [100-2806], D11T [100-3172], 25S [378-2656], 4OS [378-1843], or Schein double-end Plugger-Spreader No. 608 [100-9062])
- Pluggers (such as single end 1-4 [100-8337, 100-6578, 100-0971, 100-3095])
- Spiral filling burs (for example, 60-mm length for canine teeth and 29-mm length for premolar and molar teeth [100-3791, 100-4273])
- Barbed broaches (assorted sizes in 47-mm lengths [100-6351])
- Irrigating syringe
- Paper Point Pliers such as Schein Grooved Self-Locking [100-0264]
- Endodontic file organizer and rule [808-1013] (Fig. 11-25)
- Bead or salt sterilizer [100-2926]

Endodontic materials include the following:

- Calcium hydroxide powder (sterile USP)
- Glass mixing slab [100-4432]
- Cement-mixing spatula [100-9387]
- Dy-Cal hard setting calcium hydroxide cement kit, including ball-point applicator [222-5882]

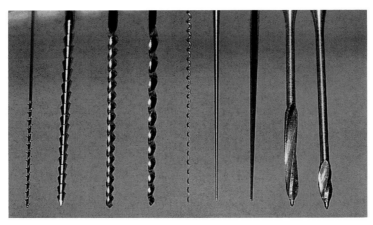

FIGURE 11-24
Endodontic instruments *(from left):* barbed broach, Hedstrom file, K-file, reamer, lentulo, endodontic spreader, endodontic plugger, Peeso reamer, Gates Glidden bur.

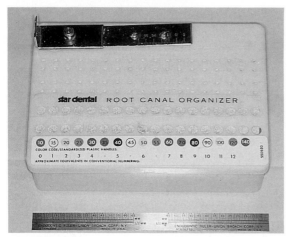

FIGURE 11-25
Endodontic file organizer and millimeter rule.

- Root canal chelating agent (such as Premier R-C Prep [378-4499])
- Sodium hypochlorite, normal household bleach
- Gutta-percha points: because 45-mm lengths are available only in limited sizes, 25-mm length gutta-percha must be used with Nos. 15 to 90 as a starting set (Endo Aide [100-8393])
- Root canal sealing cement such as zinc oxide–eugenol [100-1757, 100-4540] or Tubli-Seal, Sealapex
- Restorative materials of choice to close access site
- Paper points, assorted sizes in human (25 mm) and veterinary (55 mm) lengths [100-6590, 100-9339]

▶ RESTORATIVE EQUIPMENT, INSTRUMENTS, AND MATERIALS

Equipment is based on these considerations: if composite material will be used extensively, a light curing system is recommended; this requires a light-curing gun [100-4296] (Fig. 11-26). If amalgam or glass ionomer capsule systems are to be used, an amalgamator is used [100-2532] (Fig. 11-26). The glass ionomer capsule system also requires capsule activator

and application instruments [378-6700 or 378-6238] (Fig. 11-27).

Instruments (Fig. 11-28) include the following:
- Dental spoon excavator (for example, No. 18)
- Plastic filling instrument (for example, Schein W3 or No. PF with a round packing tip and a flat, paddle-shape "beaver-tail" tip [100-0049])
- Carver (for example, Schein No. 89/92 discoid and cleoid [100-7078])
- Amalgam plugger and carver D/E [100-0982], burnisher 28/29 [100-3450]
- Amalgam carrier, Schein double end No. 3/4 [100-1293]; retrofill amalgam carrier [317-1676]

Restorative materials include the following:
- Composite filling material (for example, Schein Chemical Cure Kit [100-1673], light Cure Caulk—Prisma APH [222-4281])
- IRM temporary cement [222-1135] or Cavit temporary cement [378-4404]
- Retraction cord [100-2020]
- Glass ionomer such as Premier Ketac System (Ketac-Fil [378-6700] or Ketac-Silver [378-6238]) if an amalgamator is available; if not, Chelon-Fil [378-5025], Chelon-Silver [378-3707], or feline restorative kit (VRx, Inc., Harbor City, Calif.) that includes conditioner and brushes
- Orthophosphoric acid etch
- Flour pumice [100-5836]

▶ IMPRESSION AND CAST EQUIPMENT AND MATERIALS

Equipment and materials include the following:
- Wax bite material
- Impression material (for example, alginate, Schein regular set [100-5292]; vinyl polysiloxane caulk such as Reprosil [222-1144])
- Impression trays [100-7884] (Fig. 11-29) and tray-forming material (for example, Formatray-Kerr [123-1551])
- Wax strips [547-0063])
- Dental stone [569-0883] (Fig. 11-32)
- Vibrator [100-4157] (Fig. 11-32)
- Flexible mixing bowl (Fig. 11-30) (small [547-4425], medium [547-4106], and large [547-3089] and spatula [365-6828])

A

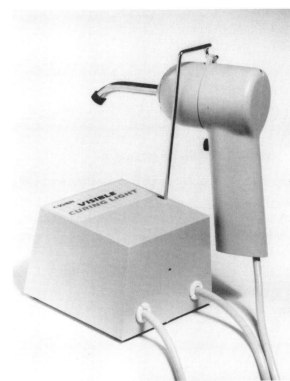

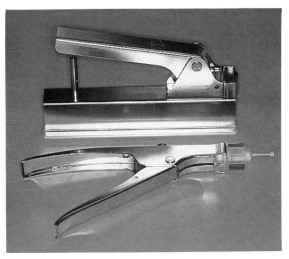

FIGURE 11-27
Capsule activator *(top)* and applicator *(bottom)* for use with glass ionomer capsule systems.

B

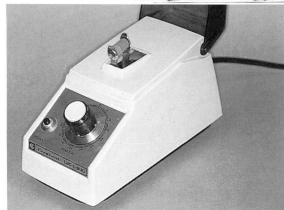

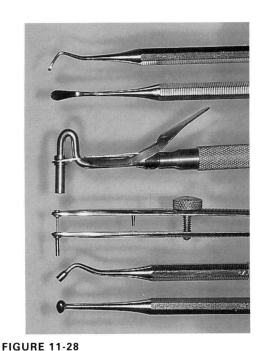

FIGURE 11-26
A, Composite light curing gun. **B,** Amalgam and glass ionomer capsule mixer.

FIGURE 11-28
Restorative instruments *(from top):* Spoon excavator, beaver tail filling instrument, amalgam carrier, retrofill amalgam carrier, amalgam plugger, amalgam burnisher.

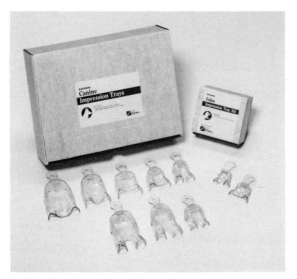

FIGURE 11-29
Canine and feline plastic impression trays.

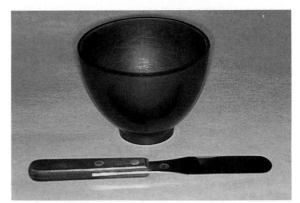

FIGURE 11-30
Flexible mixing bowl and spatula for mixing alginate and dental stone.

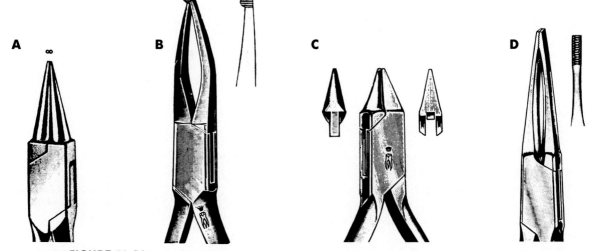

FIGURE 11-31
Orthodontic pliers *(from left):* Round nose wire bending pliers, Howe crown pliers, Angle bending pliers, Fischer flat nose pliers.

A

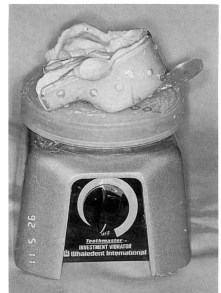

FIGURE 11-32
Dental stone being poured into an impression while the impression is vibrated on a vibrator to eliminate air bubbles. **A,** The impression on the top plate of the vibrator. **B,** The thin stone paste is poured first into the tooth impressions. **C,** A poorly performed pour and vibration of the stone causes air bubbles that distort the finished cast. The near side canine tooth *(arrow)* is not present in the cast because of air bubble, whereas the opposite canine tooth is complete.

B

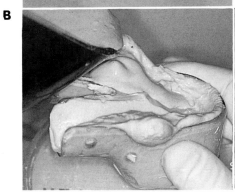

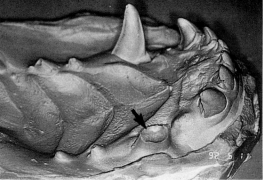

C

▶ ORTHODONTIC AND ACRYLIC SPLINT INSTRUMENTS AND MATERIALS

Instruments include the following:
- Orthodontic pliers (Fig. 11-31) (for example, McKellop No. 134 wire bending [100-2258]; Howe No. 110 [100-3929]; No. 139 angle bending [100-7712]; and Fischer No. 156 flat nose [100-5357])
- Orthodontic wire (in assorted diameters 0.018 to 0.030)

Materials include the following:
- Jet acrylic [125-1546]
- Orthodontic bonded brackets (for example, those made by Rocky Mountain Orthodontics)
- Orthodontic ligatures and Masel chain (available in assorted sizes from Rocky Mountain Orthodontics)
- Bracket bonding cement kit (for example, Comspan [222-0845], Panavia [721-1856], or Concise [777-3430])

▶ ORAL SURGERY AND EXTRACTION INSTRUMENTS

In addition to a standard surgical instrument pack, the following are needed:

- Dental extraction forceps (for example, Schein ST-5 and No. 65 [100-8266, 100-6525] for small dogs and cats)
- Dental elevators (for example, Schein ST-8, ST-9, and H-1 [100-9235, 100-3332, 100-9415])
- Dental luxators (for example, Tactile Plus, Whaledent)
- Root tip pick (for example, Schein ST-11 [100-6967])
- Rongeur (for example, Luer 6-inch [100-7453])
- Periosteal elevator (for example, Goldman Fox No. 14 and Schein ST-7 [100-8204])
- Wedelsteadt chisel [600-5525]
- Bone file (for example, Schein No. 12CA [100-0812])

▶ SUGGESTED READINGS

1. American Dental Association: *Dental materials specifications,* Chicago, The Association.
2. Golden AL: Problems with dental equipment and materials, *Problems Vet Med* 2(1):1, 1990.
3. Pattison G, Pattison AM: *Periodontal instrumentation: a clinical manual,* Reston, Va, 1992, Reston Publishing Co.

Index

Page numbers in *italic* indicate illustrations;
page numbers followed by *t* indicate tables.